Intimate Partner Violence

A Resource for Professionals
Working with Children and Families

STM **Learning,** Inc.

St. Louis

STM **Learning,** Inc.
St. Louis

OUR MISSION

To become the world leader in publishing and

information services on child abuse, maltreatment,

diseases, and domestic violence. We seek to

heighten awareness of these issues and provide

relevant information to professionals and consumers.

A portion of our profits is contributed to nonprofit organizations
dedicated to the prevention of child abuse and the care of victims of abuse
and other children and family charities.

This book is dedicated to the Institute for Safe Families (ISF) and its two founding executive directors—Martha Davis, MSS, and Sandra Dempsey, MSS, MLSP. Under their leadership, and with the support and guidance of its volunteer Board of Directors and National Advisory Board, ISF has consistently sought to inform, educate, and train professionals on the proper methods of screening clients for exposure to Intimate Partner Violence (IPV) and effectively responding to it. In addition to helping professionals, ISF has also invested countless hours and immense effort towards raising community awareness of the existence of IPV while working diligently to highlight the connection of IPV to the risks of child maltreatment.

Angelo P. Giardino, MD, PhD, MPH, FAAP

Eileen R. Giardino, PhD, RN, FNP-BC, ANP-BC

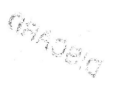

Intimate Partner Violence

A Resource for Professionals
Working with Children and Families

Angelo P. Giardino, MD, PhD, MPH, FAAP
Medical Director
Texas Children's Health Plan
Clinical Professor of Pediatrics
Baylor College of Medicine
Attending Physician
Children's Assessment Center
Texas Children's Hospital
Houston, Texas

Eileen R. Giardino, PhD, RN, FNP-BC, ANP-BC
Associate Professor
The University of Texas Health Science Center-Houston
Department of Acute & Continuing Care
School of Nursing
Houston, Texas

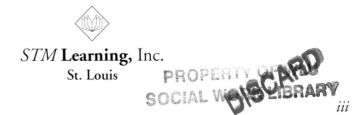

STM **Learning**, Inc.
St. Louis

Publishers: Glenn E. Whaley and Marianne V. Whaley

Design Director: Glenn E. Whaley

Managing Editor: John Wu Gabbert

Associate Editors: Christine Bauer
                                  Kieran Blasingim

Book Design/Page Layout: G.W. Graphics

Print/Production Coordinator: Heather N. Green

Cover Design: G.W. Graphics

Developmental Editor: Elaine Steinborn

Copy Editor: Amy Rosenstein

Proofreader: Suzanne Sherman

Indexer: Robert A. Saigh

Printed in Korea

Publisher:

STM Learning, Inc.
721 Emerson Road, Suite 645, St. Louis, Missouri 63141 USA
Phone: (314) 993-2728 Fax: (314) 993-2281 Toll Free: 1-800-600-0330
http://www.gwmedical.com

Library of Congress Cataloging-in-Publication Data

Intimate partner violence : a resource for professionals working with children and families / editors, Angelo P. Giradino, Eileen R. Giardino.

     p. cm.

 Includes bibliographical references and index.

  Summary: "Intimate Parter Violence includes in-depth analyses of every aspect of IPV, including contemporary concepts and research on its prevalence, nature, causes, and impact"--Provided by publisher.

 ISBN 978-1-878060-77-8 (pbk.)

 1. Intimate partner violence--United States. 2. Intimate partner violence--United States--Prevention. 3. Victims of family violence--Services for--United States. I. Giardino, Angelo P. II. Giardino, Eileen R.

 HV6626.2.I59 2009

 362.82'920973--dc22

                                2009028095

CONTRIBUTORS

Juan Carlos Areán, MM
Senior Program Manager
Family Violence Prevention Fund
Boston, Massachusetts

Janice Asher, MD, FACOG
Associate Clinical Professor
Department of Obstetrics & Gynecology
Director
Women's Health Division of Student Health Services
University of Pennsylvania
Philadelphia, Pennsylvania

Megan H. Bair-Merritt, MD, MSCE
Assistant Professor of Pediatrics
Division of General Pediatrics & Adolescent Medicine
Johns Hopkins Children's Center
Baltimore, Maryland

Sandra L. Bloom, MD
Associate Professor of Health Management and Policy
School of Public Health
Drexel University
Philadelphia, Pennsylvania

Mariana Chilton, PhD, MPH
Principal Investigator
Philadelphia GROW Project
Department of Health Management and Policy
School of Public Health
Drexel University
Philadelphia, Pennsylvania

Peter Cronholm, MD, MSCE
Assistant Professor, Director of Community Programs
Department of Family Medicine and Community Health
Senior Scholar
Center for Public Health Initiatives
Senior Fellow, Leonard Davis Institute of Health Economics
Associate
Firearm & Injury Center at Penn
Attending Physician
Hospital of the University of Pennsylvania and Penn Presbyterian Medical Center
University of Pennsylvania
Philadelphia, Pennsylvania

Lonna Davis, MSW
Director of Children Programs
Family Violence Prevention Fund
Boston, Massachusetts

Martha B. Davis, MSS
Co-Director
Institute for Safe Families
Philadelphia, Pennsylvania

Sandra H. Dempsey, MSS, MLSP
Co-Director
Institute for Safe Families
Philadelphia, Pennsylvania

Diana Faugno, MSN, RN, CPN, SANE-A, SANE-P, FAAFS
Forensic Nurse Consultant
Board Director EVAW International
Escondido, California

Joel Fein, MD, MPH
Associate Professor of Pediatrics and Emergency Medicine
University of Pennsylvania School of Medicine
Attending Physician, Emergency Medicine
The Children's Hospital of Philadelphia
Director
The Philadelphia Collaborative Violence Prevention Center
Philadelphia, Pennsylvania

Kathleen Franchek-Roa, MD, FAAP
Assistant Professor of Pediatrics
University of Utah School of Medicine
Medical Director
University Pediatric Clinic
Attending Physician
Primary Children's Hospital
Salt Lake City, Utah

Eric L. Gibson, JD
Trial Attorney
Civil Rights Division
US Department of Justice
Washington, DC

G.L. Isaacs, BS, Ed
Director of Public Safety & Security
Oral Roberts University
Tulsa, Oklahoma

Jeffrey R. Jaeger, MD, FACP
Assistant Clinical Professor of Medicine
Division of General Internal Medicine
University of Pennsylvania School of Medicine
Philadelphia, Pennsylvania

Mary Graw Leary, JD
Associate Professor
Columbus School of Law
The Catholic University of America
Washington, DC

Linda E. Ledray, RN, SANE-A, PhD, FAAN
Director, SARS
Hennepin County Medical Center
Minneapolis, Minnesota

Maria D. McColgan, MD, MEd
Director, Child Protection Program
St. Christopher's Hospital for Children
Assistant Professor of Pediatrics and Emergency Medicine
Drexel University College of Medicine
Philadelphia, Pennsylvania

JoAnn Mick, PhD, MBA, RN, AOCN, CNAA
Director, Nursing Research & Clinical Outcomes
Harris County Hospital District
Houston, Texas

Claire Nelli, RN, SANE-A
Director
Independent Forensic Services, LLC
San Diego, California

Mary Reina, RN, MSN
Director
Antelope Valley Hospital SART Center
Palmdale, California

Sharon Robinson, RN, FNB, SANE
Chief Administrative Officer
Fort Wayne Sexual Assault Treatment Center
Fort Wayne, Indiana

Patricia M. Speck, DNSc, FNP-BC, FAAN, FAAFS, DF-IAFN, SANE-A, SANE-P
Assistant Professor and Public Health Nursing Option Coordinator
University of Tennessee Health Science Center College of Nursing
Memphis, Tennessee

Joseph B. Straton, MD, MSCE
Chief Medical Officer
Penn Wissahickon Hospice
University of Pennsylvania Health System
Assistant Professor
Department of Family Medicine and Community Health
Department of Anesthesiology and Critical Care
University of Pennsylvania
Secondary Faculty Appointment
School of Nursing
University of Pennsylvania
Philadelphia, Pennsylvania

Michelle Teti, MPH, DrPH
Research Scientist
School of Public Health
Drexel University
Philadelphia, Pennsylvania

Jennifer B. Varela, LCSW
Clinical Social Worker
Director of Family Violence Services
Harris County District Attorney's Office
Houston, Texas

L. Sloane Winkes, MD
Family Physician
North Cascade Family Physicians
Mount Vernon, Washington

Marcy N. Witherspoon, MSW, LSW
Staff Adjunct
Philadelphia Department of Human Services
Director of Children & Youth
Institute for Safe Families
Philadelphia, Pennsylvania

FOREWORD

Intimate partner violence (IPV) is as old as history. According to the Minnesota Center Against Violence and Abuse, the first recorded laws governing IPV date from 753 BCE during Romulus's reign over Rome.[1] The "Laws of Chastisement" condoned wife beating. The husband could use a switch or a rod as long as the diameter of the instrument was no greater than that of the base of the man's right thumb, which is the origin of the commonly used term "rule of thumb." The authority of the husband continued in Jewish and Christian traditions. The Roman Emperor Constantine the Great had his spouse burned alive, and England's King Henry VIII was known for violently disposing of inconvenient wives.

Even in current times, intimate partner violence continues to threaten family, physical, and mental health. In many Arab and Islamic countries, domestic abuse is considered a private "family matter" rather than a problem that should be addressed by the police and medical care providers. The reputation of the family is of utmost importance, and the involvement of outside agencies and authorities is not tolerated.[2] In Western countries, laws against spousal abuse are on the books, and as a culture, intimate partner violence is not tolerated. Even so, the Department of Justice reports that each year in the United States, women experience 4.8 million assaults and rapes by intimate partners and almost 1200 women are killed by their partners.[3,4] Men can be victims of intimate partner violence as well, although it is not reported as frequently as in women (2.9 million assaults and 800 deaths yearly).[3,5]

How can we tolerate this level of family violence, with the knowledge that it causes physical and mental pain, increases medical expenses, and triggers long-term psychological harm to children who witness these events? For health care providers in particular, Towervi has identified 3 major factors that prevent effective response to intimate partner violence: 1) health care professionals' lack of knowledge about IPV that leads to failure to identify abuse; 2) personal attitudes and beliefs held by health professionals that make it uneasy for them to address IPV with patients; and, 3) a lack of time, which inhibits caregivers from responding appropriately to IPV issues.[6]

This book, edited by Giardino and Giardino, addresses these 3 barriers to identifying and caring for victims of IPV. The book distills a large body of knowledge into a readable, useful, rich resource. It is well organized and carefully annotated. The information is both theoretical and practical. The book is a single source that can educate professionals, change attitudes, and save time by having all the necessary information readily available in a single resource. The book addresses another sensitive issue in the field of IPV: the unresolved tension between advocates for children and advocates for adult IPV victims. Should children be taken away from a battered woman who is unable to separate from the batterer? Is that considered blaming the victim or protecting the children who experience secondary trauma from witnessing the abuse? The book's title, *Intimate Partner Violence: A Resource for Professionals Working with Children and Families,* reflects the editors' awareness of the need for balance and consideration for parents as well as children.

Hopefully we, as a society, are gradually recovering from millennia of family violence and realizing that these problems can be confronted with multidisciplinary efforts by health care providers, mental health professionals, victims' advocates, and law enforcement.[7]

Carole Jenny, MD, MBA
Professor of Pediatrics
Warren Alpert Medical School at Brown University
Providence, Rhode Island

REFERENCES

1. Herstory of Domestic Violence: A Timeline of the Battered Women's Movement. Minnesota Center Against Violence and Abuse. http://www.mincava.umn.edu/documents/herstory/herstory.html. Accessed June 25, 2009.

2. Douki S, Nacef F, Belhadj A, et al. Violence against women in Arab and Islamic countries. *Arch Womens Ment Health.* 2003;6:165-171.

3. Understanding Intimate Partner Violence: Fact Sheet, 2006. National Center for Injury Prevention and Control, Centers for Disease Control and Prevention. http://www.cdc.gov/ncipc/dvp/ipv_factsheet.pdf. Accessed June 25, 2009.

4. Tjaden P, Thoennes N. US Department of Justice. Extent, Nature, and Consequences of Intimate Partner Violence: Findings from the National Violence Against Women Survey. Available at http://www.ojp.usdoj.gov/nij/pubs-sum/181867.htm. Accessed June 25, 2009.

5. Fox JA, Zawitz MW. US Department of Justice. Homicide Trends in the United States. http://www.ojp.usdoj.gov/bjs/homicide/homtrnd.htm. Accessed June 25, 2009.

6. Tower M. Intimate partner violence and health care response: a postmodern critique. *Health Care Women Int.* 2007;28:438-452.

7. Dutton DG. My back pages: reflections on thirty years of domestic violence research. *Trauma Violence Abuse.* 2008;9:131.

FOREWORD

As a society, we have made significant strides to address victimization and perpetration caused by intimate partner violence (IPV) in the United States. Our approaches to addressing IPV were brought center stage in the early 1990s when the Violence Against Women Act (VAWA) 1994 became law. After significant inquiry into the extent and severity of domestic violence, sexual assault, and stalking, congress determined that there needed to be funds allocated to address the issues of intentional violence, as the problem in the US was pervasive and was having a detrimental impact on society.

This was to be a pivotal moment in the United States' history as it defined the values we choose to invest in as a nation. VAWA became a comprehensive legislative package that facilitated services for victims, strengthened local and federal laws, and promoted enforcement of protective orders. VAWA also created legal assistance for immigrants who were battered that prevented their abusers from using immigration law to control victims. The toll-free National Domestic Violence Hotline was also established through the passage of VAWA. Additionally, funds were appropriated to support battered women's shelters, DV and sexual assault education intervention, and prevention programs. The grant programs provided support to state, tribal, and local governments and community-based agencies to train staff, establish specialized domestic violence and sexual assault units, assist victims of violence, and hold perpetrators accountable. This nation could not have begun to address the depth of societal issues caused by IPV without VAWA. As I reflect on this history, I gratefully acknowledge the progress we have made while remaining equally mindful of the dire need to do more.

Much has been discovered about the effects of violence on individuals, families, and communities. It was the late Dr. Martin Luther King that summarized the effects of intentional violence so poignantly, by stating, "Violence is immoral because it thrives on hatred rather than love. Violence is impractical because it is a descending spiral ending in destruction of all. It is immoral because it seeks to humiliate the opponent rather than win his understanding; it seeks to annihilate rather than convert. Violence ends up defeating itself. It creates bitterness in the survivors and brutality in the destroyers."

Dr. King's words have resonated true in my professional experience over the past 20 years. As a nurse practitioner and sexual assault nurse examiner in a variety of clinical settings, I have repeatedly witnessed the devastating effects that intentional violence (such as IPV) has on women, children, and men. I believe that Dr. King would be proud of the progress made over the past two decades and he would, without a doubt, challenge us to do more. After all, the approaches used to address intentional violence are based on the values that we, as a society, choose to adopt. Understanding inflicted intentional violence begins with saying, "This is not right," and then asking, "What can be done?"

Intimate Partner Violence: A Resource for Professionals Working with Children and Families assists the reader in answering the latter question: "What can be done?" We now know and understand the dynamics of IPV and its effects. The literature related to IPV has grown exponentially and what sets this volume apart are its multiple interdisciplinary contributions. This book provides practical information that is needed to address intervention strategies that need to be employed in the various clinical settings. Integrating a number of disciplines in one book has great value. We have come to know and acknowledge that caring for victims of violent acts is best done is concert and that learning from each other makes us more proficient in our respective disciplines. Each chapter is written by scholars who have earned the respect of those of us working in the domestic violence community. Compiling the knowledge of these authors collectively serves novice and experts well and comprises a book that can be used in a variety of clinical and educational settings. We know that no single discipline is capable of providing all the tenants of care needed on its own—but, together, we have the capability to assist victims and their families in healing and thriving in the aftermath of violence.

Annie Lewis-O'Connor NP-BC, MPH, PhD
Assistant Professor Boston University School of Medicine
Child Protection Team- Boston Medical Center
Boston, Massachusetts

FOREWORD

For the past 15 years, I have served as the director of an intervention program for young children affected by violence. The program partnered with the Boston Police Department and was created in response to the epidemic of community violence afflicting our city (and many urban areas) in the early 1990s. Our intention was to identify the hidden victims of crime—the youngest bystanders to street and gang violence—and to provide them with developmentally informed counseling to alleviate the pernicious effects of violence.

Our first referral was a four-year-old boy who had witnessed the shooting death of his mother. The police first thought it was a random shooting; this assumption turned out to be wrong. The woman was shot and killed by her boyfriend. This unfortunate event exemplified a trend that was clear by the end of our first year of offering services, a trend that has since remained the same: the vast majority of referrals we received were for children who had witnessed violence in the home, often between the adults who provided care for them, not violence among strangers on the street. This violence, the kind that occurs behind closed doors, was much less visible than community violence. We realized, also, that it was much easier to talk about the violence in our streets than to confront the violence within our homes.

In the years since then, domestic or intimate partner violence has become a more visible and public issue. There is now increasing social acceptance for women to come forward and disclose intimate partner violence, which has been called a national epidemic and a public health crisis. Professional medical societies have issued position papers and guidelines to their members about assessing for and responding to intimate partner violence. In 1994, federal legislation, the Violence Against Women Act, was enacted that provided funding in every state to support shelter and legal services for battered women and their children.

Concurrently, unprecedented advancements have been made in the research and knowledge base about the impact of trauma on children. A finding with particular relevance to this topic comes from an analysis provided by the National Child Traumatic Stress Network of children served by its network of programs. This survey investigated the various kinds of traumatic events that were in the case histories of children referred for mental health services. Forty-six percent of children had histories of intimate partner violence. Additionally, the average age of the child's first traumatic experience was age 5. There are now hundreds of studies that explore the range of adverse effects of children's exposure to intimate partner violence. The risks include emotional and behavioral problems, learning problems, difficulties with peer relationships, juvenile delinquency, adolescent substance abuse, and adverse health outcomes in adulthood. These links are especially strong if the exposure to violence occurs in early childhood—the time when young children are the most dependent on their adult caregivers for physical and psychological protection.

The encouraging news is that we now know more about how to help victims and perpetrators, and we know that early intervention with vulnerable children makes an important difference. The single most effective approach to intervention for children is to help their adult caregivers reestablish a safe environment. The increased recognition of the devastating legacy of intimate partner violence demands that we intervene early and that we redouble our efforts to identify adult victims and offer them services.

The health care system—both adult and pediatric health services—is a critical ally in the effort to identify and intervene with families affected by intimate partner violence. It is perhaps the one service system that encounters most adults and virtually all children at some point. For adults, their health care providers are a trusted and respected source of information and a critical link to services. Although health care providers sometimes worry that these questions are unnecessary or offensive to patients, our experience proves otherwise. For example, in a recent initiative to improve screening for intimate partner violence in the pediatric Emergency Department at Boston Medical Center, a large majority of parents have expressed approval—even appreciation—when being asked about relationship violence. In order to build our capacity to identify and respond to families who struggle with intimate partner violence, it is essential that health care providers have the opportunity to increase their understanding of the issue, their knowledge of resources and collaborators in the community, and their skills in discussing this issue with patients.

Thus, the value of this book, *Intimate Partner and Domestic Violence: A Resource for Professionals Working with Children and Families,* is evident. Written by a diverse group of health care professionals, the book includes social work and mental health professionals in its audience. It is comprehensive in scope, with a concise review of the literature on screening in health care settings, 2 chapters on working with male perpetrators, and a chapter on teen dating violence. The material includes research, epidemiological data, and concrete practice suggestions. This will be a useful and accessible resource for a range of professionals who work with families and it will help each of us to ensure that children and families remain safe.

Betsy McAlister Groves, LICSW
Director, Child Witness to Violence Project
Boston Medical Center
Associate Professor of Pediatrics
Boston University School of Medicine
Boston, Massachusetts

PREFACE

This book was specifically developed to meet the information and clinical practice needs for professionals who work with children and families to identify and initially respond to intimate partner violence (IPV). Parents, mostly mothers, who bring their children in for care are willing to answer questions on a whole host of issues that may impact their children's well being, including violence in their own households. As a society, we have learned the significant negative consequences that IPV can have for the children living in its shadow. Such consequences include the ongoing stress of living in an unstable, volatile home environment, the potential for the child to be physically maltreated, and the increasingly recognized psychological damage that comes from witnessing or being exposed to violence in the home where a loved one is threatened or harmed.

In 1988, two publications helped raise awareness of IPV's overlap with child maltreatment. Both Tjaden and Thoennes' *In Harm's Way: Domestic Violence and Child Maltreatment*[1] and the statement by the American Academy of Pediatrics' (AAP) Committee on Child Abuse and Neglect, entitled, "The Role of the Pediatrician in Recognizing and Intervening on Behalf of Abused Women,"[2] provided data and policy recommendations that made clear that intervening on behalf of the victimized intimate partner was also a way to reduce risk and decrease harmful exposure for children who lived in those violent households. The AAP clearly stated that intervening on behalf of the mother who was being harmed might very well be the most effective child abuse prevention program available. All that we have learned over the past decade has reinforced the wisdom of intervention and has prompted a great deal of professional interest while calling attention to the need for increased training and attention to the signs and symptoms of abuse in the clinical setting. Despite growing awareness, many opportunities are still missed to screen, identify, and respond to parents who are being harmed by their partners. Missed opportunities in both adult and pediatric settings are evidenced by the generally low screening rates and the paucity of effective office procedures and protocols around IPV screening and intervention.

Professionals in other health care settings who deal with children and families may find this book valuable to their professional practice. The authors have kept all health care professionals in mind when writing the various chapters contained herein. We see our audience as broad while directed at physicians, nurse practitioners, physicians assistants, nurses (office, emergency department, and school), and clinical social workers. We also think the information will be beneficial for teachers, child care workers, social service workers, attorneys, law enforcement personnel, judges, and others who consider themselves child advocates.

Long ago, those of us in the child abuse field learned that it takes a whole team of professionals, each with their own expertise and professional identity, to adequately deal with the problem of child maltreatment. The same is true for IPV—no one field or agency has all the tools to help those we seek to serve. Professionals must work together, share knowledge, and forge linkages between fields, agencies, and areas of professional practice. We are fortunate that early in our careers, we came across incredibly dedicated professionals and community activists in Philadelphia who came together to form the Institute for Safe Families. The mission of the Institute for Safe Families (www.instituteforsafefamilies.org) was singularly focused on increasing the awareness of and the community's response to both those who were at risk and those who were harmed by IPV. Being part of multiple training efforts, several community initiatives, and a number of public awareness campaigns showed us one thing—

professionals will do the right thing if empowered with up-to-date knowledge and the tools to respond effectively. We saw that adequately prepared professionals who were supported by well designed community resources were not limited by the age-old "fear of opening Pandora's box," but instead, would passionately seek to screen their patients in hopes of drawing the problem of IPV out of the shadows to prevent and eliminate the harm that IPV brings.

We hope this book contributes towards that shared mission of encouraging our professional colleagues to address this multifaceted public health issue in an informed and effective manner. We all dream about the day when books such of this will no longer be necessary, but in current times, IPV causes far too much harm for us to avoid directly confronting it in our clinical work. So, we offer this work to all who want to make a difference in the lives of children and their families. Clinicians diagnose what they know just as other professionals working to prevent and end IPV work within the context of their knowledge. This is the reason why, with this book as a desk reference, professionals will be enabled to properly and authoritatively screen, identify, and respond to IPV. Together as a committed team of professionals, we can identify this problem and make effective efforts towards mitigating the negative effects that IPV has on children and families.

Angelo P. Giardino, MD, PhD, MPH, FAAP
Medical Director
Texas Children's Health Plan
Clinical Professor of Pediatrics
Baylor College of Medicine
Attending Physician
Children's Assessment Center
Texas Children's Hospital
Houston, Texas

Eileen R. Giardino, PhD, RN, FNP-BC, ANP-BC
Associate Professor
The University of Texas Health Science Center-Houston
Department of Acute & Continuing Care
School of Nursing
Houston, Texas

REFERENCES

1. U.S. Department of Health and Human Services. Children's Bureau, Administration on Children, Youth Families. Administration for Children and Families. National Clearing House on Child Abuse and Neglect Information. *In Harm's Way: Domestic Violence and Child Maltreatment.* http://www.calib.com/dvcps/facts/harmway.doc. Accessed May 23, 2008.

2. American Academy of Pediatrics Committee on Child Abuse and Neglect: The Role of the pediatrician in recognizing and intervening on behalf of abuse women. *Pediatrics.* 1998;101:1091-1092

TABLE OF CONTENTS

CHAPTER 6: THE ABUSED PATIENT: A CLINICAL RESPONSE USING THE STAGES OF CHANGE MODEL

CHAPTER 11: DOMESTIC CRIMES INVESTIGATIONS AND LAW ENFORCEMENT

CHAPTER 12: ROLE OF IPV PROFESSIONALS IN CRIMINAL PROSECUTION

Intimate Partner Violence

A Resource for Professionals
Working with Children and Families

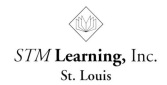

STM **Learning,** Inc.
St. Louis

Chapter 1

OVERVIEW OF THE PROBLEM

Maria D. McColgan, MD, MSEd
Sandra Dempsey, MSS, MLSP
Martha Davis, MSS
Angelo P. Giardino, MD, PhD, MPH, FAAP

When conjuring an image of intimate partner violence (IPV), most people find themselves picturing the sad face of a woman covered with bruises. But the damage and long-term effects of IPV run deeper than the visible physical injuries to its victims. These victims may experience shame, isolation, detrimental physical and mental health consequences, and financial stressors. Intimate partner violence also has dramatic effects on the families of victims, especially children, who, in addition to the increased risk of physical abuse, may experience the trauma of witnessing the violence and feeling the fear, guilt, and shame associated with it.

Intimate partner violence is commonly defined as a pattern of coercive behaviors including repeated battering and injury, psychological abuse, sexual assault, progressive isolation, deprivation, and intimidation.[1-3] Although professional literature makes use of more specific terms, such as spousal abuse, wife-battering, and domestic violence, IPV is the most inclusive referent for this phenomenon. Intimate partner violence is a pattern of coercive behavior in which an individual establishes and maintains power and control over another with whom he or she has a relationship. Intimate partner violence as described above not only includes physical abuse, but also verbal, emotional, economic, and sexual victimization, and involves intimidation, threats, and isolation. Intimate partner violence crosses all socioeconomic and ethnic groups and occurs in both heterosexual and same-sex relationships. Because most IPV incidents are not reported to the police, it is believed that available data greatly underestimate the true magnitude of the problem.[4,5]

Intimate partner violence is appropriately seen as a public health priority, in that large numbers of the population are at risk for this form of victimization. As professional understanding of IPV has increased, screening tools have emerged for health care professionals to use during the health care encounter, and intervention strategies have been developed to help ensure the victim's safety and to enable them to leave the relationship. Additionally, batterer intervention programs have emerged with the goal of decreasing the risk that perpetrators will use violence in their relationships again.

This book is directed at health care professionals who may be the first nonfamily member a victim of domestic violence turns to for help.[1] Physicians, nurse practitioners, and other clinicians are frequently in a position to observe patterns of injury, repeated injuries, adverse mental outcomes, and other indicators of IPV, but may fail to recognize them as such. Initiatives around IPV screening in the health care setting initially studied adult providers such as emergency medicine, family practice, internal medicine, and obstetrics and gynecology (OB/GYN), but these initiatives have been disseminated to pediatrics and pediatric emergency medicine as well. While progress has been made in the recognition of IPV as a health care issue, there is room for improvement in screening practices and intervention. The purpose of this book is to provide a resource for practitioners from all disciplines dealing with IPV.

SCOPE OF THE PROBLEM

Among adults 18 and over, approximately 5.3 million intimate partner victimizations occur among women and 3.2 million among men each year in the United States, resulting in nearly 2 million injuries and 1300 deaths.[4,6] Females are the most common victims, with males as the most common perpetrator. Approximately 1 in 3 to 1 in 4 adult women have experienced a physical assault by an intimate partner during adulthood.[7,8] A national study found that 29% of women and 22% of men had experienced physical, sexual, or psychological IPV during their lifetime.[9]

Although victims of IPV are more commonly female, they may be male, female, or transgender; they may be either married or unmarried, involved in heterosexual or same-sex relationships, and may be members of any ethnic or socioeconomic group.[10–12] Bragg points out that it is a myth that only poor, uneducated women are victims of IPV, and the National Coalition of Anti-Violence Programs, a coalition of 24 community-based organizations serving the lesbian, gay, bisexual, and transgender communities, has raised awareness of this problem in those communities as well.[11,12]

Controversy remains regarding the race and economic status and their relationship to IPV.[3] Some studies find no relationship between IPV and race, economic status, educational level, or insurance status. Other studies assert that lower socio-economic status conveys a higher risk for IPV. In the National Violence Against Women (NVAW) Survey, the ethnic groups most at risk are American Indian/Alaskan Native women and men, African American women, and Hispanic women.[4] Those below the poverty line are also disproportionately identified as victims of IPV.[10] The use of alcohol or drugs increases risk additionally.

While there are no proven psychological or cultural profiles that are specific to battered women, different characteristics appear to be related to a higher risk for domestic abuse. Women who are between the ages of 17 and 28, women who abuse alcohol, and pregnant women are more likely to be victims of abuse.[1] During pregnancy, 4% to 8% of women are abused at least once.[13] Other studies have identified the prevalence of IPV in pregnancy from 18% to 38%.[14,15]

Teens are also at risk for IPV. In a study of adolescents in Massachusetts, approximately 1 in 5 female high school students (20.2% in 1997 and 18.0% in 1999) reported being physically or sexually abused by a dating partner.[16] Nearly 10% of older girls reported abuse by dates or boyfriends, and 8% of high school age girls said "yes" when asked whether "a boyfriend or date has ever forced sex against your will."[17] Forty percent of girls age 14 to 17 reported knowing someone their age who had been hit or beaten by a boyfriend.[18] The college years appear to be a particularly risky time to be victimized by IPV as well. In a survey of college women, 88% of respondents had experienced at least one episode of physical or sexual abuse and 64% had experienced both.[19]

Intimate partner violence is chronic in nature. Of the women raped by an intimate partner, 51.2% were victimized multiple times by the same partner.[4] **Tables 1-1 to 1-5** summarize the data gathered by the NVAW report and provide various quantitative snapshots of the number of victims harmed by IPV based on parameters, including type of victimization, gender, type of physical assault, and ethnicity.

Table 1-1. Persons Victimized by an Intimate Partner in Lifetime, by Victim Gender, Type of Victimization, and Victim Race

| Type of Victimization | Persons Victimized in Lifetime (%) | | | | |
	White	African-American	Asian Pacific Islander	American Indian/ Alaska Native	Mixed Race
Women	(*n*=6452)	(*n*=780)	(*n*=133)	(*n*=88)	(*n*=397)
Rape[a]	7.7	7.4	3.8[b]	15.9	8.1
Physical assault[c,d]	21.3	26.3	12.8	30.7	27.0
Stalking	4.7	4.2	—[e]	10.2[b]	6.3
Total victimized[e]	**24.8**	**29.1**	**15.0**	**37.5**	**30.2**
Men	(*n*=6424)	(*n*=659)	(*n*=165)	(*n*=105)	(*n*=406)
Rape	0.2	0.9[b]	—[e]	—[e]	—[e]
Physical assault	7.2	10.8	—[e]	11.4	8.6
Stalking	0.6	1.1[b]	—[e]	—[e]	1.2[b]
Total victimized	**7.5**	**12.0**	**3.0**[b]	**12.4**	**9.1**

[a] *Estimates for American Indian/Alaska Native women are significantly higher than those for white and African-American women: Tukey's B, p≤.05.*

[b] *Relative standard error exceeds 30 percent; estimates not included in statistical testing.*

[c] *Estimates for Asian/Pacific Islander women are significantly lower than those for African-American, American Indian/Alaska Native, and mixed-race women: Tukey's B, p≤.05.*

[d] *Estimates for African-American women are significantly higher than those for white women: Tukey's B, p≤.05.*

[e] *Estimates not calculated on fewer than five victims.*

Adapted with permission: Tjaden P, Thoennes N. Extent, nature, and consequences of intimate partner violence: findings from the National Violence Against Women Survey. Washington, DC: US Dept of Justice; 2000. NCJ 181867.

Children are also affected by IPV. Approximately 3.3 to 10 million children witness the abuse of a parent or adult caregiver each year.[7,20,21] Children living in families with IPV are more likely than their peers to be victims of abuse, as there is child abuse in 30% to 60% of families experiencing IPV.[20–24]

Children who live with IPV face increased risks of exposure to traumatic events, neglect, being directly abused, and of losing one or both of their parents. Several studies have shown that exposure to domestic violence leads to an increased likelihood of experiencing a number of adult health problems, engaging in a number of risk taking behaviors, and being at risk for experiencing violence in adulthood.[20,22,25] These risks are discussed in further detail in the section below entitled, "Consequences of IPV." In addition, children who are raised in homes with IPV suffer an increased risk of experiencing violence in adulthood.

As IPV is such a pervasive problem with dramatic consequences to the health and welfare of patients, it is a problem that health care practitioners cannot afford to ignore.

Table 1-2. Number of Rape, Physical Assault, and Stalking Victimizations Perpetrated by Intimate Partners Annually, by Victim Gender

TYPE OF VICTIMIZATION	NUMBER OF VICTIMS	AVERAGE NUMBER OF VICTIMIZATIONS PER VICTIM[a]	TOTAL NUMBER OF VICTIMIZATIONS	ANNUAL RATE OF VICTIMIZATION PER 1000 PERSONS
Women				
Rape[c]	201 394	1.6[b]	322 230[b]	3.2
Physical assault	1 309 061	3.4	4 450 807	44.2
Stalking	503 485	1.0	503 485	5.0
Men				
Rape[c]	—	—	—	—
Physical assault	834 732	3.5	2 921 562	31.5
Stalking	185 496	1.0	185 496	1.8

[a] *The standard error of the mean is 0.5 for female rape victims, 0.6 for female physical assault victims, and 0.6 for male physical assault victims. Because stalking by definition means repeated acts and because no victim was stalked by more than one perpetrator in the 12 months preceding the survey, the number of stalking victimizations was imputed to be the same as the number of stalking victims. Thus, the average number of stalking victimizations per victim is 1.0.*
[b] *Relative standard error exceeds 30 percent.*
[c] *Estimates not calculated on fewer than five victims.*

Adapted with permission: Tjaden P, Thoennes N. Extent, nature, and consequences of intimate partner violence: findings from the National Violence Against Women Survey. Washington, DC: US Dept of Justice; 2000. NCJ 181867.

THE HISTORICAL PERSPECTIVE

The roots of IPV can be found throughout history, and the predominate view relates the history of IPV primarily to the status of women and how they are treated in both family settings as well as the body politic in general.[26] In many cultures throughout the world, women throughout the ages have often been considered subordinate and dependent, and have typically been given few to no civil rights or protections from violence. The occurrence of family and domestic violence is an international tragedy that remains pervasive in many societies in both the developed and in the developing world. Even today, in our modern age, conditions exist throughout the world wherein women and children are harmed by members of their families. Progress is being made—albeit too slowly for the victims—that builds awareness of IPV and has the potential to correct the situations that permit this problem to continue. According to a presentation to the UN Secretary General concerning an in-depth study on violence against women in October 2006[27]:

Violence against women is not confined to a specific culture, region, or country, or to a particular group of women within a society. Quite the reverse. Violence against women is truly a global phenomenon. Complex, pervasive, persistent, pernicious. It occurs in different settings, takes many different manifestations, and evolves and emerges in new forms. The way that women the world over experience it is influenced by a range of factors, such as age, class, disability, ethnicity, and economic status. On average, at least one in three women is subject to violence at some point in her lifetime. Let me repeat this: at least *one in three*.

Any and all violence against women is unacceptable, whether perpetrated by the State and its agents, by family members or strangers, in the public or private sphere, in peacetime or in times of conflict. Violence against women endangers women's lives, violates their rights as citizens and human beings, harms their families and communities, and poses an affront to humanity itself. It tears at the fabric of all societies. And so all societies must take responsibility to deal and do away with it. And all States have a particular obligation to protect women from violence, to hold perpetrators accountable, and to provide justice and remedies to victims.

Even in the United States, founded under the principles of justice for all, women as a group had to struggle politically for equal rights under the law. Prior to advocates taking up the cause, no help existed to protect and aid women in abusive relationships. Violence between married partners was typically considered a private matter between individuals, and law enforcement did not generally intervene. Victims of violence were forced to suffer essentially in silence because they had no recourse and felt shame and embarrassment. Until the mid-1970s violence against wives was considered a misdemeanor in most states.[1] Following a nationwide recognition of the rights of women to be safe in their homes, Pennsylvania enacted the nation's first domestic restraining law in 1976.[28] Through open discussion, it became obvious that many women were forced to stay in violent relationships because they had no legal recourse, no job skills, no control of finances, and no safe haven. In-depth case studies provided insight into the reality of the lives of battered women, leading to the establishment of shelters and programs for victims of IPV.[29]

In 1990, the first comprehensive federal legislation responding to violence against women was introduced. With the help of advocates nationwide, The Violence Against Women Act (VAWA) was signed into law in 1994 (PL-103-322).[30,31] Subsequently, programs for domestic violence victims have proliferated across the country.[14] Since 1996, the National Domestic Violence Hotline has answered more than 1 million calls.[31]

With laws protecting women from abuse, shelters as safe havens, and counseling, women are more likely to report abuse and are less fearful and more empowered to get out of the vicious cycle. **Table 1-6** summarizes several of the important laws related to IPV in the United States that have been enacted with profound effect.[11,32]

Table 1-3. Persons Physically Assaulted by an Intimate Partner in Lifetime, by Type of Assault and Victim Gender

TYPE OF ASSAULT[a]	WOMEN (%) (N=8000)	MEN (%) (N=8000)
Threw something that could hurt	8.1	4.4
Pushed, grabbed, shoved	18.1	5.4
Pulled hair	9.1	2.3
Slapped, hit	16.0	5.5
Kicked, bit	5.5	2.6
Choked, tried to drown	6.1	0.5
Hit with object	5.0	3.2
Beat up	8.5	0.6
Threatened with gun	3.5	0.4
Threatened with knife	2.8	1.6
Used gun	0.7	0.1[b]
Used knife	0.9	0.8
Total reporting physical assault by Intimate Partner	**22.1**	**7.4**

[a] *With the exception of "used gun" and "used knife," differences between women and men are statistically significant: χ^2, $p \leq .001$.*

[b] *Relative standard error exceeds 30 percent; statistical tests not performed.*

Adapted with permission: Tjaden P, Thoennes N. Extent, nature, and consequences of intimate partner violence: findings from the National Violence Against Women Survey. Washington, DC: US Dept of Justice; 2000. NCJ 181867.

Table 1-4. Persons Victimized by an Intimate Partner in Lifetime, by Victim Gender, Type of Victimization, and White/Nonwhite Status of Victim

VICTIM GENDER/TYPE OF VICTIMIZATION	VICTIMIZED IN LIFETIME (%)	
	WHITE	NONWHITE[a]
Women	(*n*=6452)	(*n*=1398)
Rape	7.7	7.8
Physical assault[b***]	21.3	25.5
Stalking	4.7	5.0
Total victimized[b**]	**24.8**	**28.6**
Men	(*n*=6424)	(*n*=1335)
Rape	0.2	0.5[c]
Physical assault[b**]	7.2	9.1
Stalking[b*]	0.6	1.1
Total victimized[b**]	**7.5**	**10.0**

[a] *The nonwhite category consists of African-American, Native American/Alaska Native, Asian/Pacific Islander, and mixed-race respondents.*

[b] *Differences between whites and nonwhites are statistically significant: χ^2, *$p \leq .05$, **$p \leq .01$, ***$p \leq .001$.*

[c] *Relative standard error exceeds 30 percent; statistical tests not performed.*

Adapted with permission: Tjaden P, Thoennes N. Extent, nature, and consequences of intimate partner violence: findings from the National Violence Against Women Survey. Washington, DC: US Dept of Justice; 2000. NCJ 181867.

It was not until the last decade of the 20th Century that the health care system became an important site for IPV programs.[14] In 1992, the authoritative Joint Commission on Accreditation of Healthcare Organizations (JCAHO) required that all accredited hospitals implement policies and procedures in their facilities to identify, treat, and refer victims of domestic violence.[1] While this mandated attention to the problem in our nation's health care facilities, most of the programmatic responses have focused on screening and identification; only a small number have focused on treatment of victims of IPV.[14]

CONCEPTUAL FRAMEWORKS

Intimate partner violence has been described as a spiral of violence in which threats, intimidation, control, and battering increase over time.[3] While the types of abuse may vary, the perpetrator is maintaining a constant state of power and control. The abuser may stop some blatant behaviors at times, as outlined in the cycle of violence theory, but will continue different oppressive tactics.

CYCLE OF VIOLENCE THEORY

In the late 1970s, *The Battered Women*, an influential book published by psychologist Lenore E. Walker, framed out a paradigm for the battering cycle. It has since been renamed the ***Cycle of Violence Theory*** and is intended to assist in the conceptualization of how the typical case of IPV unfolds.[33,34] There were originally 3 distinct stages in the cycle of violence: tension building, explosion, and the honeymoon, or contrition, period (a fourth was subsequently added). In the original description, the tension building stage denotes the period during which the abuser may use verbal threats as a means of control. Eventually, the increased tension leads to increasing violence in the explosion stage. Finally, in the honeymoon period, an attempt at reconciliation and promises of an end to the abuse are generally made. It is the honeymoon phase that encourages the victim to stay in the relationship, with the hope that the situation will improve.[35] Over time, though, these periods of reconciliation and peace diminish and the severity of the abuse and violence increases. The cycle may repeat hundreds of times, with each stage lasting anywhere from a few hours to a year or more. Often, as time goes on, the tension building and the honeymoon stages may disappear. Subsequent to the original description of the cycle theory of violence, a fourth stage was proposed by S.A. Matar Curnow, referred to as the open window phase. This stage is thought to occur between the explosion and honeymoon stages. Using interview data drawn from a qualitative study of women at a women's shelter, the open window stage was characterized as the stage immediately following an acute battering incident in which victims are most likely to see that they have been abused, seek help, learn alternatives to violence, and be receptive to intervention.[36] Hence, this stage is called the "open window" because it presents the woman with an opportunity to see ways of keeping herself safe and avoiding exposure to the abusive behavior of the perpetrator in the future. Other authors have offered additional modifications to this model over the years, but the basic structure, as originally proposed, remains intact.[35,37] **Table 1-7a** summarizes the original 3 stages of the cycle of violence theory, while **Table 1-7b** provides a summary of the additions or modifications that has been suggested over the years following its original publication.

Table 1-5. Persons Victimized by an Intimate Partner in Lifetime, by Gender, Type of Victimization, and History of Same-Sex/Opposite-Sex Cohabitation

VICTIM GENDER/ TYPE OF VICTIMIZATION	HISTORY OF SAME-SEX COHABITATION[a]	HISTORY OF OPPOSITE-SEX COHABITATION[b]
Women	(*n*=79)	(*n*=7193)
Rape	11.4[c]	4.4
Physical assault[d*]	35.4	20.4
Stalking	—[e]	4.1
Total victimized[d**]	**39.2**	**21.7**
Men	(*n*=65)	(*n*=6,879)
Rape	—[e]	0.2
Physical assault[d*]	21.5	7.1
Stalking	—[e]	0.5
Total victimized[d**]	**23.1**	**7.4**

[a] *Subsample consists of respondents who have ever lived with a same-sex intimate partner.*

[b] *Subsample consists of respondents who have ever married and/or lived with an opposite-sex intimate partner but never with a same-sex intimate partner.*

[c] *Relative standard error exceeds 30 percent; statistical tests not performed.*

[d] *Differences between same-sex and opposite-sex cohabitants are statistically significant: χ^2, *$p \leq .01$, **$p \leq .001$.*

[e] *Estimates not calculated on fewer than five individuals.*

Adapted with permission: Tjaden P, Thoennes N. Extent, nature, and consequences of intimate partner violence: findings from the National Violence Against Women Survey. Washington, DC: US Dept of Justice; 2000. NCJ 181867.

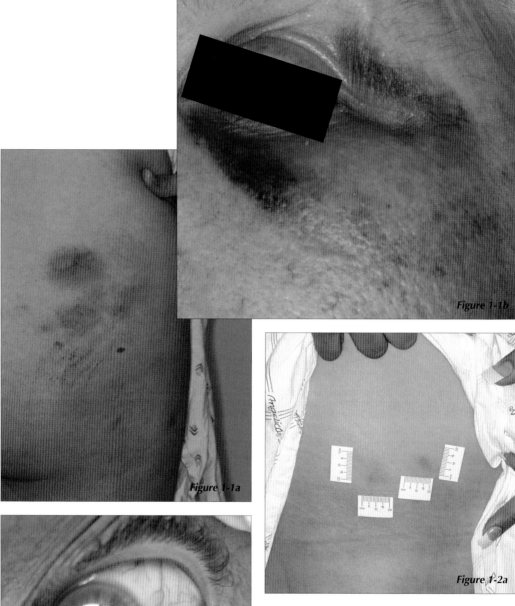

Figure 1-1a and 1-1b. Typical bruises resulting from physical violence.

Figure 1-2a. Fingertip sized bruises on the outer left thigh prove forceful grabbing as the victim attempted to flee. The bruises' yellowish hue indicates that they are not fresh.

Figure 1-2b. Upon restraining the victim, the batterer began strangling her despite the lack of petechial hemorrhages in the sclera of the eye.

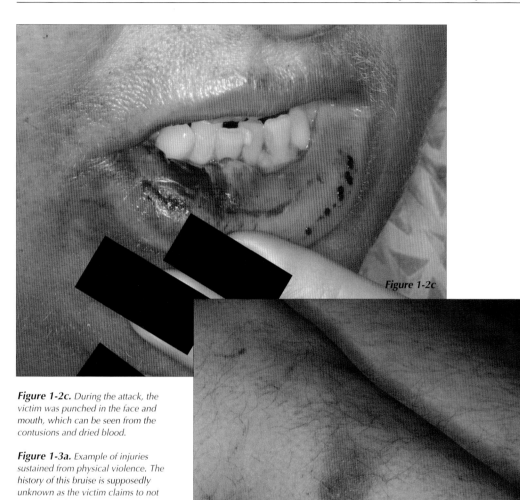

Figure 1-2c

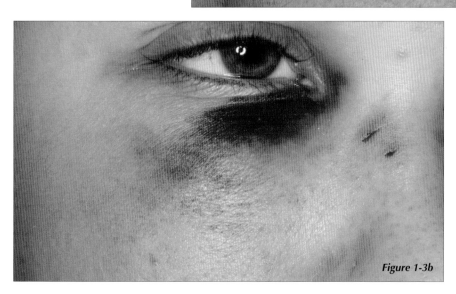

Figure 1-3a

Figure 1-2c. *During the attack, the victim was punched in the face and mouth, which can be seen from the contusions and dried blood.*

Figure 1-3a. *Example of injuries sustained from physical violence. The history of this bruise is supposedly unknown as the victim claims to not "remember how that happened."*

Figure 1-3b. *Example of injuries sustained from physical violence.*

Figure 1-3b

Table 1-6. Key Federal Domestic Violence Legislation

LEGISLATION	DESCRIPTION	NOTES
Family Violence Prevention and Services Act of 1984 (Pub L No. 98-457)	Helped states' public awareness efforts. Funded victims' shelters and other services. Grants awarded for program development and training of law enforcement and community providers.	First time IPV was addressed by Congress.
Violence Against Women Act (VAWA), Title IV of the Violent Crime Control and Law Enforcement Act (Pub L No. 103-322)	Four titles within act that address IPV, sexual assault, stalking, and protection against violence. Improved law enforcement and criminal justice system response. Increased funding for prevention, education, training, and victims' services. New protection for battered immigrant women.	Major turning point in federal government's recognition and handling of IPV. Demonstrated government commitment to the problem of IPV.
Personal Responsibility and Work Opportunity Reconciliation Act of 1996 (PRWORA) – Wellstone/Murray Amendment (Pub L No. 104-193)	PRWORA replaced AFDC with TANF. Wellstone/Murray Amendment has a provision called the "Family Violence Option." Acknowledges the safety and economic barriers of IPV victims.	States have option of exempting IPV victims from TANF time limits and work requirements of PRWORA mandates.
Victims of Trafficking and Violence Prevention Act of 2000 (VTVPA) (Pub L No. 106-386)	Primary purpose is to protect human rights of victims of human trafficking, who are primarily women and girls. Immigrant victims of domestic violence are included under legislation. U-Visas were created to allow immigrant victims of crimes to apply for legal residency where domestic violence is included under the crimes.	U-Visas have yet to be fully enacted by the federal government agency overseeing immigration. Immigrant victims of domestic violence can apply for U-Visas interim relief to obtain temporary legal status until U-Visas are available.

Adapted from Bragg HL. Child Protection in Families Experiencing Domestic Violence. Washington, DC: US Dept of Health and Human Services, Office on Child Abuse and Neglect. www.childwelfare.gov/pubs/usermanuals/domesticviolence.pdf. Accessed June 19, 2008 *and WomensLaw.org. Information for immigrants: U-Visa laws and procedures. Available at: http://www.womenslaw.org/immigrantsUvisa.htm. Accessed May 21, 2007.*

SALTZMAN'S TYPOLOGY OF INTIMATE PARTNER VIOLENCE

Saltzman describes 4 primary types of IPV[38]:

1. *Physical violence.* (**Figure 1-1a to Figure 1-3b**) The intentional use of physical force. Physical violence includes, but is not limited to, scratching; pushing; shoving; throwing; grabbing; biting; choking; shaking; slapping; punching; burning; use of a weapon; and use of restraints or one's body, size, or strength against another person.

2. *Sexual violence.* (**Figure 1-4a to Figure 1-4d**) Divided into 3 categories: 1) use of physical force to compel a person to engage in a sexual act against his or her will, whether or not the act is completed; 2) attempted or completed sex act involving a person who is unable to understand the nature or condition of the act, to decline participation, or to communicate unwillingness to engage in the sexual act, for example, because of illness, disability, or the influence of alcohol or other drugs, or because of intimidation or pressure; and 3) abusive sexual contact.

3. *Threats of physical or sexual violence.* Perpetrator uses words, gestures, or weapons to communicate the intent to cause death, disability, injury, or physical harm.

4. *Psychological/emotional violence.* Involves acts, threats of acts, or coercive tactics, such as humiliating the victim, controlling what the victim can and cannot do, withholding information from the victim, deliberately doing something to make the victim feel diminished or embarrassed, isolating the victim from friends and family, and denying the victim access to money or other basic resources.

In addition, a fifth category of behavior, stalking, can be included among the types of IPV and may be viewed as an additional fifth form.[4] **Stalking** can be defined as physically following another person in an unwelcome manner. In more legally precise terms, virtually all state definitions include language that defines a pattern of conduct that is directed at a specific person and which is intended to and may actually place the targeted person in fear for their safety.[39]

STAGES OF CHANGE APPROACH

First described by Prochaska in 1979 as it applied to smoking cessation and other areas of behavioral change, the transtheoretical model of change, commonly referred to by one of its components, the stages of change, involves a dynamic process of progression through 5 stages of change: precontemplation, contemplation, preparation, action, and maintenance.[29,44,45] There are other components to the transtheoretical model that are more fully described in chapter 6. Recently, this model has been gaining attention as a possible treatment framework for victims of IPV.[14,29] The transtheoretical model offers practitioners a conceptualization of the concerns of the victim in each stage, thereby allowing the providers to ask relevant questions and develop a plan for the best methods of helping the victim.[14] Further studies demonstrated that, through utilization of stage-matched interventions, dramatic improvements could be made in recruitment, retention, and progress in health promotion programs for at-risk populations and in helping physicians to avoid overloading the victim with information for which she is not ready.[29,44–46] We cannot force people to change.[29] Pushing a victim of abuse to do more than they are ready to do may alienate the victim.[46] Progression through the 5 stages of change (precontemplation, contemplation, preparation, action, and maintenance) is not usually linear. Once a stage is achieved, the person may regress and begin recycling through previous stages.[29] Relapse is a natural and expected part of progressing, as the person potentially learns from her mistakes.[29]

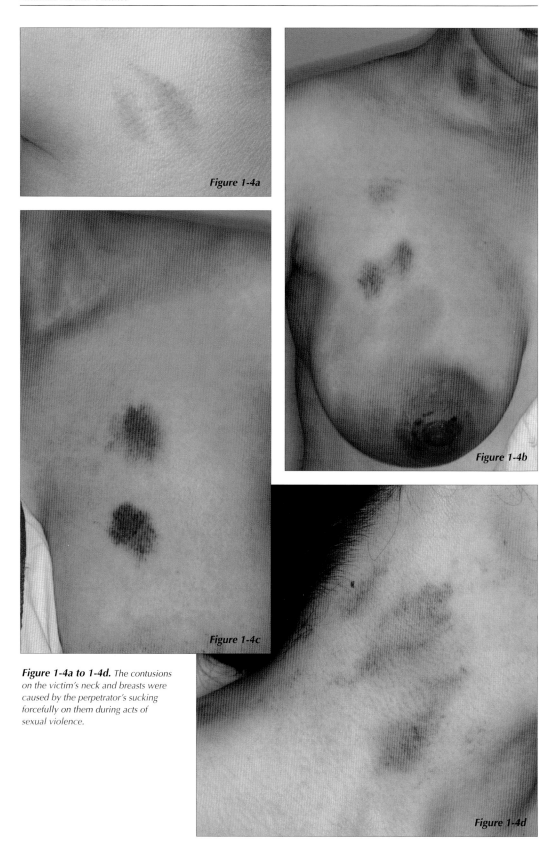

Figure 1-4a

Figure 1-4b

Figure 1-4c

Figure 1-4a to 1-4d. *The contusions on the victim's neck and breasts were caused by the perpetrator's sucking forcefully on them during acts of sexual violence.*

Figure 1-4d

Health care professionals in every specialty from pediatrics to geriatrics will encounter patients who are affected by IPV. There are an estimated 4.8 million acts of intimate partner rape and physical assault each year, with more than 2 million resulting in injury. More than 500 000 of these injuries result in medical treatment for the victim.[10] One study found that 44% of women murdered by their partner had visited an emergency department (ED) within 2 years of the homicide. Ninety-three percent of these victims had at least 1 ED visit for an injury.[47] Another study found that 37% of female patients with injury presenting to the ED were injured by their partner and that only 5% to 7% of battered women were identified by ED staff.[48] They further concluded that, without institutional policies and procedures for detecting and treating victims of domestic violence, many abused women would remain unidentified and untreated.

In addition to presenting with injuries, victims of IPV and their families were more likely to experience negative health outcomes and to have barriers to health care (**see Table 1-8**).[49,50] For example, victims of IPV were less likely to have health insurance, less likely to seek early prenatal care, and less likely to seek treatment for their injuries. Their children were less likely to have up-to-date immunizations. Victims of IPV have more migraines, frequent headaches, chronic pain, heart problems, high blood pressure, gastrointestinal problems, and arthritis. They are also more likely to engage in high-risk behaviors such as smoking and drug and alcohol use and are more likely to contract a sexually transmitted infection. For these reasons, many professional organizations, such as the American Academy of Family Practice, the American College of Obstetrics and Gynecology, the American Academy of Pediatrics, and the American Medical Association, have issued policies or treatment guidelines on identifying and treating patients who are victims of IPV.[51–53]

At present, screening for IPV occurs to a varying degree among the various medical specialties. Routine screening for IPV by OB/GYNs is the highest at 17% to 20.5%. Routine screening among family medicine physicians and pediatricians ranges from 8.5% to 12% in various state surveys.[49,54–56] Studies examining patient perception of screening show a favorable response. In the ED setting, 86% of patients surveyed felt that it was appropriate to ask all women whether they had experienced violent or threatening behavior from someone close to them.[57] Looking specifically at the pediatric ED, Duffy and colleagues conducted a cross-sectional survey of 157 mothers with children fewer than 3 years of age who visited an urban pediatric ED and found that 52% of the women reported histories of adult physical abuse and 21% reported adult sexual abuse. The perpetrators were intimate partners in 67% of the cases of adult physical abuse victimization of women and in 55% of the adult sexual victimization, again supporting the presence of DV/IPV in the families of caregivers bringing their children in for care to pediatricians and emergency departments.[58] A qualitative study that explored the perspectives of 59 mothers, 21 nurses, and 17 physicians in a pediatric ED on IPV screening found that mothers viewed DV/IPV as a common problem that warranted routine screening in the pediatric ED.[59] The study presented the following recommendations about DV/IPV practices in pediatric EDs: 1) those assigned to screen must demonstrate empathy, warmth, and a helping attitude; 2) the child's medical needs must be addressed first and screening for DV/IPV should be performed in a minimally disruptive manner; 3) a clear and organized process of determining risk to the child as a result of the IPV environment must be maintained, especially when child protective services needs to be involved; and 4) resources and referrals for women who request them must be available.[59]

Table 1-7a. Stages of Battering Cycle

STAGE	DESCRIPTION	VICTIM'S PERSPECTIVE	PERPETRATOR'S PERSPECTIVE
Phase 1: Tension Building	Characterized by minor battering incidents and tension building.	Senses tension mounting but may deny tension and abuse are escalating. Believes she can control perpetrator's behavior. Accepts responsibility for abuse. Justifies perpetrator's behavior as caused by external stressors.	Aware that victimizing behavior is inappropriate by societal standards. Fears victim is pulling away or will leave. Jealous, possessive, controlling. Believes he has the right to discipline.
Phase 2: Acute Battering	Characterized by a severe beating incident. Release of tension from tension building phase. Complete loss of control by both the victim and the perpetrator.	Under severe stress, sometimes manifesting in physical symptoms, in anticipation of acute event. Emotionally trapped. Believes that the more she resists the acute battering, the worse it will be. Feels disassociated from the attack. Feels no one can protect her from battering.	Not much is known about the perpetrator at this phase of the cycle. Rage is out of control. Wants to teach a lesson and won't stop until lesson is learned or he is exhausted. Rationalizations include things said or done in tension building phase by victim or stress from outside world.
Phase 3: Honeymoon	Characterized by perpetrator acting loving, kind, and contrite about his actions. Victim and perpetrator makeup. The most loving and fulfilling time of the relationship.	Wants to believe she will no longer suffer abuse. Believes perpetrator can change. Realizes perpetrator needs help, and believes only way he will receive it is if she stays. Believes perpetrator is showing his true self at this stage.	Believes he will never hurt the victim again and promises so. Feels he will be able to control future violence. Believes he has taught the victim a lesson. Threatens suicide or great harm if victim leaves.

Adapted from Walker LE. The Battered Woman. New York, NY: Harper & Row; 1979.

Table 1-7b. A Summary of Suggested Additions or Modifications Following Publication

STAGE	DESCRIPTION

Matar Curnow SA. The open window phase: helpseeking and reality behaviors by battered women. *Appl Nurs Res.*;1997;10:128-135.

| **Open Window** | The author suggests an *Open Window* phase as an addition to Walker's cycle theory of violence. This occurs directly after the acute battering incident and before any loving or contrite behavior of the Honeymoon phase has happened. Victims of intimate partner violence are most likely to see themselves as victims, seek help, learn alternatives to violence, and be receptive to intervention during the *Open Window* phase. |

Long GM, McNamara JR. Paradoxical punishment as it relates to the battered woman syndrome. *Behav Mod.* 1989;13:192-205.

| **Victim's Escape** | According to this author, the *Victim's Escape* is something that occurs in an abusive relationship at a time in the relationship where the honeymoon phase of Walker's cycle theory of violence has ceased to exist. This usually occurs after some length of time, when the honeymoon phase has begun to decrease in frequency or duration. This proposed addition occurs directly after the acute battering incident. The *Victim's Escape* works to reestablish the honeymoon phase in the cycle. |
| **Victim's Return** | This author proposes the addition of the *Victim's Return* directly after the contrition of the honeymoon phase. Battered women are motivated to return to the relationship because of the hypothesized reinforcement that occurs as a result of the love and contrition of the honeymoon phase. |

Copel LC. Partner abuse in physically disabled women: a proposed model for understanding intimate partner violence. *Perspect Psychiatr Care.* 2006;42:114-129.

| **Cooling Off** | The author found that Walker's cycle theory of violence did not exactly apply to the experience of women with physical handicaps. The love and contrition characterizing the honeymoon phase is absent, and in its place exists the opposite of loving, contrition, or even acknowledgement by the batterer that they had done something wrong. Rather, there is a period of separation or *cooling off* after the battering incident, the duration of which is determined by the batterer. |

Adapted from Walker LE. The Battered Woman. New York, NY: Harper & Row; 1979.

In 1998, the American Academy of Pediatrics published a statement recommending routine screening for domestic violence during pediatric visits and stated that "identifying and intervening on behalf of battered women may be one of the most effective means of preventing child abuse."[60] Siegel and colleagues screened 154 women during well-child visits over a 3-month period and found 47 (31%) of the women revealed IPV at some time in their lives, with 25 (17%) of them reporting IPV within the past 2 years and 5 of the women reporting that they were most recently injured during their most recent pregnancy.[61] Of these cases, 5 were associated with child maltreatment cases. Thus, universal screenings found unsuspected cases not associated with child maltreatment, supporting the notion that IPV screening should be done in a pediatric primary care setting.

Screening initiatives have been consistently shown to increase the identification of patients experiencing acute episodes of abuse and seeking treatment. However, sustaining screening programs has proven to be difficult.[62] At present, standard protocols for IPV screening and charting prompts for both screening and interventions are supported by evidence from a number of EDs and primary care settings.[63] Additionally, ongoing training for health care providers is necessary to initiate and maintain screening as well.

Estimates of the financial cost of IPV are huge, with 1 estimate exceeding $5.8 billion annually. These costs include nearly $4.1 billion in direct costs of medical and mental health care and nearly $1.8 billion in indirect costs such as lost productivity.[6] Studies looking at long-term costs for IPV victims found that the average health care costs for women affected by IPV exceeded those of women who had not experienced IPV by up to $1700 USD annually.[64,65] Another study looking at the utilization of medical services in women with diagnosed IPV compared with those without evidence of IPV found that victims of IPV displayed a 1.6-fold increase in the rate of all health care visits and costs compared with those without evidence of IPV.[66]

BLAMING THE VICTIM

Despite the physical and emotional abuse sustained by the battered person, victims commonly find themselves blamed for the abuse. Recurrent questions such as "Why do you put up with that?" or "Why don't you just leave?" are ego deflating and may delay the victim's pursuit of change by putting the onus of abuse on the victim.[29,40] By attempting to understand the complex nature of the battered woman's situation, we can gain insight into the victim's survival skills and the strength needed to decide to leave and act upon that decision.[40] In an effort to understand the complexities of the process of change in the battered woman's situation, imagine the difficulty faced when trying to change even simple behaviors to improve health such as dietary changes, exercise, or smoking cessation.[29] Only by considering the context of relationships, fear of bodily harm and threats, limited financial and social resources, issues of housing, children, the dangers of leaving, et cetera, can we begin to understand the dramatic issues the battered woman faces.[29]

CONSEQUENCES OF INTIMATE PARTNER VIOLENCE

In addition to the immediate risk of injury, there are many short- and long-term consequences of IPV. Women who were victims of both sexual and physical abuse as a child were more likely to become adult victims of sexual or physical abuse and were more likely to be victimized in high school.[19] Women who were victimized in high school were found to be at much greater risk of physical or sexual abuse in college.[19] In addition, physical and sexual abuse against adolescent girls in dating relationships increased the likelihood that the girl would abuse drugs or alcohol, develop an eating disorder, consider or attempt suicide, engage in risky behavior, or become pregnant.[16]

THE ADVERSE CHILDHOOD EXPERIENCES STUDIES

Over the past several years, the Adverse Childhood Experiences (ACE) studies—a series of large scale, methodologically sound studies—found associations between traumatic early childhood experiences such as physical, psychological, and sexual abuse as well as forms of family dysfunction and the presence of substance abuse, mental illness, or criminal behavior in the household; and most notably if the child's mother or stepmother was treated violently; and relatively poor later adult health status.[41] Thus, beyond the obvious immediate negative health consequences associated with being abused, the ACE studies point to significant negative health effects that extend into later life.

The connection that was uncovered by these studies between both prior maltreatment and witnessing IPV and the development in later adult life of serious physical problems (eg, ischemic heart disease, cancer, stroke, chronic bronchitis, emphysema, diabetes, hepatitis, and skeletal fractures) is indeed profound and validates the clinical observation that exposure to family dysfunction may have long-reaching health consequences. But how does an adverse childhood experience lead to adult health problems decades later? The ACE studies demonstrated that, compared with those adults who had no adverse events in their childhoods, those who had experienced 4 or more ACEs showed a fourfold to twelvefold increase in health risks for alcoholism, drug abuse, depression, and suicide attempts; a twofold to fourfold increase in risks for smoking, poor self-rated health, having a high number of sexual partners, and sexually transmitted diseases; and a 1.4-fold to 1.6-fold increase in the risk of physical inactivity and severe obesity. Additionally, there was a steadily increasing relationship between the presence of ACEs and the presence of various adult diseases.

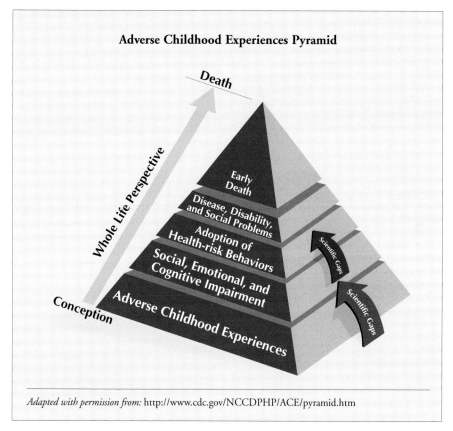

Adverse Childhood Experiences Pyramid

Death

Whole Life Perspective

Early Death

Disease, Disability, and Social Problems

Adoption of Health-risk Behaviors

Social, Emotional, and Cognitive Impairment

Adverse Childhood Experiences

Conception

Scientific Gaps

Scientific Gaps

Adapted with permission from: http://www.cdc.gov/NCCDPHP/ACE/pyramid.htm

Figure 1-5. The ACE Pyramid shows how negative experiences in childhood lead to social, emotional, and cognitive impairments.

The ACE Pyramid **(Figure 1-5)** represents the conceptual model that underlies the process by which adverse childhood experiences may have significant negative health outcomes occur well into adulthood. It systematically shows how negative experiences in childhood lead to social, emotional, and cognitive impairments that may lead to health risk behaviors and lifestyle choices that predispose the individual to develop a variety of illnesses later in life, some of which shorten life expectancy. The diagram also shows scientific gaps that future research needs to address to more fully develop the linkages between the steps in the model. For professionals working in the IPV arena, the ACE studies provide a prominent, quantitative call to action for prevention efforts

Table 1-8. Health Consequences of IPV

PARAMETER	LIFETIME HISTORY OF ABUSE	CURRENT IPV	LIFETIME HISTORY OF IPV	TEEN DATING VIOLENCE	ABUSE DURING OR AROUND PREGNANCY
Access to Health Care	Not addressed.	Most victims of IPV did not seek medical treatment for injuries.	Women with a history of IPV had health insurance coverage at a lower rate.	Abused teens reported first time prenatal care at the third trimester at a higher rate.	Abused women were more than twice as likely to seek first time prenatal care at the third trimester. Abused, older women waited longer to seek prenatal care. Abused women with more financial resources waited longer to seek prenatal care.
Immunization	Almost one third of children living at women's shelters did not have all their immunizations. The children of abused women were less likely to be up to date on their immunizations.	Not addressed.	Not addressed.	Not addressed.	Not addressed.
Injury and Violence	Not addressed.	In emergency rooms, 37% of women with violence-related injuries reported that a current or former intimate partner caused the injuries.	Not addressed.	24% of teens who had experienced dating violence reported that they had experienced severe violence (ie, rape or use of a weapon).	IPV is the leading cause of death among pregnant women.

(continued)

Table 1-8. *(continued)*

PARAMETER	LIFETIME HISTORY OF ABUSE	CURRENT IPV	LIFETIME HISTORY OF IPV	TEEN DATING VIOLENCE	ABUSE DURING OR AROUND PREGNANCY
Injury and Violence *(continued)*	Not addressed.	In an emergency room, 28% of abused women required hospitalization and 13% need major medical treatment. One-third of murdered women were killed by an intimate partner.			
Mental Health	Not addressed.	Women who experienced IPV were more likely to consider and attempt suicide. Women who experienced IPV were more likely to have been depressed, experience difficulty sleeping, anxiety, and symptoms of PTSD* compared with women who did not experience IPV.	The majority of women who are abused are diagnosed with a psychiatric disorder. Almost one third of women who attempt suicide have a history of IPV. Experiences of symptoms of depression (37%), anxiety (46%), and PTSD* (45%) occur with higher frequency in women who have a history of IPV.	Teens who have experienced dating violence are more likely to have suicidal ideation or to have attempted to commit suicide.	There is a higher risk for depression, suicide, increased stress, and lowered self-esteem among women who experience IPV related to pregnancy.
Overweight and Obesity	Morbidly obese individuals were more likely to report history of childhood abuse compared with adults who were not obese.	Not addressed.	Not addressed.	Not addressed.	Not addressed.

(continued)

19

Table 1-8. *(continued)*

PARAMETER	LIFETIME HISTORY OF ABUSE	CURRENT IPV	LIFETIME HISTORY OF IPV	TEEN DATING VIOLENCE	ABUSE DURING OR AROUND PREGNANCY
Overweight and Obesity *(continued)*	Morbidly obese individuals who lost substantial amounts of weight were more likely to regain weight with history of childhood sexual abuse compared with those without such a history. College students' abnormal eating was correlated to a history of sexual assault.				
Physical Health	Not addressed.	Not addressed.	Women who have experienced IPV have more migraines, frequent headaches, chronic pain, heart problems, high blood pressure, and arthritis. Women with a history of IPV have more gastrointestinal related issues.	Not addressed.	Women who are abused during pregnancy are at increased risk for preterm labor and chorioamnionitis. Pregnant teens that experience IPV are at an increased risk for miscarriage.
Responsible Sexual Behavior	Not addressed.	Women who are forced to have sex are at an increased risk for HIV.**	Women seeking an abortion were more likely to report a history of abuse compared with women not seeking an abortion.	High school students who experienced severe dating violence reported a history of pregnancy at higher rates compared with those who had not experienced dating violence.	Women who had experienced IPV in the past 5 years were more likely to report that a pregnancy was unwanted than women who had not experienced IPV.

(continued)

Table 1-8. *(continued)*

PARAMETER	LIFETIME HISTORY OF ABUSE	CURRENT IPV	LIFETIME HISTORY OF IPV	TEEN DATING VIOLENCE	ABUSE DURING OR AROUND PREGNANCY
Responsible Sexual Behavior *(continued)*			HIV**-positive women reported experiencing physical (68%) and sexual abuse (32%) as adults. Women who have experienced abuse were diagnosed with sexually transmitted infections at higher rates compared with women who have not experienced IPV. With a lifetime history of IPV, there are higher rates of pelvic inflammatory disease, invasive cervical cancer, and preinvasive cervical neoplasia.	Young African American females who had experienced dating violence were more likely to have an STD*** and less likely to use condoms. Half of young mothers on public assistance reported that a partner sabotaged their birth control method. Teen girls who were abused were more likely to become pregnant. Low-income teenage girls who experienced IPV were more likely to have rapid repeat pregnancies.	Women with unwanted pregnancies were 4 times more likely to experience IPV.
Substance Abuse	Not addressed.	Women who have experienced IPV in the last 12 months were more likely to report having 3 drinks at a time at least once a week than women who did not report IPV. There is an increased risk of substance abuse if a women is currently experiencing IPV.	Women who have experienced IPV were 3 times more likely to binge drink compared with women who did not report history of IPV.	High school students who experienced severe dating violence reported illegal drug use at higher rates compared with students who did not experience dating violence. Teens who have been abused were 2 times as likely to report drinking and drug use compared with girls who were not abused.	Women experiencing IPV during pregnancy were more likely to have used substances before pregnancy and while pregnant compared with women who had not experienced IPV.

(continued)

Table 1-8. *(continued)*

PARAMETER	LIFETIME HISTORY OF ABUSE	CURRENT IPV	LIFETIME HISTORY OF IPV	TEEN DATING VIOLENCE	ABUSE DURING OR AROUND PREGNANCY
Tobacco	Not addressed.	Women experiencing IPV reported current smoking at higher rates than women who did not report IPV.	Women who have experienced IPV reported current smoking at higher rates compared with women who did not report IPV. Adolescent girls who witnessed IPV were more likely to smoke compared with those who did not witness IPV.	High school students who experienced severe dating violence reported smoking at higher rates compared with those who did not experience dating violence.	Not addressed.

* PTSD, postraumatic stress disorder; ** HIV, human immunodeficiency virus; *** STD, sexually transmitted disease.

Adapted from: Chamberlain L. Making the connection: domestic violence and public health. Family Violence Prevention Fund. Available at: http://endabuse.org/programs/display.php3?DocID=344. Accessed May 21, 2007; Family Violence Prevention Fund. Intimate partner violence and healthy people 2010 fact sheet. Available at: http://www.endabuse.org/hcaddd/2003/tier4.pdf. Accessed Retrieved May 21, 2007.

directed at decreasing IPV in families and thus avoiding both the witnessing by children of violence in the home and the physical and psychological harm that may occur in those homes.

In addition, IPV is a major cause of family homelessness. Up to half of all women and children living on the streets are homeless as a result of IPV.[42,43]

THE EFFECT OF MANDATORY REPORTING LAWS

There is wide variation among states concerning what is required by health care providers regarding reporting cases of IPV to legal authorities.[67] Proponents of mandatory reporting laws for IPV cite potential benefits, including making access to victims assistance easier. Opponents voice concerns that knowing that a report will be made if one discloses IPV to a health care provider may decrease victims' likelihood of disclosing, grants another person control over the victim, and may increase the risk of the perpetrator retaliating against the victim because the report may not coincide with the victim's safety planning.[68] Abused women who are victims of IPV were significantly less likely to support mandatory reporting laws when compared with the views of nonabused women.[68] Looking at 2 states, one with a mandatory reporting law (California) and one without such a mandate (Pennsylvania), Rodriquez and colleagues conducted a cross-sectional survey among women in EDs in each state. Of IPV victims, slightly more than half supported mandatory reporting, whereas more than two-thirds of women who were not DV/IPV victims supported mandatory reporting. In an anonymous 10-question survey given to women in various EDs, Hayden and colleagues found that many of the IPV victims felt comfortable discussing IPV issues in the ED, especially if asked directly, but nearly 40% of the IPV victims would not have disclosed if they knew that the health care personnel were required to report it to legal authorities.[69] Houry and colleagues conducted an assessment of the impact of a 1995 mandatory reporting law for IPV in Colorado and found convincing evidence in their survey of 577 patients that the mandatory reporting law only rarely deterred a patient from seeking medical care.[70] In the study, only 12% of patients stated that they would be less likely to seek medical care for an IPV-related injury because of the existence of the mandatory reporting law. Thus, at this point, the overall impact of mandatory reporting laws remains unclear, but what is certain is that victimized women who have been studied are more likely to see mandatory reporting in a negative light, whereas nonvictimized women see mandatory reporting of IPV by health care providers as positive and beneficial.

PREVENTION PROGRAMS AND OTHER RESOURCES

Like many complex public health problems, prevention of IPV would be an ideal solution and one that the health care profession, along with the other professions and organizations that work with this problem, would readily embrace. Prevention of IPV is of particular importance because of the pervasive nature of the problem, because of the far-reaching consequences to the victim and to any children who may become involved, and for the community at large. Because of its complex nature, the prevention of IPV has not been an easy task, however.

Because IPV spans various dimensions of an individual's and of a family's life, the screening and intervention planning is, by its very nature, complex, and often requires the assistance of other members of a multidisciplinary team. Screening in health care is either universally applied to all patients (ie, primary prevention) or targeted to those thought to be at high risk (ie, secondary prevention). Additionally, intervening in cases where the problem has already occurred and offering treatment may be referred to as tertiary prevention, because one of the goals of the treatment is the avoidance of a recurrence of the problem. This is the case for IPV as well. Overall, rates of screening at any level have been disappointingly low among the various medical disciplines, including family medicine, emergency medicine, internal medicine, OB/GYN, and in pediatric practice (in either the primary care or emergency settings).

The US Preventive Services Task Force (USPSTF), a group of health experts who routinely review published research and make preventive health care recommendations, found insufficient evidence of routine or universal DV/IPV screening in the general population, but did find evidence to support targeted interventions in families at higher risk for abuse can reduce harm to children.[71] The USPSTF observed that potential benefits to screening for family violence include decreased disability, injury, or premature death. Potential harms included increased risk of abuse and abuse when the victims or others confronted the abuser.[72] The studies reviewed by the USPSTF were inadequate to find an effect for women, and no studies were found that directly measured potential harms of screening families for family violence. Specifically, quoting from the USPSTF guideline recommendation[72]:

The USPSTF found no direct evidence that screening for family and intimate partner violence leads to decreased disability or premature death. The USPSTF found no existing studies that determine the accuracy of screening tools for identifying family and intimate partner violence among children, women, or older adults in the general population. The USPSTF found fair to good evidence that interventions reduce harm to children when child abuse or neglect has been assessed... The USPSTF found limited evidence as to whether interventions reduce harm to women, and no studies that examined the effectiveness of interventions in older adults. No studies have directly addressed the harms of screening and interventions for family and intimate partner violence. As a result, the USPSTF could not determine the balance between the benefits and harms of screening for family and intimate partner violence among children, women, or older adults.

Building off of the cost effectiveness of targeted child abuse prevention programs, one could reasonably assume that similar cost–benefit trends will emerge in the screening and intervention programs around DV/IPV, especially when child maltreatment is prevented as a result. We must await such rigorous data, however, as the results of such studies have not been published in the literature at present.

Despite this equivocal support for screening, many professional organizations, government agencies, and advocacy groups have recommended universal screening programs based on consensus of opinion.[51–53] Several resources are available for practitioners in the area of IPV. See **Table 1-9**.

Table 1-9. Resources		
RESOURCE	ORGANIZATION	WEBSITE
National consensus guidelines on identifying and responding to domestic violence victimization in health care settings.	Family Violence Prevention Fund	www.endabuse.org
Helping children thrive, supporting abuse survivors as mothers, a resource to support parenting.	Centre for Children and Families in the Justice System	www.lfcc.on.ca

REFERENCES

1. American Medical Association. *Diagnostic and Treatment Guidelines on Domestic Violence*. Washington, DC: American Medical Association; 1992.

2. Anonymous. Emergency medicine and domestic violence. American College of Emergency Physicians. *Ann Emerg Med*. 1995;25:442-443.

3. Director TD. Linden JA. Linden, Domestic violence: an approach to identification and intervention. *Emerg Med Clin North Am*. 2004;22:1117-1132.

4. Tjaden P, Thoennes,N. Extent, nature, and consequences of intimate partner violence: findings from the National Violence Against Women Survey. Washington, DC: US Dept of Justice; 2000. NCJ 181867.

5. Centers for Disease Control and Prevention, National Center for Injury Prevention and Control. *Intimate Partner Violence: Fact Sheet*. Atlanta, Ga: Centers for Disease Control and Prevention, National Center for Injury Prevention and Control; 2005.

6. Centers for Disease Control and Prevention, National Center for Injury Prevention and Control. *Costs of Intimate Partner Violence Against Women in the United States*. Atlanta, Ga: Centers for Disease Control and Prevention, National Center for Injury Prevention and Control; 2003.

7. American Psychological Association. *Violence and the Family: Report of the American Psychological Association Presidential Task Force on Violence and the Family*. Washington,DC: American Psychological Association; 1996.

8. Tjaden P, Theonnes N. *Prevalence, Incidence, and Consequences of Violence Against Women: Findings from the National Violence Against Women Survey*. Washington, DC: US Dept of Justice; 1998:1-16.

9. Coker AL, Flerx VC, Smith PH et al. Intimate partner violence incidence and continuation in a primary care screening. *Am J Epidemiol* 2007;165:821-827.

10. Tjaden P, Theonnes N. Full *Report of the Prevalence, Incidence, and Consequences of Violence Against Women: Findings from the National Violence Against Women Survey*. Washington, DC: Dept of Justice; 2000. NCJ 181867, 2000b; NCJ183781.

11. Bragg HL. Child Protection in Families Experiencing Domestic Violence. Washington, *DC: US Dept of Health and Human Services, Office on Child Abus*e and Neglect. www.childwelfare.gov/pubs/usermanuals/domesticviolence.pdf. Accessed June 19, 2008.

12. National Coalition of Anti-Violence Programs. Lesbian, gay, bisexual and transgender domestic violence in 2002: a report of the National Coalition of Anti-Violence Programs. Available at: http://www.ncavp.org/common/document_files/Reports/2002NCAVPdvrpt.pdf. Accessed January 7, 2008.

13. Gazmararian JA, Peterson R, Spitz AM, et al Violence and reproductive health: current knowledge and future research directions. *Matern Child Health J*. 2000;4:79-84.

14. Haggerty LA, Goodman LA. Stages of change-based nursing interventions for victims of interpersonal violence. *J Obstet Gynecol Neonatal Nurs*. 2003;32:68-75.

15. Curry MA. The interrelationships between abuse, substance use, and psychosocial stress during pregnancy. *J Obstet Gynecol Neonatal Nurs*.1998;27:692-699.

16. Silverman JG, Raj A, Mucci LA, Hathaway JE. Dating violence against adolescent girls and associated substance use, unhealthy weight control, sexual risk behavior, pregnancy, and suicidality. *JAMA*. 2001;286:572-579.

17. Schoen C, Davis K, Collins KS,. *The Commonwealth Fund Survey of the Health of Adolescent Girls*. Publisher, Location: Commonwealth Fund; 1997.

18. Children Now. National Poll on Kids Health & Safety. Oakland, CA: Kaiser Permanente Poll; 1995.

19. National Institute of Justice: *Violence Against Women: Identifying Risk Factors*. Washington, DC: US Dept of Justice, Office of Justice Programs; 2004.

20. Anonymous. *Children and Domestic Violence: A Bulletin for Professionals*. Washington, DC: National Clearinghouse on Child Abuse and Neglect Information, Dept of Health and Human Services; 2003.

21. Staus MA, Gells RJ, eds. *Physical Violence in American Families: Risk Factors and Adaptations to Violence in 8,145 Families*. New Brunswick, NJ: Transaction; 1990.

22. Edelson J. The overlap between child maltreatment and woman battering. *Violence Against Women*. 1999;5:134-154.

23. Appel A, Holden GW. The co-occurrence of spouse and physical child abuse: a review and appraisal. *J Fam Psychol*. 1998;12:578-599.

24. Parkinson GW, Adams RC, Emerling FG. Maternal domestic violence screening in an office-based pediatric practice. *Pediatrics*. 2001;108:E43.

25. Corvo K, Johnson P. Does patriarchy explain intimate partner violence? State-level correlates of violence toward women and female homicide. *In*: Kendall-Tackett K, Giacomoni S, eds. *Intimate Partner Violence*. Kingston, NJ: Civic Research Institute; Chapter 5; pp 1-10.2007

26. Felitti VJ. The relationship of adverse childhood experiences to adult health: turning gold into lead. *Z Psychosom Med Psychother*. 2002;48:359-369.

27. United Nations Office of the Under-Secretary. Presentation to the Third Committee of the Secretary General's in-depth study on violence against women. New York, NY. October 2006. Available at: http://www.un.org/esa/desa/ousg/statements/2006/20061009_ga61_3rd.html. Accessed June 7, 2007.

28. Erickson RA, Hart SJ. Domestic violence: legal, practice, and educational issues. *Medsurg Nurs*. 1998;164:142-147.

29. Brown J. Working toward freedom from violence. The process of change in battered women. *Violence Against Women*. 1997;3:5-26.

30. Family Violence Prevention Fund. Family Violence Prevention Fund, 2005. www.endabuse.org/VAWA/factsheets/prevention.pdf. Accessed June 19, 2008.

31. Durose M, Harlow CW, Langan PA, Motivans M, Rantala RR, Smith EL. *Family Violence Statistics: Including Statistics on Strangers and Acquaintances*. Washington, DC: US Dept of Justice, Office of Justice Programs Bureau of Justice Statistics; 2005. NCJ 207846.

32. WomensLaw.org. Information for immigrants: U-Visa laws and procedures. Available at: http://www.womenslaw.org/immigrantsUvisa.htm. Accessed May 21, 2007.

33. Walker LE. *The Battered Woman*. New York, NY: Harper & Row; 1979.

34. Rothenberg B. The success of the battered woman syndrome: an analysis of how cultural arguments succeed. *Sociol Forum*. 2002;17:81-103.

35. Long GM, McNamara JR. Paradoxical punishment as it relates to the battered woman syndrome. *Behav Modif*. 1989;13:192-205.

36. Curnow M. The open window phase: helpseeking and reality behaviors by battered women. *Appl Nurs Res*. 1989;10:128-135.

37. Copel LC. Partner abuse in physically disabled women: a proposed model for understanding intimate partner violence. *Perspect Psychiatr Care*. 2006;42:114-129.

38. Saltzman LE, Fanslow JL, McMahon PM, Shelley GA. Intimate Partner Violence Surveillance: Uniform Definitions and Recommended *Data Elements, Version 1.0*. Atlanta, Ga: Centers for Disease Control and Prevention, National Center for Injury Prevention and Control; 2002.

39. Beatty D. Stalking legislation in the United States. Brewster MP, ed. *In: Stalking: Psychology, Risk Factors, Interventions, and Law*. 2:1-21. Kingston, NJ: Civic Research Institute; 2003:Chapter 1, pp 1-21.

40. Burman S. Battered women: stages of change and other treatment models that instigate and sustain leaving. *Brief Treatment Crisis Interv*. 2003;3:83-98.

41. Felitti VJ, Anda RF, Nordenberg D, et al. The relationship of adult health status to childhood abuse and household dysfunction. *Am J Prev Med*. 1998;14:245-258.

42. Zorza J. Woman battering: a major cause of homelessness. *Clgh Rev*. 1991;25:421.

43. The US Conference of Mayors. *A Status Report on Hunger and Homelessness in American Cities*. Washington, DC: The US Conference of Mayors; 1999.

44. Prochaska JO, Velicer WF. The transtheoretical model of health behavior change. *Am J Health Promot*. 1997;12:38-48.

45. DiClemente CC, Prochaska JO. Self-change and therapy change of smoking behavior: a comparison of processes of change in cessation and maintenance. *Addict Behav*. 1982;7:133-142.

46. Zink T, Elder N, Jacobson, J, et al. Medical management of intimate partner violence considering the stages of change: precontemplation and contemplation. *Ann Fam Med*. 2004;2(3):231-9.

47. Crandall ML, Nathens AB, Kernic MA, et al. Predicting future injury among women in abusive relationships. *J Trauma*. 2004;56:906-912; discussion 912.

48. McLeer SAnwar RA, Herman S, et al. Education is not enough: a systems failure in protecting battered women. *Ann Emerg Med*. 1989;18:651-653.

49. Chamberlain L, Perham-Hester KA. The impact of perceived barriers on primary physicians' screening practices for female partner abuse. *Women & Health*. 2002;35:55-69.

50. Family Violence Prevention Fund. Intimate partner violence and healthy people 2010 fact sheet. Available at: http://www.endabuse.org/hcadvd/2003/tier4.pdf. Accessed May 21, 2007.

51. American College Obstetricians and Gynecologists. *Guidelines for Women's Health Care*, 2nd ed. Washington, DC: American College Obstetricians and Gynecologists; 2002.

52. American Medical Association Policy Statement on Family and Intimate Partner Violence. H-515.965. Available at: http://www.ama-assn.org/apps/pf_new/pf_online?f_n=browse&doc=policyfiles/H-515.000.HTM. Accessed March 3, 2008.

53. American Academy of Family Physicians. Family Violence and Abuse. Available at: http://www.aafp.org/online/en/home/policy/policies/f/familyandintimatepartner-violenceandabuse.html. Accessed March 3, 2008.

54. Parsons LH, Zaccaro D, Wells B, Stovall TG. Methods of and attitudes toward screening obstetrics and gynecology patients for domestic violence. *Am J Obstst Gynecol.* 1995;173:381-387.

55. Erickson MR, Hill TD. Siegel RM. Barriers to domestic violence screening in the pediatric setting. *Pediatrics.* 2001;108:98-102.

56. Lapidus G, Cooke MB, Gelen E, Sherman K, Duncan M, Banco L. A statewide survey of domestic violence screening behaviors among pediatricians and family physicians. *Arch Pediatr Adolesc Med.* 2002;156:332-336.

57. Hurley KF, Bown-Maher T, Campbell T, et al. Emergency department patients' opinions of screening for intimate partner violence among women. *Emerg Med J.* 2005;22:97-98. (Survey, 514 adult ED patients).

58. Duffy SJ, McGrath ME, Becker BM, et al. Mothers with histories of domestic violence in a pediatric emergency department. *Pediatrics.* 1999;103(5 Pt 1): 1007-1013.

59. Dowd MD, McGrath ME, Becker BM, et al. Mothers' and health care providers' perspectives on screening for intimate partner violence in a pediatric emergency department. *Arch Pediatr Adolesc Med.* 2002;156:794-799.

60. American Academy of Pediatrics Committee on Child Abuse and Neglect. The role of the pediatrician in recognizing and intervening on behalf of abuse women. *Pediatrics.* 1998;101:1091-1092.

61. Siegel RM, Hill TD, Henderson VA, et al. Screening for domestic violence in the community pediatric setting. Pediatrics. 1999;104(4 Pt 1):874-877.

62. Ernst AA, Weiss SJ. Intimate partner violence from the emergency medicine perspective. *Women Health.* 2002;35(2-3):71-81.

63. Glass N, Dearwater S, Campbell J. Intimate partner violence screening and intervention: data from eleven Pennsylvania and California community hospital emergency departments. *J Emerg Nurs.* 2001;27:141-149.

64. Jones AS, Dienemann J, Schollenberger J, et al. Long-term costs of intimate partner violence in a sample of female HMO enrollees. *Women's Health Issues.* 2006;16:252-261.

65. Wiser CL, Gilmer TP, Saltzman LE, et al. Intimate partner violence against women: do victims cost health plans more? *J Fam Pract.* 1999;48:439-443.

66. Ulrich Y, Cain K, Sugg N, Rivara F, Rubanowice D, Thompson R. Medical care patterns in women with diagnosed domestic violence. *Am J Prev Med.* 2003;24:9-15.

67. Rodriguez MA, McLaughlin E, Nash, G, et al. Mandatory reporting of domestic violence injuries to the police: what do emergency department patients think? *JAMA*. 2001;286:580-583.

68. Sachs CJ, Koziol-Maclain J, Glass N, et al. A population-based survey assessing support for mandatory domestic violence reporting by health care personnel. *Women Health*. 2002;35:121-133.

69. Hayden SR, Barton ED, Hayden M. Domestic violence in the emergency department: how do women prefer to disclose and discuss the issues? *J Emerg Med*. 1997;15:447-451.

70. Houry D, Feldhaus KM, Abbott J. Mandatory reporting laws. *Ann Emerg Med*. 2000;35:404.

71. US Preventive Services Task Force (USPSTF). Screening for family and intimate partner violence. Available at: http://www.ahrq.gov/clinic/uspstf/usps famv.htm#related. Accessed March 3, 2008.

72. Nelson HD, Nygren P, McInerney Y, Klein J. Screening women and elderly adults for family and intimate partner violence: a review of the evidence for the US Preventive Services Task Force. *Ann Intern Med*. 2004;140:387-396.

Chapter 2

Screening and Identification in Health Care Settings

JoAnn Mick, PhD, MBA, RN, AOCN, CNAA

Every year, health care professionals process millions of domestic violence victims through the medical system. Their knowledge and skills in providing care make these health care professionals well situated to identify such patient problems. In addition, health care professionals have unique opportunities to recognize and assess the various physical, sexual, and psychological injuries or other presenting symptoms caused by domestic violence. Routine screening assessments used to identify domestic violence can enable health care professionals to diagnose the situation, offer resources and support, and make referrals for assistance. However, many victims are seen and discharged by health care providers without identification of the occurrence of domestic violence and without offers for education or treatment to help these victims manage their situations.[1] Health care providers' failure to recognize or respond to a domestic violence problem often results in a patient's continued experience with violence, which may progress in severity and negatively impact the patient's health status.[2]

Definitions

Intimate Partner Violence

The Centers for Disease Control and Prevention (CDC) defines intimate partner violence (IPV) as physical and sexual abuse, the threat of physical or sexual abuse, and/or emotional or psychological abuse (eg, humiliating the victim, controlling what the victim can and cannot do, isolating the victim from family and friends).[3] The person who is or was involved in an intimate relationship with the victim perpetrates these coercive behaviors.

Screening

Screening in health care refers to performing assessments, procedures, or tests that detect an illness early in an asymptomatic person.[4] With **_universal screening_**, health care providers assess all patients; with **_selective screening_**, health care providers only assess those patients who meet specific criteria (eg, injuries that suggest possible abuse; pregnancy associated with young age and low income; mental health problems, including depression, anxiety, and suicide attempts; alcohol or substance use; history of childhood sexual or physical abuse). Screening for intimate partner violence is described by Nelson and colleagues[5] as assessment in a health care setting for current harm or risk for harm in asymptomatic women or families who may be experiencing IPV.

Prevalence

Health care professionals currently practice routine screening for a number of common conditions in which the prevalence is less than or similar to that of domestic violence (eg, cancer, blood pressure, risk-related behaviors). Intimate partner violence affects 1 of every 4 women in the United States. Men also are victims, but the prevalence is 1 in every 12 men, and the degree of injury is much lower. The lifetime prevalence of IPV in the United States is 7.6% for men and 22.1% for women; the 1-year prevalence of IPV in the United States is 0.9% in men and 1.5% in women. Intimate partner violence occurs in all socioeconomic categories, among all ethnic groups, and in both heterosexual and homosexual relationships. An estimated 3.3 to 10 million children witness IPV annually in the United States.[6] Universal screening provides critical opportunities for disclosure of domestic violence and allows patients and health care providers the chance to develop safety plans and improve health outcomes.

HEALTH CONSEQUENCES

Harmful outcomes of family violence include acute trauma, death, unwanted pregnancy, long-term physical problems, and psychiatric disorders (eg, depression, posttraumatic stress disorder, somatization, substance abuse, risk for suicide).[7-12] When victims at risk for or experiencing domestic violence are identified early, a provider can intervene and help patients understand their options and develop safety plans to remain in or leave the relationship.[1]

HEALTH CONSEQUENCES TO VICTIMS

Results of a qualitative study by Taft, Broom, and Legge[13] support that IPV affects the entire family, including the children. Repeated physical assaults or chronic psychological stress may increase risk of injury or chronic diseases for all family members. All IPV victims experience significant short-term and long-term psychological and physical health problems.[14]

Victims of IPV have higher self-reported, gastrointestinal symptoms (eg, eating disorders, chronic irritable bowel syndrome). They may also report cardiac symptoms (eg, hypertension, chest pain) or psychological conditions (eg, depression, suicidal tendencies, symptoms of posttraumatic stress disorder). Health consequences related to alcohol or drug abuse are also common outcomes of IPV.[15,16]

HEALTH CONSEQUENCES TO CHILDREN

The American Academy of Pediatrics (AAP) recognizes IPV as a pediatric issue. If the mother is a victim of IPV, her children are also likely victims of the situation. Intimate partner violence can affect the emotions, self-perceptions, and social functioning of children, resulting in developmental delays and psychiatric disorders.[5] Intervening on behalf of victims may effectively prevent child abuse.[17]

HEALTH CONSEQUENCES OF CHILDHOOD EXPOSURE

Negative health outcomes found in adults are linked with childhood exposure to domestic violence, child abuse, sexual abuse, and family dysfunction (eg, a deceased parent, a parent with mental health problems, a parent who is in jail, a parent with substance abuse problems). Such health consequences can include unintended pregnancy, sexually transmitted diseases (STDs), alcohol abuse, smoking, suicide, depression, heart disease risk factors, chronic lung disease, and liver disease.[2,11,12,18]

CURRENT RECOMMENDATIONS OF PROFESSIONAL ORGANIZATIONS REGARDING US PREVENTIVE SERVICES

The American Nurses Association (ANA),[19] American Medical Association (AMA),[20] American Academy of Family Physicians (AAFP),[21] American College of Physicians (ACP),[22] and a number of other national health care organizations recommend that health care providers routinely screen for domestic violence. These organizations recognize that the health care system has historically played an important role in the early detection and prevention of widespread public health problems; therefore, health care providers are well positioned to play key roles in identifying victims and preventing domestic violence. The following list details specific recommendations made by professional organizations regarding preventive services for IPV in the United States:

— The AMA Council on Scientific Affairs[23] recommends that health care providers initiate screening for all women upon entering into the health care system whether in an office, hospital, clinic, or another care setting.

— The American College of Obstetricians and Gynecologists (ACOG) recommends that standards of practice include information about ways to identify victims and abusers as well as some knowledge of intervention strategies.[24]

— The American Psychological Association (APA)[25] recommends that standard medical and psychological examinations include routine screening for a history of domestic violence, because if the abuse goes undetected, then lasting mental health effects that hinder care could occur. When conducting such an assessment, health care providers should remember that domestic violence is a significant risk factor for depression, posttraumatic stress disorder, anxiety, and substance abuse.[16]

— *Healthy People 2010*, a comprehensive set of public health priorities for disease prevention and measurable health promotion objectives for the United States to achieve during the first decade of this new century, lists "Injury and Violence" as number 7 of 10 leading health indicators that are considered major health issues for the nation.[26]

— The Joint Commission (TJC)[27] mandates that all hospitals screen patients in clinical settings to identify victims of domestic violence.

— The Family Violence Prevention Fund (FVPF), a national domestic violence advocacy organization, also encourages all health care providers to routinely screen for domestic violence. The organization recommends routine screening for domestic violence victimization for all female patients older than 14 years within primary care, obstetric, gynecologic, family planning, in-patient, pediatric, and mental health settings as well as the emergency department. This routine screening should occur regardless of whether signs or symptoms are present or the health care provider suspects that abuse has occurred.

— Other organizations, such as the US Preventive Services Task Force (USPSTF),[28] have published position statements concluding that not enough evidence exists to recommend for or against routine screening for domestic violence among the general population. The USPSTF came to this conclusion after conducting an extensive literature review of research studies involving domestic violence screening; however, though research results were inconclusive, the USPSTF's position reinforces the necessity for health care providers to identify signs and symptoms of domestic violence, document the evidence, provide treatment for victims, and refer victims to counseling and social agencies that provide assistance.[5,29]

ASSESSING FOR INTIMATE PARTNER VIOLENCE

Routine screening to identify victims of domestic violence provides opportunities for health care providers to offer information, assist with safety plan development, and initiate referrals to advocacy services. McFarlane and colleagues[30] and Sullivan and

Bybee[31] found that a patient's prognosis and reported quality of life improved when fewer violence-related injuries occur after a health care provider has appropriately identified the patient as a victim and initiated interventions.[30,31] Health care providers must believe that these routine screenings will increase the likelihood of identifying victims of violence. Victim identification can lead to appropriate interventions and connections to support systems, which can ultimately decrease the victim's exposure to violence and related detrimental physical and psychological health consequences.[32] In addition to identifying victims of violence, universal screening creates opportunities to provide education regarding violence-free relationships.[33]

HOW TO ASK

Published literature provides guidance for how effective screening should be accomplished, preferably asked verbally by health care providers, and demonstrates the importance of conducting inquiries in private settings, using straightforward, nonjudgmental questions in a culturally competent manner. Patient safety and respect of autonomy should always be considered.[34-36] By simply raising the question about abuse and acknowledging the patient's situation, the health care provider has intervened in an important way.[37]

The health care provider must first gain the patient's confidence and establish a supportive environment during the assessment. Inappropriate disclosure of health information may violate confidentiality and threaten the patient's safety. An assessment for abuse should be conducted in private (ie, without friends, relatives, or caregivers present); exceptions to this guideline include:

— Children younger than 3 years, because they are less likely to understand any of the discussions about violence.

— An interpreter, who is not the patient's friend or a family member.

— Using a language-line service for telephone access to a culturally sensitive professional who is certified to interpret information that includes medical terminology.

By offering nonjudgmental support, the health care professional creates an opportunity for the patient to discuss the abuse and for the health care provider to gather information about associated health problems. The provider can then determine a plan of care for immediate, long-term health and safety needs as well as provide needed resources, information, and treatment.[38]

Templates and screening instruments provide health care professionals with questions that elicit patient responses that give the information needed to identify abuse. Such templates and screening instruments are available for use by individuals and organizations. When administering the domestic violence screening tools, health care providers must ensure that their patient feels a sense of trust, compassion, and support and understand that their conversation is confidential.[39] Victims must be allowed to share their personal feelings. In addition, creating opportunities for patients to ask questions or learn about resources helps achieve or maintain patient safety and can improve patient outcomes.

Routine screening for domestic violence involves a written, verbal, or computerized inquiry by health care providers for all patients or for special groups of patients (eg, young pregnant women with low income). These screenings are designed to help health care providers ask patients about their personal history with domestic violence.

A study by Gerbert and colleagues[40] asserted that tests of all methods effectively enlist patient disclosure of IPV risk factors; however, each approach has pros and cons regarding its effectiveness and use:

— Written assessments can eliminate concerns about asking questions in front of children, however, some people worry or express apprehension about "writing it down" because of legal or confidentiality concerns.

— Asking questions orally raises issues of speaking about the abuse in a location where information may be overheard, as well as needs for privacy to verbally answer inquiries.

— Computer screening tends to effectively increase victim identification because people provide more honest responses and express greater comfort with screening when answering computerized questions. Computerized questions may facilitate opportunities to confidentially disclose sensitive information that affects health; however, though results may be superior, not all settings have computers or resources to manage screening when using this method. In addition, a study by Rhodes and colleagues41 revealed that using computers to achieve higher rates of detection did not guarantee documentation and follow-up by health care providers.

Further research is needed to determine more clearly which methods are best.

Models are available to guide health care providers through steps of assessment and intervention (eg, RADAR, SAFE, SAVER, SHAPES, ABCDE) **(Table 2-1)**. For example, the RADAR model identifies several steps that need to be included in abuse assessment. This model recommends that health care providers routinely screen every patient as a part of everyday practice. In addition, this tool advises health care providers to ask questions directly and kindly, while remaining nonjudgmental. Documentation of assessment findings in the patient's medical records, using the patient's own words whenever possible, including details, and using body maps and photographs as necessary, is also recommended. Assessment should include ascertaining the patient's living situation and safety as well as asking whether the patient has a safety plan. The final step in the model is to review the patient's available options for dealing with domestic violence and provide the patient with appropriate referrals.[42]

Table 2-1. Instruments and Models for Assessment and Screening

SCREENING TOOL	DESCRIPTION
Abuse Assessment Screen (AAS)[50,51]	A 3- or 5-question screening tool to improve the capacity to identify, prevent, and reduce IPV. A 6-point Likert scale* score of 10 or greater indicates abuse. The tool was initially created for use in pregnant women, but can be modified by omitting the question with reference to pregnancy. A study by McFarlane et al[50] found that women identified as abused using AAS also scored higher on the CTS, ISA, and DAS. A study by Norton et al[52] identified more frequent detection of violence with AAS (41%) than with interview alone (14%). Screening questions include: — Have you ever been emotionally or physically abused by your partner or someone important to you? — Within the last year, have you been hit, slapped, kicked, or otherwise physically hurt by someone?

(continued)

Table 2-1. *(continued)*

Screening Tool	Description
Abuse Assessment Screen (AAS) *(continued)*	— Since you have been pregnant, have you been hit, slapped, kicked, or otherwise physically hurt by someone? — Within the last year, has anyone forced you to have sexual activities? — Are you afraid of your partner or anyone you listed above?
Abusive Behavior Inventory (ABI)[53]	A tool designed to help health care providers assess psychosocial health in pregnancy, suggested to be administered at 20 weeks' gestation.
Antenatal Psychosocial Health Assessment (ALPHA)[54,55]	A tool developed for obstetric providers to document the responses of pregnant women to 32 questions relating to maternal, family, substance use, and family violence issues. The tool guides providers in assessing antenatal factors associated with poor postpartum outcomes. Assessment is recommended after the 20th week of gestation. Topic assessment questions include: Family relationships: — My parents got along — My father scared or hurt my mother — My parents/family scared or hurt me Partner relationships: — We work out arguments with great difficulty — Arguments with my partner scare me — I have been hurt during a fight — My partner humiliates me — My partner emotionally abuses me — My partner has forced me to have sex
Abuse Screening Inventory (ASI)[56]	The ASI is a short abuse screening questionnaire with 16 items addressing 4 types of abuse: physical, psychological, and sexual abuse, and abuse in health care. Test-retest reliability ranged from 81% to 96% for separate items. No false positive answers were identified. Sensitivity ranged from 72% to 82% for abuse items.
Danger Assessment Scale (DAS)[57]	A clinical and research instrument that was designed to help battered women assess the danger of homicide. The tool includes items in common with other screening tools, such as: — The escalation of frequency and severity of violence — The availability of weapons — Violence towards others — Substance abuse — Suicide threats — Jealousy — Assaults during pregnancy
Dartmouth Primary Care Cooperative Information Project (COOP) Charts[58,59]	A tool that contains picture and word questions that were developed for general health screening. The Relationship Chart, a section of COOP, was evaluated as an IPV screen for use in primary care offices. Questions include: During the past 4 weeks, how often have problems in your household led to insulting or swearing? yelling? threatening? hitting or pushing?

(continued)

Table 2-1. *(continued)*

SCREENING TOOL	DESCRIPTION
Domestic Violence Survivor Assessment (DVSA)[60]	A tool that assists health care providers and abused women in identifying issues and feelings created by IPV. Information from the tool can be used to gain a deeper understanding of battered women's cognitive states to assist them during counseling, to effectively resolve the dilemmas of an abusive relationship, and to experience personal growth.
Humiliation, Afraid, Rape, Kick (HARK)[61]	The instrument is an adaptation of the Abuse Assessment Screen (AAS). The HARK focuses on IPV (not including that committed by a stranger), and has removed the pregnancy item so the test is applicable to all women. The AAS question, which included both emotional and physical abuse components, was separated into 2 items. The words "humiliation" and "rape" were used in the questions to incorporate familiar terminology. Estimated specificity of the instrument was 95%, 95% C.I. 91%-98% of HARK score ≥1 and sensitivity was determined at 81%, 95% C.I. 69%-90%. The author concluded that if a clinician asks 4 questions and a patient scores ≥1, 81% of women affected by IPV will be identified. The instrument has a simple scoring system and has been validated against the Index of Spouse Abuse (ISA). — Humiliation: Within the last year, have you been humiliated or emotionally abused in other ways by your partner or your ex-partner? — Afraid: Within the last year, have you been afraid of your partner or your ex-partner? — Rape: Within the last year, have you been raped or forced to have any kind of sexual activity with your partner or your ex-partner? — Kick: Within the last year, have you been kicked, hit, slapped or otherwise physically hurt by your partner or ex-partner?

Hurt, Insult, Threaten, Scream (HITS) Scale[62]	A tool that is designed for use in outpatient clinical settings. The tool consists of 4 questions and has been validated in the family practice setting. A 6-point Likert scale score of 10 or greater indicates abuse. A study by Sherin et al[62] found HITS to be internally consistent (Cronbach's α = .80). HITS and CTS results correlated (r = .85). Questions include:
	— How often does your partner:
	  — Physically hurt you?
	  — Insult you?
	  — Threaten you with harm?
	  — Scream or curse at you?

Measure of Wife Abuse (MWA)[63]	A self-report tool including a 60-item device designed to assess the type of abuse directed by a man toward his wife. The tool consists of 4 factors: physical, verbal, psychological, and sexual abuse. The tool measures the frequency of abuse (the number of times acts of abuse occurred in the couple's relationship within a 6-month period), and the emotional consequences experienced by the victim as a measure of the severity of abuse. Rodenburg and Fantuzzo[63] revealed that the total scale reliability of MWA was higher than the CTS. The physical and verbal abuse scales show high concurrent validity (P < .01).

(continued)

Table 2-1. *(continued)*

Screening Tool	Description
The Ongoing Abuse Screen (OAS) Ongoing Violence Assessment Tool (OVAT)[64,65]	The OAS, a 5-question screen, was developed to evaluate ongoing IPV. The OAS was revised as a 4-question OVAT. The OVAT takes 1 minute or less to complete and responses are easily evaluated without calculations. The scale is useful to identify immediate victims in busy settings to determine necessary interventions and referral. Sensitivity was 86% and accuracy was 84%. In a study by Ernst et al[66] the OAS has sensitivity of 30%, specificity of 100%, and positive predictive value of 100%. The OVAT questions include: — At the present time does your partner threaten you with a weapon? — At the present time does your partner beat you so badly that you must seek medical help? — At the present time does your partner act like he/she would like to kill you? — At the present time does your partner have respect for your feelings?
Partner Abuse Scale (Physical and Nonphysical) (PAS)[67]	A 25-item scale measuring the frequency with which a person has experienced specific forms of physical abuse. The respondent indicates the frequency with which she has experienced any of 25 physically abusive events. Examples of events include: "My partner slaps me in face or head" and "My partner pushes or shoves me violently."
Partner Abuse Inventory (PAI)[68]	An 11-item interview modified from the Conflicts Tactic Scale. Physical violence items are rated on a 4-point scale and the fear item is scored on a 3-point scale. A study by Pan et al,[68] identified the PAI was internally consistent (Cronbach's α = .82). Questions include asking patients if their partner has: — Thrown something at them? — Pushed, grabbed, or shoved them? — Slapped them? — Kicked, bit, or hit them with a fist? — Hit or tried to hit them with an object? — Beat them up? — Threatened them with a gun or knife? — Used a gun or knife? — Forced them to have sex when they didn't want to? — Other?
Partner Violence Interview (PVI)[69]	A 26-item structured interview adapted from the CTS that takes 25 minutes to complete. Adequate retest reliability of 2 scales demonstrated r = .70 and .85. internal consistency demonstrated by a KR20 (Kuder-Richardson Formula 20 statistical test) of .78 to .93 for each scale. Interview questions begin by asking about behaviors common in abusive relationships and progress to cover incidences of use of physical force. The 3 scales of PVI items are directed at 3 areas: violence inflicted by current partner (current partner scale); violence inflicted by previous partners (ex-partner scale), and violence inflicted by the subject toward a partner (toward partner scale).
Partner Violence Screen (PVS)[34]	A tool with 3 questions developed for use in the emergency room to evaluate occurrence of IPV. A study by Feldhaus et al[34] supported that PVS had a higher sensitivity and specificity (65%-71%) when compared to ISA (80%)

(continued)

Table 2-1. *(continued)*

Screening Tool	Description
PVS *(continued)*	and CTS (84%). A "yes" response on any item is considered positive for IPV. Questions include: — Have you been hit, kicked, punched, or otherwise hurt by someone within the past year? If so, by whom? — Do you feel safe in your current relationship? — Is there a partner from a previous relationship who is making you feel unsafe now?
Propensity for Abusiveness Scale (PAS)[70,71]	A brief nonreactive self-report measure used to assess propensity for male abusiveness of a female partner in intimate relationships (does not explicitly refer to abuse tactics). Dutton's evaluation of the PAS scale revealed a Cronbach's α of .91 and yielded 3 factors: recalled negative parental treatment, affective lability, and trauma symptoms. Dutton[70] validated the PAS with the PMWI (r = .47). Dutton et al[71] demonstrated correlation of PAS with PMWI and SVAWS. The PAS contains 29 questions: 12 questions about anger, 10 questions about the experience of punishment by a parent or guardian, and 7 symptom assessment questions, such as presence of insomnia, anxiety, fear, or respiratory distress.
Psychological Maltreatment of Women Inventory (PMWI)[72-74]	A tool designed to measure the nonphysically abusive behaviors exhibited by men who batter. Items were modified from the CTS and ISA scales. A 58-item survey was developed with versions for men and women using nearly identical phrasing. The tool focuses exclusively on emotional abuse and is designed to measure the extent and nature of abuse toward women in a relationship. The version for male perpetrators includes identical behaviors but reverses the pronouns and direction of abuse. Factor analyses were done separately for women's and men's scales revealing 2 true factors likely to exist in both analyses: emotional/verbal abuse and dominance/isolation subscales. Intracouple reliability testing revealed the domination/isolation scale scores were significantly correlated (r = .4849, P = .007). The emotional/verbal scales were not correlated (r = .3025, P = .265). Internal consistency coefficients for women's subscales were high: domination/isolation = 0.9451, emotional/verbal = 0.9292. Internal reliability for men's subscales were also high: domination/isolation = 0.9087, emotional/verbal = 0.9335.
Routine Universal Comprehensive Screening Protocol (RUCS)[75]	A screening protocol designed to raise health care providers' awareness of the need to screen all women for abuse on a routine basis and to guide the decision-making and follow-up activities. The protocol would facilitate assessment and documentation of the health effects of abuse, provide the opportunity to address immediate safety concerns, and make appropriate, woman-directed referrals.
SAFE-T[76]	An instrument developed after testing 18 questions identified in IPV literature with 2 groups: victims of IPV living in a shelter and women who were attending a seminar. Five of the 18 questions were found to discriminate between the 2 groups. Four indirect questions were linked with the steps in the SAFE model: **S**tress and safety, **A**buse, **F**riends and family, and **E**mergency

(continued)

Table 2-1. *(continued)*

Screening Tool	Description

SAFE-T *(continued)*	plans. The authors added a fifth step: **T**alking it out. The instrument was then tested in an emergency room setting using the 5 indirect questions, followed by a direct question, which asked whether the patient had been hit, kicked, punched, or otherwise hurt by a partner or spouse within the past year. Responses to the indirect questions were validated with responses to the direct question. Reliability of the instrument was $r = .79$. Sensitivity was 54% and specificity was 81%.
	— The 5 questions in the SAFE-T survey are:
	  — I feel comfortable/**S**ecure in my home/apartment.
	  — My husband/partner **A**ccepts me just the way I am.
	  — My **F**amily likes my husband/partner.
	  — My husband/partner has an **E**ven/calm disposition.
	  — If my husband/partner and I disagree, we resolve our differences by **T**alking it out.

Severity of Violence Against Women Scale (SVAWS)[77]	A 46-item questionnaire designed to measure 2 major behaviors: threats of physical violence and actual physical violence. The tool was developed to measure threatened, attempted, and completed behaviors likely to cause injury or pain. The validity of 9 factors or subscales has been demonstrated through factor analytic techniques: symbolic violence and mild, moderate, and serious threats (Threats of Violence behaviors) and mild, minor, moderate, serious, and sexual violence (Actual Violence behaviors). A clinical application of the instrument can be to assess 1 episode of violence or compare episodes of violence to assist a woman to identify that her partner is becoming more violent. There is also the possibility of differentiating between 9 types of violence that a woman may be experiencing.

Slapped, Things, Threatened (STaT)[78]	A screening tool using 3 questions to identify lifetime intimate partner violence and aid in identification of women who are abused. The tool was validated in emergency department and outpatient medical settings.
	— Questions include:
	  — Have you ever been in a relationship where your partner has pushed or **S**lapped you?
	  — Have you ever been in a relationship where your partner **T**hreatened you with violence?
	  — Have you ever been in a relationship where your partner has thrown, broken or punched **T**hings?
	The STaT score is calculated as the total number of affirmative responses to the 3 questions. The sensitivity (95% confidence intervals [95% CI]) of STaT for lifetime IPV is 96% (90%, 100%), 89% (81%, 98%), and 64% (50%, 78%) with corresponding specificity of 75% (59%-91%), 100%, and 100% (for scores of ≥ 1, ≥ 2, and 3, respectively).

Wife Abuse Inventory (WAI)[79,80]	An instrument developed by Lewis[79] as a self-report screening tool designed to identify women at risk for abuse by measuring emotional and physical abuse. The WAI was found to be internally consistent with coefficient alpha

(continued)

Table 2-1. *(continued)*

Screening Tool	Description
WAI *(continued)*	and split-half reliability of .90. A study by Poteat et al[80] revealed significant percentage classification ($P \leq .001$) of respondents when using the tool. Evidence was also obtained that supported instrument reliability (.91) and construct validity as an indicator of the potential for abuse by one's spouse.
Woman Abuse Screening Tool (WAST and WAST-Short) [81, 82]	An 8-item tool developed as a reliable and valid measure of abuse for use in the family practice setting. The WAST demonstrated construct and discriminate validity with internal consistency supported by a coefficient alpha of .95. The WAST-Short form has an advantage of using only 2 items. Construct validity has been demonstrated, and scores correlate with scores on the ARI ($r = 0.96$). In a validation study, significant differences were found between abused and nonabused women in the mean overall WAST scores ($P \leq .001$). A study by Brown et al[82] identified that WAST and ARI results were correlated ($r = .69$, $P = .01$) and WAST was internally consistent (Cronbach's α = .75). The WAST-Short correctly classified 100% of nonabused women and 91.7% of abused women. WAST questions include: — In general, how would you describe your relationship: A lot of tension, some tension, or no tension? — Do you and your partner work out arguments with: Great difficulty, some difficulty, no difficulty? — Do arguments ever result in your feeling down or bad about yourself? — Do arguments ever result in hitting, kicking, or pushing? — Do you ever feel frightened by what your partner says or does? — Has your partner ever abused you physically? — Has your partner ever abused you emotionally? — Has your partner ever abused you sexually? *The WAST-Short uses the first two questions only.*
Women's Experience With Battering Scale (WEB)[83]	A self-administered 10-item scale to measure physical markers of battering and the psychological experiences of an abusive relationship. The Smith et al[83] WEB framework describes 6 domains of women's experiences with battering: perceived threat, altered identity, managing, entrapment, yearning, and disempowerment. The WEB scale exhibits high internal consistency reliability (Cronbach's α is .99 for full sample, .93 for battered women, and .86 for non-battered women), good construct validity, and provides a valid and concise measure of relations between battering and health or health behavior. A study by Coker et al[48] identified a higher detection rate with WEB (16%) than with ISA-P (10%). A study by Smith and Martin[84] identified high internal consistency of WEB (Cronbach's α = .93) A score greater than 20 indicates battering. Items include: — He makes me feel unsafe even in my own home. — I feel ashamed of the things he does to me. — I try not to rock the boat because I am afraid of what he might do. — I feel like I am programmed to react a certain way to him. — I feel like he keeps me prisoner. — He makes me feel like I have no control over my life.

(continued)

Table 2-1. *(continued)*

Screening Tool	Description
WEB *(continued)*	— I hide the truth from others because I am afraid not to. — I feel owned and controlled by him. — He can scare me without laying a hand on me. — He has a look that goes straight through me and terrifies me.

Models	Description
ABCDE Model of Intervention[85]	A model including the following steps: — **A**sk to be alone to ensure that the survivor is able to disclose abuse if they choose to do so. A disclosure is unlikely if attending to the survivor with their partner present. — **B**elieve the disclosure. No matter how unbelievable or bizarre the story, believe it. Survivors rarely lie about the violence they have survived; if anything, they minimize it. — **C**all in resources. Be aware of agencies that can assist the survivor, for example: women's shelters, domestic violence counselors, and sexual assault referral centers. — **D**ocument history and injuries, as this documentation may be used in court to support a survivor's case. — **E**nsure safety. The safety of the survivor and any children involved is paramount. Ask the woman whether she fears for her safety or for the safety of her children. Be aware that the severity of previous violence is no indicator of future violence. Many survivors minimize the violence.
RADAR[42]	A tool to increase health care providers' awareness of IPV to help identify victims. Steps in the RADAR model include: — **R**outinely screen every patient, make screening a part of everyday practice from prenatal, postnatal, routine gynecological visits, and annual health screenings. — **A**sk questions directly, kindly, and nonjudgmentally. — **D**ocument findings in the patient's chart using the patient's own words, with details, and use body maps and photographs as necessary. — **A**ssess the patient's safety and see whether the patient has a safety plan. — **R**eview options of dealing with domestic violence with the patient and provide referrals.
SAID[86]	A mnemonic useful for recalling suggestions for IPV assessment, which includes: — **S**creening for abuse — **A**ssessing for immediate safety — **I**ntervening — **D**ocumenting

(continued)

Table 2-1. *(continued)*

MODELS	DESCRIPTION
SAFE[87]	A tool that guides the health care provider through topics for discussion during assessment, which include: — **S**afety in the relationship and ability to return home — **A**buse (physical or sexual) — **F**riend and family awareness of the situation and ability to help — **E**mergency plan
SAVER[88]	An acronym that provides a useful way to remember the following key aspects of the screening process: — **S**creen all female patients for violence — **A**sk direct questions in a nonjudgmental way — **V**alidate the patient — **E**valuate survivors and educate all female patients — **R**efer survivors
SHAPES[4]	A model outlining the following topics to include in an abuse assessment: — **S**elf-esteem — **H**itting, kicking or punching — **A**fraid — **P**hysical abuse — **E**motional abuse — **S**exual abuse

RESEARCH	DESCRIPTION
Abuse Risk Inventory (ARI)[89]	A 25-item self-report tool used in the identification of abuse in the female population. Women rate 25 items on the basis of frequency of occurrence, using a 4-point scale ranging from "rarely or never" to "always." A score of 50 or higher suggests that the respondent may be in an IPV situation. The tool has demonstrated reliability (Cronbach's α = .91).
Composite Abuse Scale (CAS)[89]	A 31-item questionnaire to measure physical, emotional, and sexual abuse by partners or ex-partners. The CAS has 4 dimensions: severe combined abuse, physical abuse, emotional abuse, and harassment.
Conflict Tactics Scale (CTS, CTS-2, and CTS2S)[49,68,90,91]	An 18-item self-report tool that measures both the extent to which partners in a dating, cohabiting, or marital relationship engage in psychological and physical attacks on each other and their use of reasoning or negotiation to deal with conflicts. The CTS was designed to measure all intrafamily violence and was one of the first instruments to identify partner violence by measuring interpersonal aggression. The tool lists distinct actions generally used during disputes (negotiation, physical assault, and psychological aggression) and asks the respondent to rate the frequency that each of the actions has been used within the past year. The modified CTS-2 has 78 items, measuring the frequency of partners' psychological and physical attacks. The CTS has strong evidence of reliability and validity. The CTS-2 has internal consistency and reliability ranges from

(continued)

RESEARCH	DESCRIPTION
Table 2-1. *(continued)*	
Conflict Tactics Scale *(continued)*	.79 to .95. The CTS2S was designed to further the utility of the CTS2 by making it available in a 20-question short form. The CTS2 takes approximately 10 to 15 minutes to complete, the CTS2S takes approximately 3 minutes to complete.
Index of Spouse Abuse-Physical Scale (ISA-P) and Nonphysical Scale (ISA-NP)[72,92]	A 30-item self-report measure, with 2 subscales designed to measure the severity or magnitude of 11 types of physical spousal abuse and 19 types of nonphysical spousal abuse. The tool includes a self-report scale designed to be administered to the female victim to assess verbal, emotional, sexual, and physical aggression. The ISA determines a severity of physical abuse score (ISA-P) and also a severity of nonphysical abuse score (ISA-NP). Tolman[72] evaluated that the ISA has good evidence for construct validity, and each subscale has high internal consistency. Compared with the CTS, the ISA-NP has more items that attempt to measure nonphysical aspects of abuse. An identified limitation of the tool was that it is written for women's reports only and includes a small sample of nonphysically abusive behaviors.

A Likert scale is a type of psychometric response scale often used in questionnaires and is the most widely used scale in survey research. When responding to a Likert questionnaire item, respondents specify their level of agreement to a statement.

Injuries caused by physical abuse are commonly found in areas of the body covered by undergarments. Burns, bruises, and scars may be in various stages of healing. Therefore, when performing a physical assessment, the health care professional should examine all skin surfaces. The presence of multiple or bilateral injuries, symmetrical bruising, pattern injuries, or bruises with an obvious shape should initiate further inquiry about the cause. During an assessment, a patient may complain of vague or chronic conditions (eg, back pain, neck pain, headaches, pelvic pain). Gastrointestinal symptoms may include complaints of frequent indigestion, constipation, diarrhea, peptic ulcers, and irritable bowel syndrome. Noting a flat affect, complaints of chronic fatigue, significant weight loss or gain, insomnia, depression, suicidal ideation, low self-esteem, and other vague somatic symptoms may also be indicators of prolonged stress caused by abuse.[43]

Assessment of more subtle or indirect signs may include observations of fear (eg, a visual appearance of distress, hand or voice tremors, lack of eye contact, visible shaking, flinching, showing signs of discomfort when being touched during the examination). If a health care provider notices that the patient's partner seems overprotective of the patient, interrupts, controls or dominates the assessment interview, and refuses to leave the patient alone with the health care provider during a clinical exam, these are other potential signs of abuse. The patient may seem overly anxious if being assessed with the partner present.[38] If the partner is present during the clinical examination, the health care provider should defer from asking questions about IPV. Asking the patient such questions while in the presence of the partner may place that patient at greater risk. A partner who discovers that a patient has sought information or care may respond with further violence in retaliation to any comments the patient may make.[37]

If obtaining privacy becomes difficult, the health care provider needs to attempt to create a situation to be alone with the patient so an abuse assessment can be completed. For example, walking the patient to the bathroom to obtain a specimen may create an opportunity to inquire about the patient's situation, assess for safety, and provide information about IPV and available resources. If the patient denies IPV, but the health care provider suspects that the patient may be at risk, the provider should discuss the specific risk factors that created concern and offer information and available resources.[37]

TOOLS FOR SCREENING

In an effort to identify more domestic violence victims, numerous screening tools have been developed for use in different clinical settings. For example, effective assessment strategies and reliable, culturally relevant screening tools can be located at the Violence Against Women Network (VAWnet),[44] a national online resource that supports effective prevention and education activities by identifying and addressing factors that perpetuate and increase risk of domestic violence. Most screening tools ask patients to report about the frequency, severity, and type(s) of abuse experienced in past and current relationships. Expert opinion suggests that identification through screening and interventions by health care providers in situations of domestic violence may lead to reduced morbidity and mortality.[45] Models or protocols developed to prevent other chronic health problems may also be effectively applied to prevent domestic violence.[1]

Evidence-based health care practice requires not only research-tested interventions, but also reliable assessment tools that are valid for use in practice.[46] As previously discussed, many written and verbal screening tools are available to facilitate the identification of domestic violence victims. Such screening tools include questions in written medical histories that patients complete during routine visits as well as verbal questions that health care providers can ask all patients to detect the presence of violence in the patients' current relationships. Some organizations use protocols requiring a simple notation on the patient's chart, assessment form, intake form, medical form, or social history form.

The most obvious signs of domestic violence include evidence of severe, recurring, or life-threatening physical abuse[47]; however, screening tools for assessment can often help detect even the more subtle symptoms of domestic violence. Health care providers need validated screening tools to efficiently and reliably screen patients for domestic violence. Some available screening tools assess physical violence and injury without considering the chronic experience of battering and the psychological consequences associated with the experience of violence.[48] Other screening tools are considered too long for effective use in practice.

The Conflicts Tactics Scale[49] (CTS) was the first instrument created to identify partner violence and used for assessment of the presence of domestic violence by measuring interpersonal aggression. In addition, the CTS measures the extent to which partners in a dating, cohabiting, or marital relationship engage in psychological and physical attacks on one another, as well as their use of reasoning or negotiation skills to deal with conflicts.

REVIEW OF SELECTED DOMESTIC VIOLENCE ASSESSMENT/SCREENING INSTRUMENTS AND MODELS

Twenty-five assessment tools and 6 models were identified during a literature search for available screening tools and models that health care providers can use to assess IPV. In addition, several research tools used to validate clinical tools were found (ie, ARI, CTS, ISA, and CAS) **(Table 2-1)**. The RADAR, SAFE, SAVER, SHAPES, and ABCDE models review steps that a health care provider can include in the assessment process. A variety of instruments were designed for use in specific settings (eg, hospitals, outpatient clinics, obstetric and general practice offices, emergency room settings). The Abuse

Assessment Screen, Abusive Behavior Inventory, and the Antenatal Psychosocial Health Assessment were specifically designed for abuse risk assessment of pregnant women. The Danger Assessment Scale is a clinical and research instrument designed to help battered women assess the danger of homicide.

Most assessment tools evaluate physical, emotional, verbal, and psychological abuse and many include the assessment of both actual violence and threats of violence. Several tools included assessment of sexual abuse. Short, easy-to-use instruments include AAS, HITS, PVS, and WAST. The Woman's Experience with Battering Scale and Abusive Behavior Inventory help identify psychological abuse. The Partner Abuse Scale (Physical and Nonphysical) measures various types of physical abuse. The Domestic Violence Survivor Assessment helps health care providers and victims identify issues and feelings created by domestic violence. Information identified by using the DVSA can be used to gain a deeper understanding of a battered victim's cognitive state. This understanding better helps the health care provider assist the victim during counseling so the victim can more effectively resolve the dilemmas of an abusive relationship and experience personal growth.

WHAT TO DO

Potentially effective interventions can include health care provider referrals to counseling, family support services, special police programs focused on IPV, shelters, and postshelter advocacy, personal, or vocational counseling.[93,94] The lack of rigorous studies to support improved outcomes for victims identified as at risk by IPV screening creates a quality issue for some providers. Questions have arisen regarding the investment of time for screening when there are no proven interventions. Further research is recommended to identify whether screening, counseling, and referrals result in a decrease in violence against women.[95,96] In contrast, the inclusion of questions about domestic violence when conducting routine assessments is supported by the high prevalence of undetected abuse, the potential value of screening to identify a need to provide information to at-risk patients, and the low costs and low risks associated with screening. Routine screening can effectively detect domestic violence and increase referrals to community resources, thereby resulting in improved outcomes related to quality of life and fewer violence-related injuries for victims.[97]

During screenings, health care providers can display negative, positive, or equivocal responses. ***Negative responses*** discourage the patient from seeking information or assistance. ***Positive responses*** affirm and validate the presence of domestic abuse and the victim's experiences. ***Equivocal responses*** provide information simply by commenting that domestic violence is a common issue or talking about knowing someone who has experienced intimate partner violence during the conversation with the victim. Helping identify the resources available to patients and offering free materials for them to take and share with a friend provides an opportunity for patients to access information without disclosing their personal situation.

Health care providers often find the issue of nondisclosure frustrating. Although victims of IPV may recognize the relationship as abusive, they may be unwilling or unable to disclose their situation to others. Victims of abuse may make decisions or do things that they dislike or that make them feel badly; this may seem wrong or "crazy" to others who do not know the details of the victims' situation. Leaving an abusive relationship presents many risks, including economic and social consequences as well as a loss of what was valued in the relationship for the victims and their children. Fear of making their situation worse often causes nondisclosure.[98] Victims may be threatened by death for revealing the abuse, which makes disclosure of the situation very frightening.

Existing data support that leaving an abusive relationship is a process that may take months or years of planning and often involves a pattern of leaving and returning to a relationship 5 to 7 times before leaving permanently.[99] Sometimes the initial purpose of leaving is for the victim to test whether the abuser will seek help or stop the violence, other times the initial purpose is to gather resource information for development of a plan to leave the relationship permanently.[38]

SAFETY PLAN

Health care providers must understand that only the victim can know when the right time to leave a relationship is, because the victim knows the abuser better than anyone else. Even though victims do not have control over the violence in their lives, many victims develop routines to remain as safe as possible. Deciding to leave an abusive partner and the actual act of leaving increases the risk of violence. Planning for safety during this time period is extremely important.[38,43]

When developing a safety plan for leaving an abuser, victims need to determine when they can most safely leave and where they will go. They need to consider whom they can trust and to whom they can disclose their plan to leave. Victims need to plan how they will travel to and from work or school and how to pick up their children after school. A pamphlet provided by the health care provider that includes written information about available resources and phone numbers is helpful in developing these plans.

Even when victims decide to stay with a batterer, safety planning remains important. Victims need to consider what works best to keep them safe during an emergency. They should also consider resources they can call when in a crisis. Victims should plan escape routes and identify a place to go if the violence starts again. In addition, victims need to develop plans concerning having important papers (eg, birth certificates, social security cards, marriage and driver's licenses, insurance information, health and school records) and some money or a credit card available if they should find the need to leave quickly. Clothing, keys, medications, and phone numbers should also remain readily accessible.[1]

MANDATED REPORTING

In the United States, laws vary from state to state regarding when a physician needs to report a suspected case of IPV. The following list details some examples[1,5,100]:

— California, Colorado, and Kentucky mandate the reporting of suspected IPV.

— Forty-two states require the reporting of injuries caused by firearms, knives, or other weapons; these reports may include some IPV cases.

— Twenty-three states require the reporting of injuries that result from crime.

— Seven states require reporting injuries that result from IPV.

Most states mandate the reporting of child abuse to protective services. Hospital and practice protocols, policies, and procedures should link to services and resources in the community, police departments, the judicial system, and social service agencies.[101]

ONGOING MANAGEMENT

The primary responsibilities for health care providers include conducting an assessment to identify and acknowledge the occurrence of abuse, remaining sensitive and non-judgmental while providing support, documenting the findings of abuse assessments in the medical record, and providing referrals and information about available resources. Health care providers must continue to express concerns about patient safety and also offer assistance in a supportive, empowering manner. Providing support prevents patients from feeling pressured to initiate steps with which they are uncomfortable or not yet ready to take. This support also allows these patients to negotiate necessary stages of precontemplation, contemplation, nondisclosure, and safety assessment planning before leaving a relationship.[102] Once the victim has developed a plan for safety, including plans for a job, childcare, and housing, they may finally leave their abuser for the last time. Most victims of IPV do eventually leave the abusive relationship.[38]

RESEARCH RECOMMENDATIONS

Research funded by the Agency for Healthcare Research and Quality (AHRQ) has identified gaps in research regarding domestic violence, which indicates the need for a stronger evidence base for screening, detecting, and treating victims.[103] Several screening instruments have demonstrated good internal consistency (eg, HITS, PAI, PMWI, WAI, WEB, WAST), which indicates that all the items on the instrument are consistent with one another. Further research is needed, however, to determine the best methods to administer screening instruments in various settings. Further research is also needed for the development of valid and effective screening tools for use with the general population. Such screening tools would provide helpful information that could be used to develop programs that can improve health outcomes and reduce violence, decrease abuse outcomes, and reduce the health-related consequences of family violence and IPV. Finally, research assessing the outcomes of health care providers' time and efforts to screen and assist patients experiencing IPV may support improved interventions and recommendations for screening to identify victims in relationships that involve IPV.

REFERENCES

1. Family Violence Prevention Fund. *Preventing Domestic Violence: Clinical Guidelines on Routine Screening.* San Francisco, Calif: Family Violence Prevention Fund; 1999. Available at: http://endabuse.org/programs/healthcare/files/screpol.pdf. Accessed September 4, 2007.

2. Cohn F, Rudman WJ. Fixing broken bones and broken homes: domestic violence as a patient safety issue. *Jt Comm J Qual Saf.* 2004;30:636-646.

3. Saltzman LE, Fanslow JL, McMahon PM, Shelley GA. *Intimate Partner Violence Surveillance: Uniform Definitions and Recommended Data Elements.* Atlanta, Ga: National Center for Injury Prevention and Control, Centers for Disease Control and Prevention; 1999.

4. Ontario College of Family Physicians. Screening for domestic violence. In: *Violence Against Women Modules.* Toronto, Canada: Ontario College of Family Physicians; 2004. Available at: http://www.ocfp.on.ca/local/files/VAW/WAST%20Screen_facilitator%20notes.pdf. Accessed September 4, 2007.

5. Nelson HD, Nygren P, McInerney Y, Klein J, for the US Preventive Services Task Force. Screening women and elderly adults for family and intimate partner violence: a review of the evidence for the US Preventive Services Task Force. *Ann Intern Med.* 2004;140:387-396.

6. Tjaden P, Thoennes N. Extent, *Nature, and Consequences of Intimate Partner Violence: Findings From the National Violence Against Women Survey.* Washington, DC: National Institute of Justice, Centers for Disease Control and Prevention; 2000.

7. Anda RF, Chapman DP, Felitti VJ, et al. Adverse childhood experiences and risk of paternity in teen pregnancy. *Obstet Gynecol.* 2002;100:37-45.

8. Campbell JC, Lewandowski LA. Mental and physical health effects of intimate partner violence on women and children. *Psychiatr Clin North Am*. 1997;20:353-374.

9. Coker AL, Smith PH, Thompson MP, McKeown RE, Bethea L, Davis KE. Social support protects against the negative effects of partner violence on mental health. *J Womens Health Gend Based Med*. 2002;11:465-476.

10. Diaz A, Simantov E, Rickert VI. Effect of abuse on health: results of a national survey. *Arch Pediatr Adolesc Med*. 2002;156:811-817.

11. Dube SR, Anda R, Felitti VJ, Chapman DP, Williamson DF, Giles WH. Childhood abuse, household dysfunction, and the risk of attempted suicide throughout the life span: findings from the Adverse Childhood Experiences Study. *JAMA*. 2001;286:3089-3096.

12. Felitti VJ, Anda RF, Nordenberg D, et al. Relationship of childhood abuse and household dysfunction to many of the leading causes of death in adults: The Adverse Childhood Experiences (ACE) Study. *Am J Prev Med*. 1998; 14:245-258.

13. Taft A, Broom DH, Legge D. General practitioner management of intimate partner abuse and the whole family: qualitative study. *BMJ*. 2004;328:618-621.

14. Coker AL, Davis KE, Arias I, et al. Physical and mental health effects of intimate partner violence for men and women. *Am J Prev Med*. 2002;23:260-268.

15. Campbell JC. Health consequences of intimate partner violence. *Lancet*. 2002; 359:1331-1336.

16. Golding JM. Intimate partner violence as a risk factor for mental disorders: a metaanalysis. *J Fam Violence*. 1999;14:99-132.

17. Wright RJ, Wright RO, Isaac NE. Response to battered mothers in the pediatric emergency department: a call for an interdisciplinary approach to family violence. *Pediatrics*. 1997;99:186-192.

18. Kitzmann KM, Gaylord NK, Holt AR, Kenny ED. Child witnesses to domestic violence: a meta-analytic review. *J Consult Clin Psychol*. 2003;71:339-352.

19. American Nurses Association. *Position Statement on Physical Violence Against Women*. Washington, DC: American Nurses Association; 1994. Available at: http://www.nursingworld.org/MainMenuCategories/HealthcareandPolicyIssues/ ANAPositionStatements/social/scviolnw14518.aspx. Accessed September 4, 2007.

20. Violence against women. Relevance for medical practitioners. Council on Scientific Affairs, American Medical Association. *JAMA*. 1992;267:3184-3189.

21. Family and intimate partner violence and abuse. American Academy of Family Physicians Web site. 2004. Available at: http://www.aafp.org/online/en/home/ policy/policies/f/familyandintimatepartner-violenceandabuse.html. Accessed September 4, 2007.

22. American College of Physicians. *Domestic Violence: Position Paper of the American College of Physicians*. Philadelphia, Pa: American College of Physicians; 1986.

23. American Medical Association diagnostic and treatment guidelines on domestic violence [erratum in *Arch Fam Med*. 1992;1:287]. Arch Fam Med. 1992;1:39-47.

24. Jones RF III, Horan DL. The American College of Obstetrics and Gynecologists: a decade of responding to violence against women. *Int J Gynaecol Obstet*. 1997;58:43-50.

25. American Psychological Association. *Violence and the Family: Report of the American Psychological Association Presidential Task Force on Violence and the Family*. Washington, DC: American Psychological Association; 1996.

26. US Department of Health and Human Services. *Healthy People 2010: Understanding and Improving Health*. 2nd ed. Washington, DC: US Government Printing Office; 2000. Available at: http://www.healthypeople.gov/document/pdf/uih/2010uih.pdf. Accessed September 4, 2007.

27. Joint Commission on Accreditation of Healthcare Organizations. Standard PC.3.10; RI.2.150. *2007 Comprehensive Accreditation Manual for Hospitals: The Official Handbook*. Chicago, Ill: Joint Commission Resources; 2007.

28. US Preventive Services Task Force. Screening for family and intimate partner violence: recommendation statement. *Ann Intern Med*. 2004;140:382-386.

29. US Preventive Services Task Force. Screening for family and intimate partner violence: recommendation statement. *Ann Fam Med*. 2004;2:156-160.

30. McFarlane J, Parker B, Soeken K, Silva C, Reel S. Safety behaviors of abused women after an intervention during pregnancy. *J Obstet Gynecol Neonat Nurs*. 1998;27:64-69.

31. Sullivan CM, Bybee DI. Reducing violence using community-based advocacy for women with abusive partners. *J Consult Clin Psychol*. 1999;67:43-53.

32. Ramsay J, Richardson J, Carter YH, Davidson LL, Feder G. Should health professionals screen women for domestic violence? Systematic review. *BMJ*. 2002; 325:314.

33. Gillespie CA. Domestic violence: what clinicians should know. *Internet J Acad Physician Assist [serial online]*. 2004;4. Available at: http://www.ispub.com/ostia/index.php?xmlFilePath=journals/ijapa/vol4n1/violence.xml. Accessed September 4, 2007.

34. Feldhaus KM, Koziol-McLain J, Amsbury HL, Norton IM, Lowenstein SR, Abbott JT. Accuracy of 3 brief screening questions for detecting partner violence in the emergency department. *JAMA*. 1997;277:1357-1361.

35. McFarlane J, Christoffel K, Bateman L, Miller V, Bullock L. Assessing for abuse: self-report versus nurse interview. *Public Health Nurs*. 1991;8:245-250.

36. Parker B, McFarlane J. Nursing assessment of the battered pregnant women. *MCN Am J Matern Child Nurs*. 1991;16:161-164.

37. U.S. Department of Health and Human Services. 2003. *Recognizing child abuse and neglect: Signs and symptoms*. Available at: http://www.childwelfare.gov/pubs/factsheets/signs.pdf. Accessed September 4, 2007.

38. Fleck-Henderson A. *Domestic Violence Training Curriculum*. Boston, Mass: Simmons College School of Social Work; 2004. Available at: http://www.simmons.edu/ssw/dvtraining/index.htm. Accessed September 4, 2007.

39. McCauley J, Yurk RA, Jenckes MW, Ford DE. Inside "Pandora's Box": abused women's experiences with clinicians and health services. *J Gen Intern Med*. 1998; 13:549-555.

40. Gerbert B, Bronstone A, Pantilat S, McPhee S, Allerton M, Moe J. When asked, patients tell: disclosure of sensitive heath-risk behaviors. *Med Care.* 1999;37:104-111.

41. Rhodes KV, Lauderdale DS, He T, Howes DS, Levinson W. "Between me and the computer": increased detection of intimate partner violence using a computer questionnaire. *Ann Emerg Med.* 2002;40:476-484.

42. Massachusetts Medical Society. *RADAR Action Steps Developed by the Massachusetts Medical Society.* New York State Office for the Prevention of Domestic Violence; 1992. Available at: http://www.massmed.org/AM/Template.cfm?Section= Search&section=Public_Health_Materials_for_Physicians&template=/CM/Content Display.cfm&ContentFileID=493. Accessed September 4, 2007.

43. Intimate partner violence: fact sheet. National Center for Injury Prevention and Control Web site. Available at: http://www.cdc.gov/ncipc/factsheets/ipvfacts.htm. Accessed September 4, 2007.

44. Violence Against Women Network (VAWnet), the National Online Resource Center on Violence Against Women Web site. Available at: http://www.vawnet.org. Accessed September 4, 2007.

45. Saltzman LE, Salmi LR, Branche CM, Bolen JC. Public health screening for intimate violence. *Violence Against Women.* 1997;3:319-331.

46. Vermeersch P, Beavers J. Appraisal of tools to enhance evidence-based clinical practice. *Clin Nurse Spec.* 2004;18:186-191.

47. Bedke RD. Domestic violence: signs, symptoms, and resource basics. American Bar Association Web site. 2005. Available at: http://www.abanet.org/yld/tyl/ Nov2000/violence.html. Accessed September 4, 2007.

48. Coker AL, Pope BO, Smith PH, Sanderson M, Hussey JR. Assessment of clinical partner violence screening tools. *J Am Med Womens Assoc.* 2001;56:19-23.

49. Straus M. Measuring intrafamily conflict and violence: the Conflict Tactics (CT) scales. *J Marriage Fam.* 1979;41:75-88.

50. McFarlane J, Parker B, Soeken K, Bullock L. Assessing for abuse during pregnancy. Severity and frequency of injuries and associated entry into prenatal care. *JAMA.* 1992;267:3176-3178.

51. Soeken KL, McFarlane J, Parker B, Lominack MC. The Abuse Assessment Screen: a clinical instrument to measure frequency, severity, and perpetrator of abuse against women. In: Campbell JC, ed. *Empowering Survivors of Abuse: Health Care for Battered Women and Their Children.* Thousand Oaks, Calif: Sage Publications; 1998:195-203.

52. Norton LB, Peipert JF, Zierler S, Lima B, Hume L. Battering in pregnancy: an assessment of two screening methods. *Obstet Gynecol.* 1995;85:321-325.

53. Shepard MF, Campbell JA. The abusive behavior inventory: a measure of psychological and physical abuse. *J Interpers Violence.* 1992;7:291-305.

54. Midmer D, Biringer A, Carroll JC, et al. *Reference Guide for Providers: The ALPHA Form—Antenatal Psychosocial Health Assessment Form.* 2nd ed. Toronto, Canada: Department of Family and Community, University of Toronto; 1996.

55. Midmer D, Carroll J, Bryanton, J, Stewart D. From research to application: the development of an antenatal psychosocial health assessment tool. *Can J Public Health*. 2002;93:291-296.

56. Swahnberg K, Wijma K. Validation of the Abuse Screening Inventory (ASI). *Scand J Public Health*. 2007; 35(3):330-4.

57. Campbell JC. Nursing assessment for risk of homicide with battered women. ANS *Adv Nurs Sci*. 1986;8:36-51.

58. Wasson JH, Jette AM, Johnson DJ, Mohr JJ, Nelson EC. A replicable and customizable approach to improve ambulatory care and research. *J Ambul Care Manage*. 1997;20:17-27.

59. Wasson JH, Jette AM, Anderson J, Johnson DJ, Nelson EC, Kilo CM. Routine, single-item screening to identify abusive relationships in women. *J Fam Pract*. 2000;49:1017-1022.

60. Dienemann J, Campbell J, Landenburger K, Curry MA. The domestic violence survivor assessment: a tool for counseling women in intimate partner violence relationships. *Patient Educ Couns*. 2002;46:221-228.

61. Sohal H, Eldridge S, Feder G. The sensitivity and specificity of four questions (HARK) to identify intimate partner violence: a diagnostic accuracy study in general practice. *BMC Family Practice*. 2007;8(1):49.

62. Sherin KM, Sinacore JM, Li XQ, Zitter RE, Shakil A. HITS: a short domestic violence screening tool for use in a family practice setting. *Fam Med*. 1998;30:508-512.

63. Rodenburg FA, Fantuzzo JW. The measure of wife abuse: steps toward the development of a comprehensive assessment technique. *J Fam Violence*. 1993;8:203-227.

64. Ernst AA, Weiss SJ, Cham E, Hall L, Nick TG. Detecting ongoing intimate partner violence in the emergency department using a simple 4-question screen: the OVAT. *Violence Vict*. 2004;19:375-384.

65. Weiss SJ, Ernst AA, Cham E, Nick TG. Development of a screen for ongoing intimate partner violence. *Violence Vict*. 2003;18:131-141.

66. Ernst AA, Weiss SJ, Cham E, Marquez M. Comparison of three instruments for assessing ongoing intimate partner violence. *Med Sci Monit*. 2002;8:CR197-201.

67. Attala JM, Hudson W, McSweeney M. A partial validation of two short-form Partner Abuse Scales. *Women Health*. 1994;21:125-139.

68. Pan HS, Ehrensaft MK, Heyman RE, O'Leary KD, Schwartz R. Evaluating domestic partner abuse in a family practice clinic. *Fam Med*. 1997;29:492-495.

69. Boris NW, Heller SS, Sheperd T, Zeanah CH. Partner violence among homeless young adults: measurement issues and associations. *J Adolesc Health*. 2002;30:355-363.

70. Dutton DG. A scale for measuring propensity for abusiveness. *J Fam Violence*. 1995;10:203-221.

71. Dutton DG, Landolt MA, Starzomski A, Bodnarchuk M. Validation of the propensity for abusiveness scale in diverse male populations. *J Fam Violence*. 2001; 16:59-73.

72. Tolman RM. The development of a measure of psychological maltreatment of women by their male partners. *Violence Vict*. 1989;4:159-177.

73. Tolman RM. Psychological abuse of women. In Campbell JC, ed. *Assessing the Risk of Dangerousness*. Newbury, Calif: Sage Publishers; 1992; 291-309.

74. Tolman RM. The validation of the Psychological Maltreatment of Women Inventory. *Violence Vict*. 1999;14:25-37.

75. Task Force on the Health Effects of Woman Abuse. *Task Force on the Health Effects of Woman Abuse–Final Report*. London, England: Middlesex-London Health Unit; 2000.

76. Fulfer JL, Tyler JJ, Choi NJ, et al. Using indirect questions to detect intimate partner violence: the SAFE-T questionnaire. *J Interpers Violence*. 2007;22:238-249.

77. Marshall LL. Developing of the severity of violence against women scales. *J Fam Violence*. 1992;7:103-121.

78. Paranjape A, Liebschutz J. STaT: a three-question screen for intimate partner violence. *J Womens Health (Larchmt)*. 2003;12:233-239.

79. Lewis BY. The wife abuse inventory: a screening device for the identification of abused women. *Soc Work*. 1985;30:32-35.

80. Poteat GM, Grossnickle WF, Cope JG, Wynne DC. Psychometric properties of the wife abuse inventory. *J Clin Psychol*. 1990;46:828-834.

81. Brown JB, Lent B, Brett PJ, Sas G, Pederson LL. Development of the woman abuse screening tool for use in family practice. *Fam Med*. 1996;28:422-428.

82. Brown JB, Lent B, Schmidt G, Sas G. Application of the Woman Abuse Screening Tool (WAST) and WAST-short in the family practice setting. *J Fam Pract*. 2000;49:896-903.

83. Smith PH, Earp JA, DeVellis R. Measuring battering: development of the Women's Experience with Battering (WEB) scale. *Womens Health*. 1995;1:273-288.

84. Smith M, Martin F. Domestic violence: recognition, intervention, and prevention. *Medsurg Nurs*. 1995;4:21-25.

85. Royal Darwin Hospital—Accident and Emergency Dept. Domestic Violence Reference Card in Family and Domestic Violence Training Package. 1997; page 32. Available at: http://www.health.wa.gov.au/publications/documents/fdvtrainingparticipantskit.doc. Accessed September 4, 2007.

86. Lassen D, Bunting D. Teaching medical students and residents about domestic violence: uncovering a hidden and potentially lethal problem. *Around the State*. Winter 2006;7; Pearls for Preceptors section. Available at: http://www.medicine.uiowa.edu/oscep/mededucation/newsletter/documents/Pearls7-1.pdf. Accessed September 4, 2007.

87. Neufeld B. SAFE questions: overcoming barriers to the detection of domestic violence. *Am Fam Physician*. 1996;53:2575-2580, 2582.

88. Stevens L. Improving screening of violence for women: basic guidelines for healthcare providers: SAVER—an acronym to remember [CME/CE activity]. *Medscape* [serial online]. August 2005. Available at: http://www.medscape.com/viewprogram/4397. Accessed September 4, 2007.

89. Yegidis BL. *Abuse Risk Inventory Manual*. Palo Alto, Calif: Consulting Psychologist Press; 1989.

90. Straus MA, Hamby SL, Boney-McCoy S, Sugarman DB. The revised Conflict Tactics Scales (CTS2): development and preliminary psychometric data. *J Fam Issues*. 1996;17:283-316.

91. Straus MA, Douglas EM. A short form of the Revised Conflict Tactics Scales, and typologies for severity and mutuality. *Violence Vict*. 2004;19:507-520.

92. Hudson WW, McIntosh SR. The assessment of spouse abuse: two quantifiable dimensions. *J Marriage Fam*. 1981;11:873-888.

93. MacMillan HL, Wathen CN. *Prevention and Treatment of Violence Against Women: Systematic Review and Recommendations*. London, Canada: Canadian Task Force on Preventive Health Care; 2001.

94. Wathen CN, MacMillan HL. Prevention of violence against women: recommendation statement from the Canadian Task Force on Preventive Health Care. *CMAJ*. 2003;169:582-584.

95. Rhodes KV, Levinson W. Interventions for intimate partner violence against women: clinical applications. *JAMA*. 2003;289:601-605.

96. Lachs MS. Screening for family violence: what's an evidence-based doctor to do? *Ann Intern Med*. 2004;140:399-400.

97. Punukollu M. Domestic violence: screening made practical. *J Fam Prac*. 2003; 52:537-543.

98. The role of the pediatrician in recognizing and intervening on behalf of abused women. American Academy of Pediatrics: Committee on Child Abuse and Neglect. *Pediatrics*. 1998;101:1091-1092.

99. Brown J. Working toward freedom from violence: the process of change in battered women. *Violence Against Women*. 1997;3:5-26.

100. Houry D, Sachs CJ, Feldhaus KM, Linden J. Violence-inflicted injuries: reporting laws in the fifty states. *Ann Emerg Med*. 2002;39:56-60.

101. Kaur G, Herbert L. Recognizing and intervening in intimate partner violence. *Cleve Clin J Med*. 2005;72:406-409, 413-414, 417.

102. Zink T, Elder N, Jacobson J, Klostermann B. Medical management of intimate partner violence considering the stages of change: precontemplation and contemplation. *Ann Fam Med*. 2004;2:231-239.

103. Agency for Healthcare Research and Quality. More research is needed on screening and treating domestic violence victims [Impact of AHRQ Research]. In: *Women and Domestic Violence: Programs and Tools That Improve Care for Victims*. Rockville, Md: US Dept of Health & Human Services; 2004. Research in Action, Issue 15. Available at: http://www.ahrq.gov/research/domviolria/domviolria.pdf. Accessed September 4, 2007.

Chapter 3

DATING VIOLENCE AMONG HIGH SCHOOL AND COLLEGE STUDENTS

Eileen R. Giardino, RN, MSN, PhD, MSN, FNP-BC

Dating violence is defined as psychological, sexual, or physical violence within a dating relationship.[1] Dating violence may occur at first meeting, during the dating relationship, and even after the dating relationship has ended. The definition of dating violence may vary to include physical violence only or physical violence along with emotional and psychological components of dating interactions as well. The implications of dating violence affect all aspects of the victim's health and well being. Health care providers must be aware of the problems associated with dating violence while knowing how to identify and treat victims in health care settings.

This chapter first addresses facts about dating violence among high school and college-aged people and then implications for practice of medical and mental health care providers. It is important for those who work with teenagers and young adults to know the prevalence of dating violence as well as the associated risk behaviors among those who report dating violence. The more providers know to ask about dating violence, the more likely one is to ask the right questions, make appropriate interventions, and reduce the likelihood of further victimization.

DATING VIOLENCE DEFINED

Dating violence occurs between people who are dating (both heterosexual and same-sex couples) and have or may move towards an intimate relationship, but does not apply to people who are living together without such a relationship. Dating violence is an effort to control the partner and involves a spectrum or pattern of behaviors that may include physical or psychological injury.[2]

There are many behaviors that comprise dating violence. One may experience a single incidence of violence, such as date rape or sexual assault. There may also be a repeated pattern of mistreatment or abusive behavior that escalates over time within a relationship. A perpetrator usually tries to exert power and control over their victim and may use a variety of tactics to exert that control. Patterns may include psychological abuse, physical injury, the threat of injury, progressive social isolation from friends and family, control over what someone wears, sexual assault, deprivation, stalking, threats, insults, intimidation, and even murder.[3,4]

TYPES OF DATING VIOLENCE

Table 3-1 shows behaviors that may exist in the different types of physical dating violence. The following descriptions of victimization provide examples of types of interactions and abusive acts that may occur in a dating relationship.[4,5]

Table 3-1. Types of Behaviors Seen in Different Forms of Dating Violence.[4]

Physical Violence	— Restraining — Shaking — Pushing or shoving — Throwing something hard — Kicking — Hitting or slapping — Hair pulling — Biting — Choking — Burning or scalding — Beating

Sexual Harassment	— Making lewd comments or gestures to cause embarrassment.
	— Behaviors, actions or words that are:
	  — Sexual in nature
	  — Likely to offend or humiliate
	  — In relation to a person's sex, sexuality or body parts, or are repeated even after the person has been told to stop

Sexual Coercion	— Pressure to engage in sexual acts by taunting, belittling, making fun of, or harassing — Lying to someone, or threatening to tell lies about someone (eg, to damage their reputation) in order to get sex — Exploiting or taking sexual advantage of someone, including victims who are younger or intoxicated (this includes using the Internet or date rape drugs to prey on someone for sex)
Sexual Assault	— Any form of kissing, fondling, touching, oral sex, or sexual intercourse without consent — Not stopping sexual contact when asked to — Forcing someone to engage in sexual intercourse or any other sexual act
Psychological Violence	— Being cruel, deceitful, or manipulative — Ridiculing, name calling, or making insulting comments — Constant criticism — Excessive jealousness and possessiveness — Not allowing someone to have friends or talk to or be with others — Threatening to hurt the partner, their loved ones, or their property if they do not obey — Harassing behaviors after relationship has ended through obsessive phone calls, stalking, or making threats — Bullying behaviors such as swearing, name calling, breaking things, vandalizing property, or spreading gossip or rumors about the person

— ***Physical violence.*** Involves the use of force. This may or may not result in physical injury or involve the use of a weapon. There is often a pattern of behaviors that are abusive and harmful.

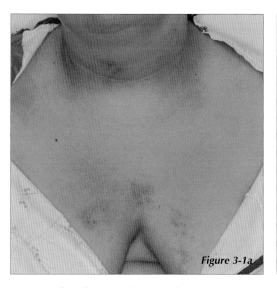
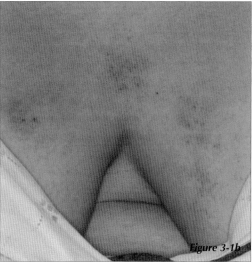

Figure 3-1a *Figure 3-1b*

— **Sexual violence.** Includes all forms of sexual harassment, sexual coercion, or sexual assault. Sexual harassment is a pattern of unwelcome or unwanted sexual words, behavior, or actions. Sexual coercion involves manipulating a situation or person unfairly in order to get sex. Sexual assault includes any form of sexual activity without gaining the partner's consent.

— **Psychological violence.** Involves the use of words or actions to intimidate, isolate, or control someone. The intent of this form of victimization is to damage one's sense of integrity or self-worth.

Figure 3-1a and 3-1b. This victim's suck mark injuries to the right and left inner top breast area exemplify a common form of sexual violence.

INCIDENCE AND PREVALENCE

A high incidence of dating violence is reported by high school and college students ranging from 9% to 57%. However, differences in estimates of the incidence and prevalence of teen dating violence vary due to the ways in which researchers collect data about the problem.[6,7] Much of dating violence data comes from studies, rather than police reports, that ask respondents to report incidences of dating violence. The data has been collected in different ways and on different sample ages that may mix study populations of middle school, high school and college-aged students. Studies that estimate the rates of dating violence are often based on convenience samples among specific groups of people of different ages. Such samples usually limit the generalizability of the findings to broader populations.

A 2003 nationwide Youth Risk Behavior Survey (YRBS) of students in grades 9 through 12 asked one question regarding physical dating violence (PDV): "During the past 12 months, did your boyfriend or girlfriend ever hit, slap, or physically hurt you on purpose?" Of 14 956 students, 8.9% reported experiencing PDV. The prevalence of PDV victimization was similar for males (8.9%) and females (8.8%) and similar by grade level (range: 8.1%-10.1%) [**See Table 3-2**]. There was a higher reported prevalence of PDV victimization among blacks (13.9%) than whites (7.0%) and Hispanics (9.3%). The prevalence of PDV victimization was less among white males (6.6%) than black males (13.7%), and less among white females (7.5%) and Hispanic females (9.2%) than among black females (14.0%).[1]

The incidence of dating violence is widespread, with 85% to 90% of victims being female adolescents and adult women.[8] A study of women 14 to 26 years of age who visited a family planning clinic reported 43% experienced 1 or more episodes of

Table 3-2. Prevalence of physical dating violence victimization* among high school students, by sex and selected characteristics–United States, 2003.[76]

CHARACTERISTIC	TOTAL %	TOTAL (95% CI[†])	MALE %	MALE (95% CI)	FEMALE %	FEMALE (95% CI)
Overall	**8.9**	**(7.9-9.9)**	**8.9**	**(7.7-10.2)**	**8.8**	**(7.9-9.8)**
Grade level						
9	**8.1**	**(7.0-9.5)**	7.8	(6.3-9.5)	8.6	(6.7-10.8)
10	**8.8**	**(7.0-10.9)**	9.3	(7.3-11.8)	8.2	(6.4-10.3)
11	**8.1**	**(6.9-9.6)**	7.9	(6.5-9.6)	8.2	(6.7-10.1)
12	**10.1**	**(8.5-12.0)**	10.1	(7.8-13.0)	10.2	(8.4-12.4)
Race/Ethnicity						
White, non-Hispanic	**7.0**	**(6.2-7.9)**	6.6	(5.8-7.5)	7.5	(6.2-9.0)
Black, non-Hispanic	**13.9**	**(12.3-15.5)**	13.7	(11.8-16.0)	14.0	(11.8-16.5)
Hispanic	**9.3**	**(7.6-11.3)**	9.2	(6.7-12.6)	9.2	(7.7-11.1)
Geographic region[§]						
Northeast	**10.6**	**(8.4-13.2)**	10.8	(8.7-13.3)	10.4	(7.8-13.7)
Midwest	**7.5**	**(5.8-9.7)**	8.3	(6.2-10.9)	6.5	(4.9-8.5)
South	**9.6**	**(8.3-11.1)**	9.3	(7.6-11.4)	9.9	(8.6-11.5)
West	**6.9**	**(5.2-9.1)**	6.1	(3.7-10.0)	7.8	(6.3-9.5)
Self-reported grades						
Mostly A's	**6.1**	**(5.0-7.4)**	6.6	(4.9-8.9)	5.7	(4.6-7.1)
Mostly B's	**7.7**	**(6.8-8.7)**	7.4	(6.3-8.7)	8.0	(6.7-9.6)
Mostly C's	**11.2**	**(9.8-12.8)**	10.4	(8.8-12.3)	12.3	(10.3-14.8)
Mostly D's or F's	**13.7**	**(11.1-16.7)**	13.0	(10.1-16.7)	14.9	(10.7-20.4)

*Defined as a response of "yes" to a single question: "During the past 12 months, did your boyfriend or girlfriend ever hit, slap, or physically hurt you on purpose?"
†Confidence interval.
§Northeast: Connecticut, Maine, Massachusetts, New Hampshire, New Jersey, New York, Pennsylvania, Rhode Island, and Vermont. Midwest: Illinois, Indiana, Iowa, Kansas, Michigan, Minnesota, Missouri, Nebraska, North Dakota, Ohio, South Dakota, and Wisconsin. South: Alabama, Arkansas, Delaware, District of Columbia, Florida, Georgia, Kentucky, Louisiana, Maryland, Mississippi, North Carolina, Oklahoma, South Carolina, Tennessee, Texas, Virginia, and West Virginia. West: Alaska, Arizona, California, Colorado, Hawaii, Idaho, Montana, Nevada, New Mexico, Oregon, Utah, Washington, and Wyoming.

IPV.[9] The US Department of Justice estimates that more than 90% of dating violence victims are female, while most perpetrators are male. Approximately 10% of men are also victims; however, this low percentage may actually be higher as male victims underreport their own victimization. Women are 5 to 8 times more likely than men to be victimized by an intimate partner.[10] Other sources cite that teenage girls in heterosexual relationships are more likely to suffer from sexual abuse than teenage boys.[11,6] Because the rates for dating violence against men are far less than those experienced by females, the focus of research and practice is more often toward the effects of abuse on women. In practice, the health care provider (HCP) should always consider that a male might also be the victim of dating violence and abuse.

Table 3-3. Statistics on Dating Violence.[16,77-79]

— About 1 in 3 high school students have been or will be involved in an abusive relationship.

— In 1995, 7% of all murder victims were young women who were killed by their boyfriends.

— One in 5 dating couples reports some type of violence in their relationship.

— A survey of adolescent and college students revealed that date rape accounted for 67% of sexual assaults.

— More than half of young women raped (68%) knew their rapist either as a boyfriend, friend, or casual acquaintance.

— Six out of 10 rapes of young women occur in their own home or a friend or relative's home, not in a dark alley.

— Between 39% and 54% of dating violence victims remain in physically abusive relationships.

— Sixty percent of acquaintance rapes on college campuses occur in casual or steady dating relationships.

— In 1 year, more than 13% of college women indicated they had been stalked, 42% by a boyfriend or ex-boyfriend.

— Fifty-one percent of college males admit perpetrating 1 or more sexual assault incidents during college.

— One in 11 adolescents reports being a victim of physical dating violence.

— Dating abuse occurs more frequently among black students (13.9%) than among Hispanic (9.3%) or white (7.0%) students.

— Seventy-two percent of eighth and ninth graders reportedly "date"; by the time they are in high school, 54% of students report dating abuse among their peers.

Although the literature shows that women experience forms of dating violence at a much higher rate than males, men also experience various forms of violence in their relationships. Price and colleagues (2000) studied 1700 youths (11 to 20 years old) regarding dating violence. Twenty-two percent of females and 12% of males reported experiencing dating violence, and 19% and 4%, respectively, for sexual abuse. There were significant differences between the percentages of adolescent girls and boys experiencing psychological or physical abuse. Overall, 13% of boys and 29% of adolescent girls in the sample reported some abuse in their dating relationships.[12] Statistics in 2003 show the highest per capita rate of IPV is in women between ages 16 to 24,[8] while IPV by current or former boyfriends, girlfriends, or spouses accounted for 20% of all nonfatal violence against females aged 12 or older in 2001.[13] Up to 92% of the perpetrators in those assaults were an acquaintance or a date.[14,15] A study of eighth and ninth graders found that 25% indicated they had been victims of dating violence, and 8% disclosed being sexually abused.[16] See **Table 3-3** for more statistics.

Studies of IPV show that lesbian, gay, bisexual, and transgender (LGBT) relationships experience violence in the same way that heterosexual relationships do. However, the phenomenon has not been studied in the LGBT population to the extent of the study of heterosexual women.[17] The prevalence of dating violence among gay, lesbian and bisexual (GLB) adolescents is similar to that of heterosexuals. A substantial proportion of gay, lesbian, bisexual, and heterosexual adolescents have experienced abuse in a dating relationship, and the prevalence of dating violence was similar among males and females.[18] A survey of men in same-sex relationships found that the prevalence of IPV was not as high as in heterosexual couples.[17]

HIGH SCHOOL STUDENTS

Of female high school students, 20% experienced physical or sexual violence by a dating partner,[7] and some figures indicate that forced sex was experienced by 8% of high school girls.[19] According to the 1997 South Carolina Youth Behavior Survey, 9.7% of girls in grades 9 through 12, reported being beaten by a boyfriend, while 21.3% reported being sexually assaulted.[20]

A 1997 study of high school students found factors that predicted dating violence. Findings showed males were more likely to inflict violence against a partner when they believed that male-female dating violence was justifiable; had witnessed more violence among and between parents; were the recipients of dating violence; used alcohol/drugs; or experienced more conflict in their dating relationships. Conversely, females were more likely to be violent toward a dating partner when they were the recipients of dating violence; believed that female-to-male dating violence was justifiable and that male-to-female violence was not justifiable; experienced more conflict in the dating relationship; used alcohol or drugs; or felt the relationship was more serious **(Table 3-4)**.[21]

The infrequent reporting of dating violence to others by teenagers is a concerning situation. Studies show that teenagers are less likely to report incidents of dating violence against them than any other age group.[11,22] One study found that 88% of victims of teenaged dating violence told no one about their victimization; 22% told a peer rather than a parent.[23]

Table 3-4. Possible Signs of a Teenager or Young Adult Who May be Experiencing Dating Violence.[16,77-79]

— Physical signs of injury

— Missing classes, dropping out of school

— Academic problems and grade failures

— Inability to make decisions

— Mood or personality changes

— Start or ongoing use of drugs/alcohol

— Pregnancy

— Emotional outbursts/Personality changes

— Withdrawal from social interactions

COLLEGE STUDENTS

White and Koss studied a national sample of college students and found that 32% of the women experienced physical dating violence from age 14 through their college years (the average age of the women was 21.4 years).[24]

The Smith and colleagues (2003) study of college women indicated that physical and sexual dating violence is a common experience. Eighty-eight percent of the 18 to 19 year old college age women (in the study) reported at least 1 incident of physical or sexual victimization from adolescence through the fourth year of college, with victimization broadly defined. Study findings showed that women physically victimized in high school were at significantly greater risk in college for physical victimization (revictimization). Also, there was a significant co-victimization risk, with either physical or sexual victimization increasing the risk of the other type of victimization. The group of women most likely to be physically or sexually victimized or co-victimized across the 4 years of college were those with a history of both childhood victimization (any type) and physical victimization in adolescence. The percentage remained high (66%) even when analyses were limited to more severe forms of sexual (attempted or completed rape) or physical (hitting, pushing, throwing something) victimization.[2]

Young people victimized by dating violence are at increased risk for victimization by violence in their intimate relationships, marriages, and family lives. A longitudinal study of students across 4 years of college at a North Carolina University found that the women most likely to be physically or sexually victimized or co-victimized were those with a history of both physical victimization during adolescence and any type of childhood victimization. The group at the second greatest risk was women who were physically victimized in adolescence, but not in childhood. Higher proportions of this group of women experienced subsequent victimization than that of women who were victimized in childhood but not in adolescence. Those women who experienced neither childhood nor adolescent victimization were at the lowest risk.[25,4]

IMPLICATIONS OF DATING VIOLENCE

Dating violence is a serious and pervasive problem facing high school and college age adolescents and young adults. Teenagers and young adults are maturing and benefit from understanding that violence and intimidation in dating relationships is unacceptable. Implications of dating violence among high school and college-aged women are paramount. Studies show that women who are victimized are at a higher risk for re-victimization than women who were not victimized during their younger years.[25] Smith and colleagues (2003) found that women who have experienced violence remained at greater risk each following year for re-victimization than those who were not.[25] A woman who has been assaulted in any year is significantly more likely to be sexually assaulted at a later time. Adolescent victimization was a better predictor of college victimization than was childhood victimization.[25] Consequently, programs that address dating violence prevention/intervention in high school and college may help reduce re-victimization.

ROLE OF THE HEALTH CARE PROVIDER

Health care providers can assist in helping to identify the problem by being aware of early warning indicators of dating violence, asking appropriate screening questions, offering support, and encouraging victims to seek out further help.

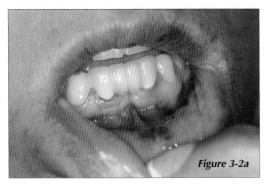

Figure 3-2a

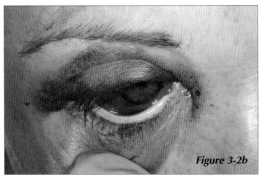

Figure 3-2b

Figure 3-2a. The lip trauma was caused by the perpetrator shoving his fingers into the victim's mouth.

Figure 3-2b. As a result of strangulation, this victim's eyes suffered massive bruising.

HEALTH RISK FACTORS AND HEALTH PROBLEMS RELATED TO DATING VIOLENCE

There are a number of immediate and long-term health consequences associated with dating violence that affect both victims and their families. Dating violence may harm victims psychologically, physically, and sexually and may damage an individual's confidence, sense of safety, and self-esteem. Social functioning and development are affected as well.[4]

The prevention agenda of *Healthy People 2010* describes a connection between women who experience IPV and the presence of 8 out of the 10 leading health indicators (LHI). This translates into the fact that IPV is a significant risk factor for chronic health problems and health risk behaviors.[2] Women who have experienced IPV and children who grow up in homes where violence is present are more likely to experience an array of physical and mental health problems.[26,27]

Survey data show that adolescent girls who report a history of experiencing dating violence are more likely to exhibit other serious health risk behaviors. Silverman and colleagues (2001) found a high association between physical and sexual dating violence against adolescent girls and increased risk of substance use, unhealthy weight control behaviors (eg, use of laxatives or vomiting), sexual risk behaviors (eg, first intercourse before age 15 years), pregnancy, and attempted suicide.[7] High school victims were 4 to 6 times more likely than their nonabused peers to become pregnant and 8 to 9 times more likely to have attempted suicide during the previous year. Unhealthy sexual behaviors that can lead to sexually transmitted infections (including human immunodeficiency virus or unintended pregnancy) are associated with dating abuse.[7]

In the population of women who have experienced forms of dating violence or IPV, there are stronger associations with an increased prevalence of physical and mental health problems, depression,[28,29] posttraumatic stress disorder,[30,31] and anxiety.[28,29] Poor development of self-esteem and body image can result from dating abuse.[32] It is important to recognize these signs and symptoms in the adolescent population.

Regarding alcohol use in physical dating violence, the 2003 Youth Risk Behavior Survey (YRBS) reported higher levels of episodic heavy drinking during the 12 months preceding the survey in those who reported PDV victimization.[1] In studies reporting IPV, alcohol use is a common factor that emerges as a link in the incidence of victimization. A study of 1600 women found that those who experienced IPV were more likely to have consumed on average 3 or more alcoholic drinks per occasion at least 1 time per week in the previous year, as opposed to women who did not disclose IPV.[33] Another study of 557 women who experienced IPV showed that they were

3 times more likely to binge drink (5 or more drinks per day) than those who reported no instances of violence.[17] A 1997 study found that girls who reported physical or sexual abuse were more than twice as likely as nonabused girls to report drinking (22% versus 12%), using illegal drugs (30% versus 13%), or smoking (26% versus 10%).

A sample of 5414 public high school students found that 52.8% of those who reported severe dating violence (SDV) were also current smokers, as compared to 34.2% of students who did not disclose SDV.[2] Furthermore, 32% of girls who had been abused reported binging and purging, as compared with 12% of those who had not been abused.[19]

A study of 863 college women between 18 and 25 years of age from a southern black university and a private mid-Atlantic college found injuries from incidences of dating violence included scratches, welts, black eyes, swelling, or lip trauma **(Figures 3-2a to 3-5b)**. Sore muscles, sprains, or pulls were the most commonly reported injuries. Concurrently, scores on tests for depression, anxiety, somatization, interpersonal sensitivity, hostility, and global severity index were significantly higher for victims than nonvictims. Victims who experienced multiple forms of dating violence had significantly higher mental health scores and reported greater numbers of injuries than victims of a single form of violence. The study found that less than half of those who reported injuries to the questionnaire sought health care and fewer than 3% saw a mental health professional.[34]

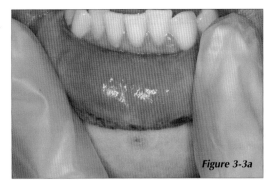

Figure 3-3a

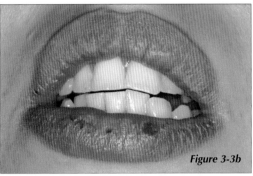

Figure 3-3b

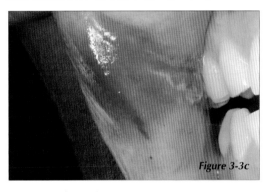

Figure 3-3c

Figure 3-3a to 3-3c. Typical lip trauma, abrasions to the lower and outer lip, as evidenced by dried blood around battered victim's mouth.

Other links between dating abuse and poor health are increased injuries and visits to emergency departments.[16,35] Dating violence is more highly associated with binge drinking, suicide attempts, physical fights, and sexual activity.[1] Girls who report physical or sexual dating violence are more than twice as likely to use drugs, alcohol, and tobacco than those who do not report abuse.[36] The 2003 Youth Risk Behavior Survey (YRBS) showed that higher levels of PDV victimization related to lower self-reported grades in school; 6.1% of students reporting mostly A's reported PDV victimization, compared with 13.7% of students receiving mostly D's or F's.[1] Dating violence may affect young women differently than young men. A research review indicates that women physically abused by their dating partners tend to suffer more physical and emotional harm than abused men.[4] Another sequela of dating violence is that victims may have a greater possibility of experiencing intimate partner violence (IPV) victimization in adulthood.[1,25] In the United States, an estimated 5.3 million women experience IPV incidents each year, resulting in approximately 2 million injuries and 1300 deaths.[37]

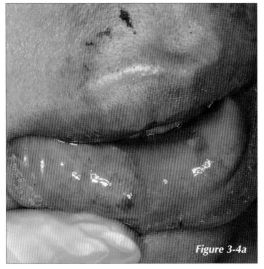

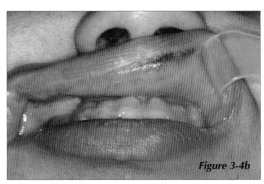

Figure 3-4b

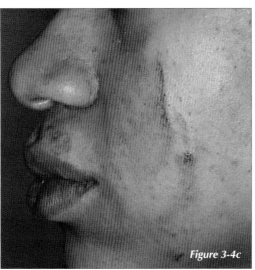

Figure 3-4a

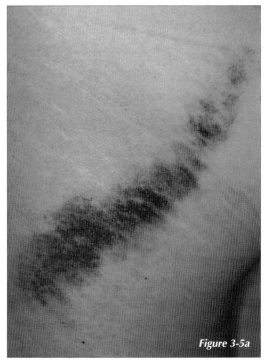

Figure 3-4c

Figure 3-5a

Figure 3-4a. *Victim was punched in the mouth, which caused the swelling abrasions on the upper lip. Upon being questioned, the victim intimated that "he [the perpetrator] has done this to me before."*

Figure 3-4b. *Lip retractors are being used to expose the victim's abrasion on the upper lip.*

Figure 3-4c. *The linear scratch mark to the left cheek was swabbed for contact DNA.*

Figure 3-5a. *The victim suffered this large bruise from her left outer buttock to her left thigh when she "was grabbed and thrown around the room numerous times" by the perpetrator.*

Figure 3-5b. *The yellow color in the bruised area displays a healing circular abrasion on the left upper back.*

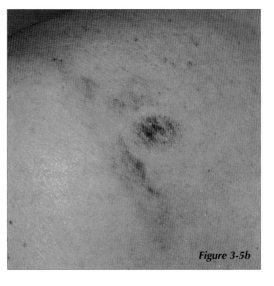

Figure 3-5b

SCREENING FOR DATING VIOLENCE IN PRACTICE

Because of the many health problems related to dating violence, the HCP must take the first step in ending abuse: identify that it is happening.[38] An organized approach to asking questions and an environment where patients feel safe to disclose such information are needed. Health care professionals are in an ideal situation to look for signs of IPV, screen for domestic violence, follow up with the right questions, and help prevent future battering by providing safety, information, resources, and support. Olsen, Rickert, and Davidson (2004) believe the question is not "*if* young women should be screened for dating violence," but rather *how* the providers can ask the questions and then *what* appropriate responses they can give to the people in their care.[39] Although much of the research on screening for IPV has focused on the adult population, it is appropriate to take that information and utilize the findings for the adolescent population. This is accomplished by being aware of the language used in the questions asked about violence that may elicit difficult answers. Future research can focus on the specifics of screening in the younger population.

Consistent screening for dating violence at every visit in the health care system provides a way to increase accurate diagnosis of violence in a timelier manner for the abused woman. Women are hesitant to report violence in their lives, so consequently HCPs only uncover about 5% of battered women. A concerning fact is that there are women who might have admitted to an abusive situation but were never asked by any member of the health care team.[40,41] Vigilant case finding helps address the range of psychological illness, general medical injuries, and social problems associated with dating violence. Consistent screening increases the time frame in which prevention, education, and treatment can begin.[42]

Health care providers are in an excellent place to uncover issues of abuse because of the relationship that one can develop with the patient, even in a short period of time. The American Medical Association stated that a female victim of violence prefers to disclose issues of abuse with her physician over any other person. So there is a great opportunity to discuss issues of dating violence, and this begins with an appropriate history.[43]

Because approximately 5% of victims are men, it is important to also include such questions when treating the adolescent male population. The key to discussing difficult issues is to make the patient comfortable, to be culturally sensitive, and to discuss issues in a way that is understandable to the client.

Health care providers in all practice settings come into contact with patients and clients who are victims of physical dating violence and IPV. Screening for all forms of violence is possible when there is a systematic focus to uncovering such experiences in a client's life. Major health care professional organizations recommend screening as well. These include the American Medical Association,[43] the American Nursing Association,[44] the US Preventive Services Task Force,[45] the American College of Obstetricians and Gynecologists,[46] and the Family Violence Prevention Fund.[3] The American Academy of Pediatrics recommends screening for "exposure to violence in the home (domestic violence or child abuse),"[47] because from a pediatric perspective, "the abuse of women is a pediatric issue."[48] The Practice Guidelines of the American Medical Association recommend partner violence screening at all levels of entry into the health care system.[43] The Joint Commission on Accreditation of Healthcare Organizations mandates universal screening for domestic violence.

Kimberg (2001) evaluated IPV from a primary care perspective and recommended that providers (internal medicine, family practice, obstetrics/gynecology, and pediatrics) screen *all* adolescent girls and women for past and present intimate partner violence.[49] All evidence of good clinical practice points consistently to the recommendation to screen for IPV at all clinical interactions with women.

There are many specialized practice areas where HCPs can routinely screen for dating violence. School nurses are in an ideal situation to routinely ask questions of students and provide education for parents of adolescents on dating violence. Health care providers, counselors, and health educators in college settings are also in excellent positions to screen and educate students about dating violence.

Given the high percentage of adolescent women in the United States who have experienced IPV, the question regarding screening is how providers can ask questions in the best possible way. The incidence of health care professionals in different clinical settings screening for domestic violence is generally found to be inconsistent to non existent.[50,51] One study found that provider behavior caused both positive and negative consequences when screening for IPV. Participants described positive consequences of screening that helped change their thoughts, attitudes, and feelings. Negative consequences from the screening process included feeling the provider was judgmental; increased anxiety about the unknown; feeling that the intervention protocol was awkward or intrusive; and disappointment in the provider's response.[52]

A multifocused emergency department study sought to both screen and provide follow-up care for women regarding IPV, a model that could be adopted for dating violence. The first approach to identification of IPV was universal screening of all women regardless of their chief complaint. The second component was an on-site IPV advocacy intervention by a local human service agency, which dispatched someone to the emergency department within 30 minutes to conduct a crisis intervention, and encouraged the patient to follow up with a case manager. The third phase was telephone-based counseling by an IPV case manager to help the client reduce her exposure to additional violence. The desired outcome was the client's self-report of a life free of violence. The outcomes were patient cooperation with the emergency department intervention and subsequent follow-up with the community-based agency.[53] Krasnoff and Moscati (2002) found that 475 (84%) of the 528 women identified as IPV victims agreed to speak to the advocate, and 258 (54% of those seen by the advocate) accepted case management follow-up. After the case management process, lasting 3 to 6 weeks, 127 women reported that they no longer believed they were at risk for violence from their abuser. This study showed that universal screening of all women was instrumental in identifying a large number who were experiencing IPV.[53]

Health care providers need to be well informed about the problem of dating violence for welfare of the patient or victim of violence as well as to inform parents about the incidence of violence in relationships. Depending on the age of the child victim, the HCP may not be able to inform a parent directly about suspected or confirmed violence. However, educating parents about the high incidence may clue a parent in to the need to watch for signs in a child's life. Parents and other caregivers are often unaware of the problem facing the adolescents in their families despite the common occurrence of dating violence among high school and college-aged people. An opinion survey of parents revealed that 81% either believe teenager dating violence is not an issue or admit they do not know if it is an issue. Fifty-four percent of those surveyed reported they had not spoken to their child about dating violence.[54]

Study findings of the low reporting of dating violence to law enforcement or HCPs underline the need for routine screening and assessment of all young women for psychological, physical, and sexual violence and stalking. Uncovering violence in a young person's life will increase the number of appropriate referrals for treatment and mental health support.[34,55]

Health care providers can help in the primary prevention of dating violence by being involved in curricula that are taught in schools and universities. A curriculum needs to be explicit about the issues and problems facing young people in the middle school and high school populations. Curricula also need to address how adolescents negotiate dating relationships and sexual practices. On college campuses, HCPs can be involved in the curricula established for all levels of the campus, such as classrooms, student-life programs, sororities and fraternities.

BARRIERS TO PHYSICIAN SCREENING AND VICTIM REPORTING

Professional organizations are consistent in recommending that health care professionals screen clients for dating violence and IPV in all types of professional practices. Despite widespread support for screening practices, there are barriers in place that prevent HCPs from asking questions as well as barriers that keep clients from disclosing information or answering questions openly about the presence of violence in their relationships.

Studies show there are HCP inadequacies that interfere with uncovering abuse. Barriers to screening for violence range from providers feeling that the patient would be uncomfortable with the screening questions to the concern that providers themselves are uncomfortable with asking difficult questions about IPV.[56-60] Barriers to pediatric residents asking about dating violence include lack of time and insufficient training.[61]

Some physicians did not ask about abuse because they did not believe it was a problem in their patient population.[62] Other research found that providers may not ask appropriate questions because of frustration that they would not be able to help their clients, a lack of formal training about abuse issues, and fear of offending patients.[59,62] Furthermore, providers felt they lack the time it takes to deal with the issues and responsibilities that arise when abuse is uncovered.[63]

Health care providers add to the problem of inconsistent screening for IPV because they have misguided beliefs regarding a victim's desire to disclose and a lack of information related to the prevalence, duration, and severity of partner violence.[64] Generally, studies indicate that patients want to be asked about IPV and that screening is a good thing to do.[65-67]

From the patient's perspective, people often protect themselves by hiding embarrassing situations from public view.[68] The victim faces barriers when deciding whether to disclose partner violence because of embarrassment, shame, or fear of disclosing personal battering or abuse.[64] Women's disclosure of abuse has been met with disbelief from family, acquaintances, and, unfortunately, HCPs to whom they have confided.[40]

Teenagers may be reluctant to report dating violence because they fear that no one will believe them, because they have either tried and been ignored, or they have difficulty describing the event effectively. It could be that an event occurred while acting against their parents' wishes, or when seeing someone the parents did not want their child to see. There is also fear of intimidation or retaliation by other teenagers or a perpetrator. [69,70]

Mandatory reporting laws may become a barrier or deterrent to teenager reporting of abuse because the teenager may want to keep the abuse confidential. They may know that once information is disclosed to a professional, that professional may be required to report the disclosed crime. Mandated reporting requires that specified adults such as HCPs, teachers, social workers, counselors, mental health professionals, and law enforcement officers in all states report child abuse or neglect. Some states require that all violence toward minors younger than 18 years be reported as child abuse.[71]

Some abused women are concerned that reporting an abusive partner may escalate violence and put themselves or other family members in further danger. Reluctance to disclose abuse or press charges may be due to victims' economic dependence or emotional ties to perpetrators .[72]

Questions for Screening for Intimate Partner Violence in Practice

There are a variety of screening tools that have been developed and tested for efficacy in practice. Most have been developed specifically for adults rather than adolescents. However, it is possible to use the tools in various settings with high school students as a way to explore issues of IPV with them.

Paranjape and Liebschutz (2003) compared IPV screening questions to determine a combination of questions that would have a high sensitivity for uncovering IPV. The study concluded that 3 simple questions could effectively identify lifetime IPV when used together and could aid clinician effort to identify abuse in women. The questions are[73]:

— "Have you ever been in a relationship where your partner has pushed or slapped you?"

— "Have you ever been in a relationship where your partner threatened you with violence?"

— "Have you ever been in a relationship where your partner has thrown, broken or punched things?"

Weiss and colleagues (2003) developed a 5-question Ongoing Abuse Screen (OAS) to evaluate ongoing IPV. They compared the OAS to the Index of Spouse Abuse (ISA) and the Abuse Assessment Screen (AAS). They sampled 856 patients and found that the OAS was more accurate, had a better positive predictive value, and was 3 times more likely to detect victims of ongoing intimate partner violence than the AAS. By the end of the study, the researchers developed a new screen titled the Ongoing Violence Assessment Tool (OVAT) because they felt the OAS was not accurate enough.[74] **Table 3-5** shows questions the interviewer can ask to uncover dating violence.[49]

Limits of Confidentiality

Finally, reporting by the adolescent presents unique challenges within the legal arena. For example, mandatory reporting takes away the adolescent's choice in reporting. Further, an adult must represent the adolescent within the legal system. In other words, the adolescent is not legally able to press charges against someone because they are not of legal age. Another complication is that, in 15 US states, dating violence is not protected under the Violence Against Women Act. Health care providers can advocate for change.

It is important to understand legal parameters of the state(s) in which one practices. There are confidentiality issues when screening for dating violence regarding the screening for and possible identification of abuse in adolescents and adults. All states require providers to report child abuse when a minor is victimized. However, each state varies in the definitions and laws regarding such reporting.[49] Health care providers must familiarize themselves with the state laws that govern their practice. Regarding what other services are available when abuse is disclosed, the health care provider should also be aware of child protective services resources available in the state, city, or town in which one practices.

Table 3-5. Screening Questions to Uncover Dating Violence and Intimate Partner Violence.[49]

Direct Questions
— Has your partner (may use boyfriend/girlfriend) ever hit you, hurt you, or threatened you in any way?

— Has your partner ever forced you to have sex when you didn't want to?

— Are you ever frightened of your partner?

— Has anyone ever hit you, hurt you, or threatened you in the past?

— Do you ever have screaming or yelling fights?

Indirect Questions
— What happens when you and your partner disagree? How do you settle disagreements?

— How do you feel your partner/family members treat you?

— Tell me more about your home environment.

— Do you feel safe at home?

Framing Questions
— I ask all my patients about violence in their relationships; does your partner ever hit you, hurt you, or threaten you?

— I want to make sure that each of my patients is safe in her/his relationships. Does anyone you know ever hit you, hurt you, or threaten you?

— Feeling that a person close to you does not respect you or treat you well can be so difficult. How do your partner/family members treat you?

The HCP must discuss confidentiality issues with adolescent patients as well as their parents at the first medical encounter. Relaying the details of legal implications and mandated reporting to the adolescent and parents is so important because of client trust issues. Information conveyed includes the protections and limits of confidentiality. A major implication for the adolescent client is that information may be disclosed that the HCP must report to parents or law enforcement. Conversely, if the adolescent is beyond the age of reporting, a parent must understand that the HCP is not able to report findings back to the parent no matter what the implications of the disclosure are. The adolescent could regard disclosure of health information to parents or legal authorities as a violation of trust, which could cause the teenager to distrust the HCP and the health care system[75] (**Table 3-6**).

Adult patients are under a different reporting structure. The mandated reporting of abuse does not apply, and adults may choose whether to report abuse to law enforcement. The HCP must also be aware of the age at which mandated reporting ends in their particular state. The American Medical Association ethics council believes it is unethical to violate the confidentiality of patient–provider disclosures or to force an intervention on an adult patient *without patient consent* in cases where the patient is not at immediate risk of losing life or limb.[43,75]

> **Table 3-6. Legal and Ethical Considerations of Consent and Confidentiality in Dating Violence Cases.**[49]
>
> — Inquire into the feasibility of parental involvement when treating a minor
>
> — Ask which other adults are important in their life, so that they could be involved in the care
>
> — Encourage open communication and parental involvement, whenever possible
>
> — Be aware of the laws in your state
>
> — Know and respect the rights of the adolescent
>
> — Advocate for what you think is best for the adolescent

Teenagers do not usually hold the same legal status and rights as adults. Therefore, legal options open to adults may not be the same for a teenager who experiences dating violence. While adults can request a protective order against an abuser, teenagers may not have that option and may not be able to file on their own behalf depending on the state in which one resides. Therefore, it is important for HCPs to be knowledgeable of the laws within their state regarding reporting, as well as the rights that teenagers have regarding dealing with abusive situations.[70]

CONCLUSION

Dating violence among adolescents is highly prevalent. Health care professionals play an important role in dealing with the issues of dating violence among high school and college-aged students. The high incidence of the problem in the population reflects that HCPs will have patients who are or who have experienced these phenomena. Efforts are needed to properly prepare HCPs to deal with this common adolescent health risk. The more that the HCP knows and understands about the problem, the more astute he or she will be in identifying victims and treating them in health care settings. The more providers know to ask about dating violence, the more likely one is to ask the right questions, make appropriate interventions to counseling, and reduce the likelihood of further victimization.

REFERENCES

1. Centers for Disease Control and Prevention. Physical dating violence among high school students—United States, 2003. *MMWR Morb Mortal Wkly Rep*. 2006b;55:532-535.

2. Intimate partner violence and Healthy People 2010 fact sheet. Family Violence Prevention Fund Web site. Available at: http://www.endabuse.org/hcadvd/2003/tier4.pdf. Accessed February 28, 2007.

3. Family Violence Prevention Fund. *Preventing Domestic Violence: Clinical Guidelines on Routine Screening*. San Francisco, CA: Family Violence Prevention Fund; 1999. Available at: http://endabuse.org/programs/healthcare/files/screpol.pdf. Accessed February 28, 2007.

4. Dating violence: a fact sheet from the Department of Justice Canada. Department of Justice of Canada Web site. Available at: http://www.justice.gc.ca/en/ps/fm/datingfs.html. Accessed February 28, 2007.

5. Lavoie F, Robitaille L, Hébert M. Teen dating relationships and aggression: an exploratory study. *Violence Against Women*. 2000;6:6-36.

6. Kaiser Family Foundation, YM Magazine. *National Survey of Teens: Teens Talk about Dating, Intimacy, and Their Sexual Experiences*. Pt 3. Menlo Park, CA: Kaiser Family Foundation; 1998. Available at: http://www.kff.org/youthhivstds/1373-datingrep3.cfm. Accessed February 28, 2007.

7. Silverman JG, Raj A, Mucci LA, Hathaway JE. Dating violence against adolescent girls and associated substance use, unhealthy weight control, sexual risk behavior, pregnancy, and suicidality. *JAMA*. 2001;286:572-579.

8. Rennison CM. Bureau of Justice Statistics Special Report. *Intimate Partner Violence and Age of Victim, 1993-99*. (2001). Bureau of Justice Statistics Special Report.

9. Rickert VI, Wiemann CM, Harrykissoon SD, Berenson AB, Kolb E. The relationship among demographics, reproductive characteristics, and intimate partner violence. *Am J Obstet Gynecol*. 2002;187:1002-1007.

10. Greenfeld LA, Rand MR, Craven D, et al. *Violence by Intimates: Analysis of Data on Crimes by Current or Former Spouses, Boyfriends, and Girlfriends*. US Dept of Justice, Office of Justice Programs; 1998. NCJ 167237. Bureau of Justice Statistics Factbook.

11. Jezl DR, Molidor CE, Wright TL. Physical, sexual, and psychological abuse in high school dating relationships: prevalence rates and self-esteem issues. *Child Adoles Social Work J*. 1996;13:69-87.

12. Price EL, Byers ES, Sears HA, Whelan J, Saint-Pierre M. *Dating Violence Amongst New Brunswick Adolescents: A Summary of Two Studies*. Fredericton, New Brunswick, Canada: Muriel McQueen Fergusson Centre for Family Violence Research; 2000. Research Paper Series, No. 2.

13. Rennison CM. *Intimate Partner Violence, 1993-2001*. US Dept of Justice, Office of Justice Programs; February 2003. NCJ 197838. Bureau of Justice Statistics Crime Data Brief. Available at: http://www.ojp.usdoj.gov/bjs/pub/pdf/ipv01.pdf. Accessed February 27, 2007.

14. Benson D, Charlton C, Goodhart F. Acquaintance rape on campus: a literature review. *J Am Coll Health*. 1992;40:157.

15. Rickert VI, Vaughan RD, Wiemann CM. Adolescent dating violence and date rape. *Curr Opin Obstet Gynecol*. 2002;14:495-500.

16. Foshee VA, Linder GF, Bauman KE, et al. The Safe Dates Project: theoretical basis, evaluation design, and selected baseline findings. *Am J Prev Med*. 1996;12(5 suppl):39-47.

17. McNutt LA, Carlson BE, Persaud M, Postmus J. Cumulative abuse experiences, physical health and health behaviors. *Ann Epidemiol*. 2002;12:123-130.

18. Freedner N, Freed LH, Yang YW, & Austin SB. (2002). Dating Violence Among Gay, Lesbian, and Bisexual Adolescents: Results From a Community Survey. *Journal of Adolescent Health, 31*, 469-474.

19. Schoen C, Davis K, Collins KS, Greenberg L, Des Roches C, Abrams M. *The Commonwealth Fund Survey of the Health of Adolescent Girls*. New York, NY: The Commonwealth Fund; November 1997.

20. White JW, Humphrey JA. A longitudinal approach to the study of sexual assault. In: Schwartz MD, ed. *Researching Sexual Violence Against Women: Methodological and Personal Perspectives.* Thousand Oaks, CA: Sage Publications; 1997:22-42.

21. O'Keefe M. Predictors of dating violence among high school students. *J Interpers Violence.* 1997;12:546-568.

22. Roscoe B, Kelsey T. Dating violence among high school students. *Psychol Q J Hum Behav.* 1986;23:53-59.

23. Koss MP. Defending Date Rape. *J Interpers Violence.* 1992;7:121-126.

24. White JW, Koss MP. Courtship violence: incidence and prevalence in a national sample of higher education students. *Violence Vict.* 1991;6: 247-256.

25. Smith PH, White JW, Holland LJ. A longitudinal perspective on dating violence among adolescent and college-age women. *Am J Public Health.* 2003;93:1104-1109.

26. Coker AL, Smith PH, Bethea L, King MR, McKeown RE. Physical health consequences of physical and psychological intimate partner violence. *Arch Fam Med.* 2000;9:451-457.

27. Campbell JC, Lewandowski LA. Mental and physical health effects of intimate partner violence on women and children. *Psychiatr Clin North Am.* 1997; 20:353-374.

28. McCauley J, Kern DE, Kolodner K, et al. Clinical characteristics of women with a history of childhood abuse: unhealed wounds. *JAMA.* 1997;277:1362-1368.

29. Jaffe P, Wolfe DA, Wilson S, Zak L. Emotional and physical health problems of battered women. *Can J Psychiatry.* 1986;31:625-629.

30. Astin MC, Ogland-Hand SM, Coleman EM, Foy DS. Posttraumatic stress disorder and childhood abuse in battered women: comparisons with maritally distressed women. *J Consult Clin Psychol.* 1995;63:308-312.

31. Schaaf KK, McCanne TR. Relationship of childhood sexual, physical, and combined sexual and physical abuse to adult victimization and posttraumatic stress disorder. *Child Abuse Negl.* 1998;22:1119-1133.

32. Ackard DM, Neumark-Sztainer D. Date violence and date rape among adolescents: associations with disordered eating behaviors and psychological health. *Child Abuse Negl.* 2002;26:455-473.

33. Lemon SC, Verhoek-Oftedahl W, Donnelly EF. Preventive healthcare use, smoking, and alcohol use among Rhode Island women experiencing intimate partner violence. *J Womens Health Gend Based Med.* 2002;11:555-562.

34. Amar AF, Gennaro S. Dating violence in college women: associated physical injury, healthcare usage, and mental health symptoms. *Nurs Res.* 2005;54:235-242.

35. Foshee VA. Gender differences in adolescent dating abuse prevalence, types and injuries. *Health Educ Res.* 1996;11:275-286.

36. Plichta SB. Violence and abuse: implications for women's health. In: Falik MM, Collins KS, eds. *Women's Health: The Commonwealth Survey.* Baltimore, Md: Johns Hopkins University Press; 1996.

37. National Center for Injury Prevention and Control. *Costs of Intimate Partner Violence Against Women in the United States*. Atlanta, GA: Centers for Disease Control and Prevention; 2003.

38. Price S, Baird K. Domestic violence in pregnancy. *Pract Midwife*. 2001;4:12-14.

39. Olson EC, Rickert VI, Davidson LL. Part II: screening for dating violence: should we screen or not? *J Pediatr Adolesc Gynecol*. 2004;17:131-136.

40. Wright RJ, Wright RO, Isaac NE. Response to battered mothers in the pediatric emergency department: a call for an interdisciplinary approach to family violence. *Pediatrics*. 1997;99:186-192.

41. McFarlane J, Greenberg L, Weltge A, Watson M. Identification of abuse in emergency departments: effectiveness of a two-question screening tool. *J Emerg Nurs*. 1995;21:391-394.

42. Valente SM. Evaluating intimate partner violence. *J Am Acad Nurse Pract*. 2002;14:505-513.

43. American Medical Association diagnostic and treatment guidelines on domestic violence. *Arch Fam Med*. 1992;1:39-47.

44. American Nurses Association. *Position Statement on Physical Violence Against Women*. Silver Spring, MD: American Nurses Association; 1994. http://www.nursingworld.org/MainMenuCategories/HealthcareandPolicyIssues/ANAPositionStatements/social/viowomen14525.aspx. Accessed July 14, 2008.

45. *Put Prevention Into Practice: Clinician's Handbook of Preventive Services*. 2nd ed. Washington, DC: US Dept of Health & Human Services, Public Health Service, Office of Public Health & Science, Office of Disease Prevention & Health Promotion; 1998.

46. American College of Obstetricians and Gynecologists. Anonymous. Domestic Violence. August, 1995. ACOG Technical Bulletin #209.

47. The role of the pediatrician in youth violence prevention in clinical practice and at the community level. American Academy of Pediatrics Task Force on Violence. *Pediatrics*. 1999;103:173-181.

48. The role of the pediatrician in recognizing and intervening on behalf of abused women. American Academy of Pediatrics, Committee on Child Abuse and Neglect. *Pediatrics*. 1998;101:1091-1092.

49. Kimberg L. Addressing intimate partner violence in primary care practice. *MedGenMed* [serial online]. 2001;3.

50. Elliott L., Nerney M., Jones T., & Friedmann P.D. (2002). Barriers to Screening for Domestic Violence. Journal of General Internal Medicine, 17, 112-116.

51. Parsons, L., Zaccaro,D.M., Wells,B., & Stovall,T.G.M. (1995). Methods of and attitudes toward screening obstetrics and gynecology patients for domestic violence. American Journal of Obstetrics & Gynecology, 173, 381-386.

52. Chang JC, Decker M, Moracco KE, Martin SL, Petersen R, Frasier PY. What happens when health care providers ask about intimate partner violence? A description of consequences from the perspectives of female survivors. *J Am Med Womens Assoc*. 2003;58:76-81.

53. Krasnoff M, Moscati R. Domestic violence screening and referral can be effective. *Ann Emerg Med*. 2002;40:485-492.

54. Charron PR, Cappello D, Wiseman R. *A Parent's Guide to Teen Dating Violence: 10 Questions to Start the Conversation*. New York, NY: Liz Claiborne; 2001. Available at: http://www.loveisnotabuse.com/pdf/10questions_hand.pdf. Accessed February 26, 2007.

55. Amar AF. Prevalence estimates of violence in the dating experiences of college women. *J Natl Black Nurses Assoc*. 2004;15:23-31.

56. Rodriguez MA, Bauer HM, McLoughlin E, Grumbach K. Screening and intervention for intimate partner abuse: practices and attitudes of primary care physicians. *JAMA*. 1999;282:468-474.

57. Gerbert B, Caspers N, Bronstone A, Moe J, Abercrombie P. A qualitative analysis of how physicians with expertise in domestic violence approach the identification of victims. *Ann Intern Med*. 1999;131:578-584.

58. McGrath ME, Bettacchi A, Duffy SJ, Peipert JF, Becker BM, St Angelo L. Violence against women: provider barriers to intervention in emergency departments. *Acad Emerg Med*. 1997;4:297-300.

59. Sugg NK, Inui T. Primary care physicians' response to domestic violence. Opening Pandora's box. *JAMA*. 1992;267:3157-3160.

60. Sugg NK, Thompson RS, Thompson DC, Maiuro R, Rivara FP. Domestic violence and primary care. Attitudes, practices, and beliefs. *Arch Fam Med*. 1999;8:301-306.

61. Forcier M, Patel R, Kahn JA. Pediatric residents' attitudes and practices regarding adolescent dating violence. *Ambul Pediatr*. 2003;3:317-323.

62. Parsons LH, Zaccaro D, Wells B, Stovall TG. Methods of and attitudes toward screening obstetrics and gynecology patients for domestic violence. *Am J Obstet Gynecol*. 1995;173:381-386.

63. Violence against women. Relevance for medical practitioners. Council of Scientific Affairs American Medical Association. *JAMA*. 1992;267:3184-3190.

64. Griffin MP, Kossn MP. Clinical screening and intervention in cases of partner violence. *Online J Issues Nurs*. 2002;7:3.

65. McCauley J, Yurk RA, Jenckes MW, Ford DE. Inside "Pandora's Box": abused women's experiences with clinicians and health services. *J Gen Intern Med*. 1998;13:549-555.

66. Caralis PV, Musialowski R. Women's experiences with domestic violence and their attitudes and expectations regarding medical care of abuse victims. *South Med J*. 1997;90:1075-1080.

67. Friedman LS, Samet JH, Roberts MS, Hudlin M, Hans P. Inquiry about victimization experiences. A survey of patient preferences and physician practices. *Arch Intern Med*. 1992;152:1186-1190.

68. Jecker NS. Privacy beliefs and the violent family: extending the ethical argument for physician intervention. *JAMA*. 1993;269:776-780.

69. National Center for Victims of Crime. Anonymous. *Breaking Silence, Building Trust. Helping Teenage Victims of Crime.* Washington, DC: National Center for Victims of Crime; 2003. Available at: http://www.ncvc.org/ncvc/AGP.Net/Components/documentViewer/Download.aspxnz?DocumentID=38812.

70. Joyce E. Teen dating violence: facing the epidemic. *Networks.* Winter 2004:1-9.

71. Gutierrez LM. *Teen Dating Violence: An Ignored Epidemic.* Newton, MA: Gender and Diversities Institute; 2002.

72. Brookoff D, O'Brien KK, Cook CS, Thompson TD, Williams C. Characteristics of participants in domestic violence. Assessment at the scene of domestic assault. *JAMA.* 1997;277:1369-1373.

73. Paranjape A, Liebschutz J. STaT: a three-question screen for intimate partner violence. *J Womens Health (Larchmt).* 2003;12:233-239.

74. Weiss SJ, Ernst AA, Cham E, Nick TG. Development of a screen for ongoing intimate partner violence. *Violence Vict.* 2003;18:131-141.

75. Diaz A, Neal WP, Nucci AT, Ludmer P, Bitterman J, Edwards S. Legal and ethical issues facing adolescent health care professionals. *Mt Sinai J Med.* 2004;71:181-185.

76. Centers for Disease Control and Prevention. Anonymous. Dating Abuse Fact Sheet. http://www.jwi.org/atf/cf/%7B3B767476-EF52-4EE7-A902-F97E1597F B88%7D/041708%20Dating%20Abuse%20Fact%20Sheet0907.pdf. Accessed July 2007.

77. Rennison, CM. Bureau of Justice Statistics Special Report. Intimate Partner Violence and Age of victim: 1993-2001. United States Department of Justice. (2003 Oct).

78. Jaffe PG, Sudermann M, Reitzel D, Killip SM. An evaluation of a secondary school primary prevention program on violence in intimate relationships. *Violence Vict.* 1992;7:129-146.

79. Dating Violence Resource Center. Campus dating violence fact sheet. National Center for Victims of Crime Web site. Available at: http://www.ncvc.org/ncvc/AGP.Net/Components/documentViewer/Download.aspxnz?DocumentID=38056. Accessed February 27, 2007.

80. Centers for Disease Control and Prevention. Dating Violence Warning Signs. The National Youth Violence Prevention Resource Center. Available at: http://www.safeyouth.org/scripts/faq/datingwarning.asp. Updated December 27, 2007. Accessed July 8, 2008.

Chapter 4

Intimate Partner Violence and Child Abuse

Megan H. Bair-Merritt, MD, MSCE
Joel A. Fein, MD, MPH

In 1998, the American Academy of Pediatrics (AAP) published guidelines, The Role of the Pediatrician in Recognizing and Intervening on Behalf of Abused Women, which state that "identifying and intervening on behalf of battered women may be one of the most effective means of preventing child abuse."[1] This statement leads to a number of related questions:

— Are child abuse and intimate partner violence (IPV) interrelated and, if so, how?

— Who perpetrates the child abuse in families with both forms of violence?

— What impact does this "double-whammy"[2] (child abuse and IPV exposure) have on children?

— How should providers manage child abuse and IPV within the same family?

This chapter addresses these questions by exploring the theoretical and historical context of child abuse and IPV, describing epidemiology and impact on children, and reviewing screening and management issues.

This chapter focuses predominantly on violence perpetrated by men against women. The authors recognize, however, that IPV is a complex phenomenon. National crime survey data support that most IPV is male-perpetrated, but some population-based surveys report high levels of female-perpetrated and bidirectional violence.[3-6] In addition, IPV occurs not only in heterosexual, but also in homosexual relationships.[7] Further study of IPV epidemiology will facilitate the development of screening and intervention protocols addressing female perpetration and IPV in same-sex couples.

Theoretical Models of Intimate Partner Violence and Child Abuse

Prior research provides an integrated conceptualization of the etiology of co-occurring IPV and child maltreatment within a given family.[6,8-10] Proposed theoretical frameworks describing this overlap include (though are not limited to) the following[8-10]:

— ***Social cognitive theory.*** In IPV research, *social cognitive theory* proposes that a triadic relationship exists between behavior, the person, and the environment. Within this dynamic relationship, each facet actively affects the other two (ie, reciprocal determinism).[11] Considering the etiology of family violence, social cognitive theory suggests that those exposed to violence (eg, men in their families of origin, women assaulted by their partners) model this behavior as a means to resolve conflict. The perpetrator then learns through operant reinforcement that the violence works, thereby reinforcing further abusive acts.[8,10]

— ***Ecological theory.*** According to *ecological theory,* violence in the home is rooted within the greater context of societal violence. Stressors combined with a lack of protective factors lead to family violence.[10]

— ***Antisocial personality or genetics theory.*** The origin of family violence in *antisocial personality theory or genetics theory* lies with a usually male perpetrator afflicted with an antisocial personality disorder.[10]

— ***Family systems theory.*** The *family systems theory* maintains a bidirectional view. This theory asserts that all family members contribute to general conflict within a family. Those espousing this view emphasize, though, that each individual, in particular the perpetrator, is accountable for his or her own behavior.[10]

— ***Feminist theory.*** The *feminist theory* states that both forms of violence originate from conflict about gender roles and men's need for power and control.[12]

Cited references provide a more thorough description of the above theoretical frameworks for interested readers. Alone, none of these models fully explains the complicated underpinnings of family violence; however, when taken together, they offer a rich foundation for better understanding the complexity of a child abuse–IPV association.

HISTORICAL CONTEXT OF INTIMATE PARTNER VIOLENCE AND CHILD ABUSE

Until the 1990s, the IPV and child abuse research and policy-making communities functioned separately with differing, and often conflicting, agendas and priorities. Historically, government agencies took responsibility for protecting maltreated children and used state and local sites (ie, child protective services [CPS]) to administer federal policies. In an effort to mandate improved well being for maltreated children, legislators passed the Child Abuse Prevention and Treatment Act (CAPTA) in 1974, Adoption Assistance and Child Welfare Act of 1980, and Adoption and Safe Families Act of 1997.[13] Those involved in protecting maltreated children recognized IPV as an important risk factor but expressed concern that IPV advocates focused on women and inadvertently neglected the safety needs of children.[13-15]

In contrast to government-based child maltreatment services, IPV programs arose from grassroots efforts of women's groups during the 1970s. Concurrent with the feminist movement, women shared their abuse experiences at the hands of their partners. In response, community-based shelters emerged throughout the United States.[13] Government recognition of IPV as an important societal problem advanced with the passage of the 1994 Violence Against Women Act, which provided significant funding to IPV shelters and organizations.[13] Though IPV advocates have long been aware of the impact of IPV on children, these advocates were reluctant to join forces with CPS. They feared that the child-based system of CPS would blame mothers for "failing to protect" the children.[13,15]

In recent years, response to concurrent IPV and child abuse has improved. In 1999, the National Council of Juvenile and Family Court Judges published *Effective Interventions in Domestic Violence & Child Maltreatment Cases: Guidelines for Policy and Practice.*[13] These guidelines offer recommendations for creating a joint response to child abuse cases with concurrent IPV. Suggestions include cross-training about IPV and child abuse among workers in community agencies, routine inquiry about IPV in CPS cases, and creating responses that avoid blaming the nonabusive parent.[13] In 2000, federal funds were allocated to 6 sites across the country to implement these recommendations.

EPIDEMIOLOGY

Multiple studies, as well as the reviews assembled from the data of these studies, point toward a significant rate of overlap between child maltreatment and IPV.[6,10,14,16] Given the complexity of studying this problem, the precise percentage of simultaneously occurring child abuse and IPV remains unknown. In a systematic review, Appel and Holden addressed this question.[10] The studies included in this review provided rates from either battered women's shelters or from the parents of abused children. The authors concluded that the median co-occurrence of child abuse and IPV was 40%.[10] However, Appel and Holden cautioned that the studies in their review had methodological flaws that included inconsistent definitions of child abuse and reliance upon self-report by mothers.[10]

Edleson similarly summarized the existing literature regarding the simultaneous occurrence of child abuse and IPV.[14] He found that most studies documented concurrent rates ranging from 30% to 60%. Like Appel and Holden, however, Edleson cautioned that limitations to the existing research preclude an exact estimation of the underlying rates.[14]

A subsequent study used the US Army Family Advocacy Program's central database of reported abuse and neglect. This study found that the adjusted relative risk for child abuse in families with IPV was twice that of families without IPV.[16] Slep and O'Leary also examined rates of IPV and child maltreatment in a community-based sample.[6] Within families disclosing any form of physical violence, most reported the presence of multiple forms of violence, including an elevated risk for child abuse among families reporting IPV.

CHILD ABUSE IN FAMILIES WITH INTIMATE PARTNER VIOLENCE

In homes with both forms of violence, both abuse victims and batterers have been implicated as the perpetrators of child abuse. Some studies conclude that batterers are the more likely perpetrators of all forms of abuse in these families.[12,15,17] With regard to sexual abuse, McCloskey determined that children of abused mothers were significantly more likely than controls to be victims of sexual abuse by the mother's partner.[18] Other authors, however, report that the victim often abuses her children.[19] Still other studies find that *both* partners involved in an abusive relationship commonly maltreat their children. Using a community-based sample, Slep and O'Leary found that instances of sole perpetrators within a family were rare; the more common scenario involved aggression by both men and women against each other and against the children.[6]

OUTCOMES FOR CHILDREN

Separately, child abuse and exposure to IPV have each been associated with deleterious outcomes for children, with both groups suffering from social-emotional health problems more often than their peers.[20-23] The impact of comorbid child maltreatment and IPV exposure may be particularly detrimental, having been referred to as a "double-whammy."[2] One study compared child witnesses with children who had witnessed IPV and were abused themselves; this study found that the latter group had significantly more externalizing behavior problems (eg, aggression) than the former.[26] Kernic determined that abused children exposed to IPV were more likely than their peers to have a cumulative grade point average of less than 1.0, to have been held back a grade, and to have been suspended from school.[27] Other studies, however, have not supported this concept that interaction between these forms of violence leads to poorer outcomes than either exposure alone.[28,29]

An additional area of concern in families with both forms of violence is the risk of child homicide. While this area has not been well studied, a report of Oregon's child fatalities indicated that IPV occurred in the families of 41% of children who had been critically injured or killed because of an inflicted injury.[14] Similarly, in Massachusetts, 43% of child fatality cases occurred in families in which the mothers were abused.[14]

INTIMATE PARTNER VIOLENCE SCREENING IN THE PEDIATRIC SETTING

Health care providers are in a unique position to detect family violence and offer resources to mitigate the resulting negative outcomes.[30] Universal screening for IPV ideally should be the standard of care.[1] Inquiry about IPV is particularly important, though, in all cases when a health care provider suspects child abuse. Conversely, when a patient's caregiver discloses IPV, the health care provider should conduct a careful assessment for child abuse. The safest and most effective way to ask about IPV remains controversial. The ensuing discussion, which focuses upon screening for IPV in a pediatric environment, raises the major issues and offers some suggestions.

Before initiating a conversation about IPV, health care providers should know the laws in their state regarding reporting. Some states have specific laws mandating that health care providers report IPV and childhood exposure to IPV. Other states interpret childhood exposure to IPV as falling within the definition of child abuse, thereby requiring a CPS report. Web sites such as the Child Information Gateway* offer assistance regarding the state laws about child abuse and IPV. If practicing in a state with mandated reporting for IPV or childhood exposure to IPV, the provider should tell the woman this requirement prior to screening.[31] Although this may inhibit disclosure, this information also empowers her to consider the safety of divulging IPV.

Defining "childhood exposure to IPV" as "child maltreatment" remains controversial. Proponents cite the negative impact of IPV on children's health. Opponents fear that considering childhood exposure to be "child maltreatment" incorrectly assumes that all children are equally affected, punishes the mother by implying that she failed to protect the child, discourages disclosure to health care providers, and overburdens an already stressed CPS system.[31]

When initiating a conversation about IPV, framing the discussion helps normalize the topic. Examples of appropriate statements prior to screening include the following[31,32]:

— Because violence is so common in many women's lives, I have begun to ask patients' caregivers about it routinely.

— The safety of moms can affect the safety of children, so I ask all my patients' caregivers some questions about violence.

When the woman is the patient rather than the patient's caregiver, recommended screening questions should be specific and behaviorally anchored. For example, Heron recommended the following IPV instrument based upon the Universal Violence Prevention Screening Protocol[33]:

— Have you been in a relationship with a partner in the past year?

— If yes, within the past year, has a partner:

  — Slapped, kicked, pushed, choked or punched you?

  — Forced or coerced you to have sex?

* *htttp://www.childwelfare.gov*

— Threatened you with a knife or gun to scare or hurt you?

— Made you afraid that you could be physically hurt?

— Repeatedly used words, yelled, or screamed at you in a way that frightened you, threatened you, put you down, or made you feel rejected?

Similarly, McFarlane validated the following screening questions[34]:

— Have you ever been hit, slapped, kicked, or otherwise physically hurt by your male partner?

— Have you ever been forced to have sexual activities?

Though this type of direct questioning is preferable in adult health care venues, a modified approach is recommended in the pediatric setting. Zink and Jacobson interviewed a group of abused women with the specific objectives of determining their feelings about being screened for IPV in front of their children, safety considerations for screening in the pediatric setting, and preferred questions.[35] In these discussions, abused women expressed concern that providers would ask them specific and direct IPV questions in the presence of their verbal children. They feared that older children (ie, children older than 3 years) might later inadvertently disclose the conversation to the perpetrator; they also expressed concern that the IPV discussion would be traumatic for their children.[35]

A resulting recommendation from Zink and Jacobson's work is that an attempt be made to screen the female caregiver alone if children older than 3 years are present.[31,35] Nursing and support staff members can facilitate this by taking these children for vision and hearing screens or for a height and weight check while their mother is questioned. If the health care provider has time alone with the caregiver, direct questions, such as those previously listed, are the most appropriate and most likely to result in a forthright response.

If the caregiver cannot be separated from the children, then the health care provider should ask general questions first. Such questions, recommended by Zink and Jacobson, include the following[35]:

— Do you feel safe in your current relationship?

— Do you and your partner handle arguments with great difficulty, some difficulty, or no difficulty?

— In general, would you describe your relationship as having a lot of tension, some tension, or no tension?

Health care providers should carefully note both verbal and nonverbal responses to these questions. Based on these responses, if the health care provider becomes concerned about IPV, an attempt should be made to separate the caregiver from the children to engage in a more detailed discussion.

DOCUMENTATION

Just as IPV screening differs between pediatric and adult medical settings, so does documentation. In adult environments, the abused woman is the patient. As such, she is the only person with access to her medical records; careful documentation may help should she seek legal action against the perpetrator. In the pediatric setting, however, both parents can access the child's chart; if the perpetrator is the child's father, he can obtain these records. Documentation of IPV in the pediatric setting is controversial as a result, since an abuser reading about an IPV discussion may lead to increased violence.[31] Nevertheless, careful and thoughtful documentation in a pediatric chart may assist women in future legal endeavors (eg, custody suits). Female caregivers should be made aware of the potential risks and benefits of documentation; in addition, health care providers should respect the female caregiver's preferences about documentation. One alternative to full documentation in the child's chart includes having providers develop a code that is known within the practice (eg, "+MIPV" means "positive for maternal IPV") and that is not accompanied by further explanation. In settings in which both children and adults are patients, the health care provider can open a separate chart for the female caregiver and document the details of their discussion within this record rather than in the child's record.

MANAGEMENT OF INTIMATE PARTNER VIOLENCE AND CHILD ABUSE

Disclosure of IPV should be followed by validating statements such as "You don't deserve to be treated that way" or "You are not to blame."[32] Such assertions from a trusted provider send an important message to women that the violence is not okay and that help is available. Women should be encouraged to discuss the violence, and the practitioner should listen nonjudgmentally.[31]

A careful safety assessment is also essential. Health care providers should ask questions about substance abuse, the woman's perception of increasing violence and risk, and the presence of weapons in the house. Often, when IPV occurs, a woman must make difficult decisions about safety and must weigh the advantages and disadvantages of leaving the perpetrator. Issues that contribute to these decisions are the following:

— Knowledge that the violence generally escalates when a woman tries to leave

— Concern about obtaining the necessary financial resources and provisions for the children

— Fear that the children may be removed from her custody

A frank, but sensitive, discussion of the woman's considerations and plans may help her to take actions that increase her own and her children's safety.

Similarly, providers should ask direct questions about whether the children are being or have ever been abused and whether the woman believes that the children are in immediate danger. Also crucial is for the health care professional to conduct a thorough physical examination of the child to look for findings consistent with abuse. Discussing the effects of violence on children often motivates women to leave the relationship; giving, if needed, mental health resources for the children may help improve child outcomes even if the woman is unable to leave. Health care providers should offer help from local and national IPV agencies. Additionally, if available, assistance from social workers practicing in the provider's setting can be invaluable.

Further management varies somewhat depending upon the presence or absence of concurrent child abuse as well as upon the state's mandated reporting laws **(Table 4-1)**. Health care providers should, therefore, consider the following scenarios:

— Response to concurrent child abuse and IPV

— Response to IPV without concurrent child abuse in a state in which providers are mandated reporters of childhood exposure to IPV

— Response to IPV without concurrent child abuse in a state that does not require practitioners to report childhood exposure

Table 4-1. Items to Consider or Perform When Evaluating a Family in Which IPV Exists

Child Abuse Present	State-Mandated Child IPV Esposure Reporting	Report to CPS (Encourage Mother to Make Report)	Validate the Mother's Experience	Provide IPV Resources	Provide CPS Resources	Safety Planning	Community Mental Health Services for Child
-	-		X	X	X	X	X
+	-	X	X	X		X	X
-	+	X	X	X		X	X
+	+	X	X	X		X	X

+/- Denotes presence or absence of concurrent child abouse and state-mandated child IPV exposure reporting laws.

Without exception, health care providers are mandated reporters of child abuse. Therefore, if concern exists for child maltreatment, the health care provider must file a CPS report. Whenever possible, the health care provider should support and encourage the woman (provided obviously that she is not the alleged perpetrator) to make a report since this may help her with future court and CPS decisions about child placement.[31] The health care providers should tell the CPS worker who receives the report about the concurrent IPV.

Because of the historically disparate agendas of CPS and IPV agencies, reporting concurrent IPV and child abuse can raise concerns about the ways that both the woman and her children's safety will be preserved. As discussed previously, recent efforts of these agencies to work together facilitate the protection of both women and children. Additionally, safety planning in the health care provider's office should investigate whether the woman and her children can return home safely, and where the woman and children might go if the violence escalates.

Management of cases in which the children are not abused but the state law mandates reporting of childhood exposure is similar to the management of concurrent child abuse and IPV previously described. Encouraging the woman to make the report herself may be beneficial, and careful safety planning is essential.[31]

In IPV cases without concurrent child maltreatment, and in which the provider is not a mandated reporter of IPV or childhood exposure, the options are more flexible. Providers should validate the mother's experience; provide her with IPV, child mental health, and CPS resource numbers; and help with her safety planning. Frequent visits for the child with the primary pediatrician are important to assess the situation and any related changes.

CONCLUSIONS AND FUTURE DIRECTIONS

Multiple forms of violence (eg, child abuse and IPV) often occur within the same family. Health care providers must be vigilant about considering both types of violence in their patients and in their patients' families. Future research will guide the development of evidence-based screening and intervention protocols targeted at improving the well being of families with concurrent IPV and child abuse.

REFERENCES

1. The role of the pediatrician in recognizing and intervening on behalf of abused women. American Academy of Pediatrics Committee on Child Abuse and Neglect. *Pediatrics*. 1998;101:1091-1092.

2. Hughes H, Parkinson D, Vargo M. Witnessing spouse abuse and experiencing physical abuse: a "double whammy?" *J Fam Violence*. 1989;4:197-209.

3. Melton H, Belknap J. He hits, she hits: assessing gender differences and similarities in officially reported intimate partner violence. *Crim Justice Behav*. 2003;30:328-348.

4. Straus MA. Women's violence toward men is a serious social problem. In: Loseke DR, Gelles RJ, Cavanaugh MM, eds. *Current Controversies on Family Violence*. 2nd ed. Thousand Oaks, Calif: Sage Publications; 2005:55-78.

5. Loseke DR, Kurz D. Men's violence toward women is the serious social problem. In: Loseke DR, Gelles RJ, Cavanaugh MM, eds. *Current Controversies on Family Violence*. 2nd ed. Thousand Oaks, Calif: Sage Publications; 2005:79-96.

6. Slep AM, O'Leary SG. Parent and partner violence in families with young children: rates, patterns, and connections. *J Consult Clin Psychol*. 2005;3:435-444.

7. Renzetti CM. *Violent Betrayal: Partner Abuse in Lesbian Relationships*. Thousand Oaks, Calif: Sage Publications; 1992.

8. Slep AM, O'Leary SG. Examining partner and child abuse: are we ready for a more integrated approach to family violence? *Clin Child Fam Psychol Rev*. 2001; 4:87-107.

9. Tajima E. The relative importance of wife abuse as a risk factor for violence against children. *Child Abuse Negl*. 2000;24:1383-1398.

10. Appel AE, Holden GW. The co-occurrence of spouse and physical child abuse: a review and appraisal. *J Fam Psychol*. 1998;12:578-599.

11. Baranowski T, Perry CL, Parcel GS. How individuals, environments, and health behavior interact: social cognitive theory. In: Glanz K, Rimer BK, Lewis FM, eds. *Health Behavior and Health Education: Theory, Research and Practice*. 3rd ed. San Francisco: Jossey-Bass; 2002:165-184.

12. Stark E, Flitcraft AH. Women and children at risk: a feminist perspective on child abuse. *Int J Health Serv*. 1988;18:97-118.

13. Schechter S, Edleson JL. *Effective Intervention in Domestic Violence and Child Maltreatment Cases: Guidelines for Policy and Practice*. Reno, Nev: National Council of Juvenile and Family Court Judges; 1999.

14. Edleson JL. The overlap between child maltreatment and woman battering. *Violence Against Women*. 1999;5:134-154.

15. McKay MM. The link between domestic violence and child abuse: assessment and treatment considerations. *Child Welfare*. 1994;73:29-39.

16. Rumm PD, Cummings P, Krauss MR, Bell MA, Rivara FP. Identified spouse abuse as a risk factor for child abuse. *Child Abuse Negl*. 2000;24:1375-1381.

17. Ross SM. Risk of physical abuse to children of spouse abusing parents. *Child Abuse Negl*. 1996;20:589-598.

18. McCloskey LA, Figueredo AJ, Koss MP. The effects of systemic family violence on children's mental health. *Child Dev*. 1995;66:1239-1261.

19. Gayford JJ. Wife battering: a preliminary survey of 100 cases. *Br Med J*. 1975;1:194-197.

20. Kitzmann KM, Gaylord NK, Holt AR, Kenny ED. Child witnesses to domestic violence: a meta-analytic review. *J Consult Clin Psychol*. 2003;71:339-352.

21. Kolbo JR, Blakely EH, Engleman D. Children who witness domestic violence: a review of empirical literature. *J Interpers Violence*. 1996;11:281-293.

22. Wolfe DA, Crooks CV, Lee V, McIntyre-Smith A, Jaffe PG. The effects of children's exposure to domestic violence: a meta-analysis and critique. *Clin Child Fam Psychol Rev*. 2003;6:171-187.

23. Lamphear VS. The impact of maltreatment on children's psychosocial adjustment: a review of the research. *Child Abuse Negl*. 1985;9:251-263.

24. Fantuzzo JW, DePaola LM, Lambert L, Martino T, Anderson G, Sutton S. Effects of interparental violence on the psychological adjustment and competencies of young children. *J Consult Clin Psychol*. 1991;59:258-265.

25. Kilpatrick KL, Williams LM. Post-traumatic stress disorder in child witnesses to domestic violence. *Am J Orthopsychiatry*. 1997;67:639-644.

26. O'Keefe M. Predictors of child abuse in maritally violent families. *J Interpers Violence*. 1995;10:3-25.

27. Kernic MA, Holt VL, Wolf ME, McKnight B, Huebner CE, Rivara FP. Academic and school health issues among children exposed to maternal intimate partner violence. *Arch Pediatr Adolesc Med*. 2002;156:549-555.

28. Sternberg K, Lamb ME. Effects of domestic violence on children's behavior problems and depression. *Dev Psychol*. 1993;29:44-52.

29. Mahoney A, Donnelly WO, Boxer P, Lewis T. Marital and severe parent-to-adolescent physical aggression in clinic-referred families: mother and adolescent reports on co-occurrence and links to child behavior problems. *J Fam Psychol*. 2003;17:3-19.

30. Campbell JC. Child abuse and wife abuse: the connections. *Md Med J*. 1994;43:349-350.

31. McAlister Groves B, Augustyn M, Lee D, Sawires P. *Identifying and Responding to Domestic Violence: Consensus Recommendations for Child and Adolescent Health*. 2nd ed. San Francisco, Calif: Family Violence Prevention Fund; 2004.

32. Institute for Safe Families, Pennsylvania Chapter American Academy of Pediatrics. *RADAR for pediatrics*. Philadelphia, Pa: Institute for Safe Families; 2002.

33. Heron SL, Kellermann AL. Screening for intimate partner violence in the emergency department: where do we go from here? *Ann Emerg Med*. 2002;40:493-495.

34. McFarlane J, Greenberg L, Weltge A, Watson M. Identification of abuse in emergency departments: effectiveness of a two-question screening tool. *J Emerg Nurs*. 1995;21:391-394.

35. Zink TM, Jacobson J. Screening for intimate partner violence when children are present: the victim's perspective. *J Interpers Violence*. 2003;18:872-890.

36. Dowd MD, Kennedy C, Knapp JF, Stallbaumer-Rouyer J. Mothers' and health care providers' perspectives on screening for intimate partner violence in a pediatric emergency department. *Arch Pediatr Adolesc Med*. 2002;156:794-799.

Chapter 5

INTERVENTION FOR WOMEN: ANSWERS TO THE QUESTION "WHY DOESN'T SHE JUST LEAVE?"

L. Sloane Winkes, MD

"Why doesn't she just leave?" is perhaps the most frequently asked question regarding violent relationships and the battered women involved. Clearly the answer to ending intimate partner violence (IPV) is simply ending the abusive relationship; however, neither the answer to the frequently asked question nor the strategies for ending IPV are quite that simple. In fact, the reasons women remain in their abusive relationships and the successful strategies used to end IPV are extraordinarily complex.

The subtext underlying the question about why an abused woman does not leave the situation is that many people have difficulty empathizing with victims of IPV. Some people believe that if a woman were truly afraid of her partner, she would just leave him, or they think that the woman may somehow be responsible for the abuse.[1] Follingstad and colleagues examined the sympathy of college students toward women in abusive relationships. This study found that the degree of physical threat and the lack of access to help or resources generated the most sympathy from the college students. Even under these dire circumstances, however, most observers did not have strong sympathy for battered women.[1] A study by Nicolaidis, Curry, and Gerrity that gauged health care workers' attitudes toward victims of IPV discovered that most health care providers found it difficult to empathize with a battered woman who was well educated, healthy, or financially secure. In addition, health care workers had unrealistic expectations for getting a victim of abuse to a shelter right away, which increased their difficulty to empathize with the victim.[2] Studies such as these help demonstrate the struggles professionals who work with victims of IPV may experience when trying to empathize with their clients.

This chapter strives to improve the understanding of battered women's reasons for staying in abusive relationships and the barriers these women often face when they decide to leave the relationship. In addition to discussing the barriers to leaving a violent relationship, a brief review of several learning theories used to explain the psychology of battered women's decisions to leave is also presented. Hopefully, by better understanding this important and complex aspect of victims' lives, empathy toward women living with violence will improve, thereby enhancing the quality of services provided to them.

Ninety-five percent of IPV cases involve victimized women and male perpetrators.[3-5] As a result, this chapter focuses on female victims. However, IPV can happen to men in either heterosexual or homosexual relationships as well. In fact, in couples seeking marital therapy, 85% of couples who reported violence in their marriage indicated that the violence was bidirectional.[6,7] Regardless, the motivation for and consequences of the violence appear to differ based upon gender, thereby creating different experiences of victimization for men and women. Studies show that women who are abused by their male partners are more likely to suffer more severe violence and sustain more injuries than men whose female partners have been violent.[6,7] Related to the increase in severity of violence and injuries sustained, women report experiencing more fear in their violent relationships than men.[8,9] Women are also more likely to report that their use of violence was in self-defense, whereas men were more likely to report violence against their partner as a means of controlling or dominating the partner.[7,8,10-13] Interestingly, though violence may be perpetrated by both partners, the experience of violence by each partner and the power and control dynamics of the relationship remain unequal.[7,8] In addition, in same-sex relationships the incidence of IPV appears to be similar to IPV in heterosexual ones.[4]

Another troubling problem with the "why doesn't she just leave?" question is that this question focuses on what the IPV victim is or is not doing to change her situation. As a result, this question suggests that the victim is to blame for a situation over which she may have no control given the power and control dynamics in violent relationships. Equally or perhaps more relevant questions would be "why does the batterer hit his partner?" or "why doesn't he stop?"

Studies show that there are few legal consequences for abusing one's partner. Arrest rates and prosecution for IPV remain low, despite the fact that IPV is a crime throughout the United States.[14,15] In fact, men are more likely to serve jail time for assaulting a stranger than for assaulting their partners, and recidivism rates when batterers attend court-mandated batterer treatment programs can be as high as 40% to 60%.[15,16] Completion of batterer treatment programs, in conjunction with court and community sanctions against batterers, does contribute to reduced rates of IPV.[16]

Though the sociocultural reasons that the criminal justice system fails to hold batterers accountable remain many and beyond the scope of this chapter, it is important to note that, upon hearing about an IPV case, most people will ask "why doesn't she leave?" more than any question about why the batterer was abusive. Although it may take several attempts to do so, as many as 70% of battered women do eventually leave their abusive partners.[15,17] As previously mentioned, to support women in the process of leaving their abusers, knowledge of the barriers to their leaving remains vitally important.

BARRIERS TO LEAVING

A woman may stay in a relationship with her abusive partner for many reasons. Grigsby and Hartman's Barriers Model portrays the victim as a central entity surrounded by 4 concentric rings representing barriers to leaving. These barriers include environmental barriers (ie, a lack of access to resources and support), family and social role expectations, the psychological impact of the abusive relationship on the victim, and the role of childhood abuse and neglect issues.[18,19]

Hamby identifies the following 5 categories of obstacles a woman faces when trying to leave a violent relationship[20,21]:

1. The batterer's behavior

2. Socioeconomic issues

3. Institutional issues

4. Social network issues

5. Personal values

With these 2 models in mind, the first level of focus should be on the victim herself as well as personal barriers she may face, and then more broadly consider barriers she confronts in her home, community, and socioeconomic contexts. As also emphasized in the models, these contexts exist as a whole for any given woman trying to decide whether or when to leave a violent relationship. A woman may need to overcome any or all of these barriers to leave successfully.

Personal Context

A woman may face a number of victim-centered barriers when trying to leave an abusive relationship. Such barriers include the victim's personal value system, her emotional attachment to the batterer, the societal values imposed on her, and the psychological effects of the abuse.

Personal Values

Most violent relationships do not start out that way. Both violent and nonviolent relationships develop over time, so a battered woman may have many reasons to stay committed to that relationship, such as sharing a home or having children together. Commitment to the relationship or family can make a woman stay in an abusive relationship.[22,23] If a woman is pregnant or already has children with her abuser, she may consider and place a number of issues above the importance of her personal safety. Such issues may include[20,21,24]:

— Her belief that her partner is a good father

— Her idea that her child or children need a father figure

— Her knowledge that leaving may require her to obtain childcare

— Her need for increased financial support if she leaves the situation

— Her need for emotional support if she leaves the situation

In addition, a woman may feel strongly that she must do everything she can to preserve her marriage or relationship. She may have been told directly by family members, clergy members, or counselors, and even indirectly by society at large, that she must maintain her relationship and keep the family together. She may have religious values that prohibit divorce under any circumstances or cultural beliefs that the couple or family must stay together no matter the circumstances.[20,21]

A battered woman may fear leaving the relationship, because that would signal her failure as a wife or partner. Being a wife, partner, or mother are important roles for women, and in these roles the burden of family unity and harmony is generally placed on the woman; therefore, the woman may view a failed relationship as her fault.[25,26] Despite the abuse, a woman may perceive her role as wife or partner, especially when her relationship is viewed as successful by outsiders, as rewarding and this contributes to her satisfaction in the relationship.[26] She may also have been socialized from a young age to believe in "true" or "perfect" love. As a result, she may feel that she should do anything to keep the relationship together once she finds her true or perfect love, regardless of the violent reality of that love.[27]

The victim may also feel that she is to blame for the violence; that is, if she did things right, then the abuse would not happen, or that if she loved her partner enough, he would change.[27,28] If she has also perpetrated violence or emotional abuse toward her partner, she may feel more to blame for the violence directed toward herself or she may feel guilty; both issues could make it difficult for her to justify leaving.[7,29]

Emotional Attachment

A woman's emotional attachment to the relationship and her abuser may be one reason she stays in the abusive relationship. In traumatic bonding theories of attachment the very nature of violent relationships (ie, relationships in which there exists intermittent abuse and power imbalance) may serve to increase a battered woman's attachment.[30] Studies focusing on the reasons women return to abusive relationships found that women are more likely to return if they have a long-term relationship or legal commitment with the abuser.[31,32] According to these studies, other frequently cited reasons for returning to the abusive relationship include the woman's ongoing, emotional attachment to the batterer; the batterer's promises to change; his expressions of remorse; and other signs of his commitment to the relationship and to improving the relationship.[32] In Barret and Lopez Real's 1985 interviews with battered women, the most frequently cited reason for remaining in an abusive relationship was the woman's hope for change.[1,28,33] Another study by Gordon, Burton, and Porter showed that some women reported that their forgiveness of their abusive partners was a reason they returned to the relationship. In fact, the less severe the violence, and the less the victim perceived her partner's behavior as malicious or intentional, the more likely the woman is to forgive her batterer and return.[34] Yet another study by Anderson and colleagues determined that the most frequently reported reasons women remain in or return to abusive relationships is that the partner promises to change (ie, 70% of instances) or he apologizes for the abuse (ie, 60% of instances).[19] A battered woman's belief that her partner will change his violent behavior is called *learned hopefulness*.[28,35] Batterers fuel this hope for change by reinforcing the positive aspects of the relationship during nonviolent periods; such behavior may increase a woman's emotional attachment and commitment to the relationship.[28,30,36]

In addition, the real possibility exists that, in spite of the violence, the woman may still love her partner. Studies of community samples indicate that love is the primary reason both partners in violent relationships provide for staying in the relationship.[29,33,37] This sense of love may be reinforced for the IPV victim during periods of nonviolence within the relationship. Walker describes a cyclical pattern of IPV involving a "honeymoon period" after an abusive incident.[36] During this honeymoon period, the guilt-ridden batterer may apologize and act more lovingly toward his partner in an effort to make up for the violence. During these periods, the batterer may also become the loving, nonviolent, "fantasy" partner the victim hopes for, which may reinforce her desire to remain in the relationship.[30,36] During times of tension or violence, she may remember the better times or the honeymoon periods and believe that these times will happen again or hope that her partner will change and become more like the person he seems to be during these honeymoon periods.[20,21,36] She may not want the relationship to end, just the violence.[38]

Societal Values

Societal values and norms imposed on women may contribute to a battered woman remaining in an abusive relationship. From childhood, gender identity and sex-role socialization create different views of men and women. Men are seen as more aggressive, independent, and powerful, while women are more nurturing, interdependent, and vulnerable.[28] The power and control that a batterer exerts over his partner can be seen as an extension of broader societal and cultural views of male dominance over women, which are essential to definitions of masculinity, sexism, and patriarchal societies.[28,38] As women grow up in a patriarchal society, they learn to give up parts of themselves to be accepted; in addition, women are trained to look to male figures to validate their identities.[18,39] Consequently, women have been socialized to believe that to have value as a person, they need a man in their lives.[18] Women are often defined by or define themselves within the context of their social relationships, specifically marriage and family.[18,28,40] Therefore, society's expectations of a woman and her relationship encourage the woman's attachment to and emotional dependence upon her partner and that relationship, thereby increasing her commitment to her partner and relationship. This does not seem pathological by societal norms until the relationship becomes abusive. A battered woman's strong desire for a successful relationship and family (ie, successful in the eyes of outsiders and society at large) may result from being raised to achieve and value such success. This desire may be so strong that she minimizes or hides the abuse.

Another societal value that may contribute to women remaining with an abusive partner is that society generally views relationship failure as the woman's fault.[25,26] As a direct result of sex-role socialization, the woman may strongly believe that she is responsible for the success of the relationship since she is the primary caretaker of her relationship and family.[19,20,21,41] Not only does she believe that her responsibility is to remain in an abusive relationship, but that she must also try to improve her relationship. As a result, the battered woman simultaneously feels profound shame about her abusive situation and unable to change the situation, which creates feelings of even more shame and humiliation.[4]

To add to the problem, most community services available to battered women (eg, domestic violence hotlines, shelters) are designed so that the victim is expected to leave the home, not the perpetrator.[20,21] While societal norms encourage battered women to stay, they also expect victims to leave the situation to end the violence, thereby sending conflicting messages. So, rather than addressing the issues surrounding the reasons women are being abused in the first place or what steps can be taken to stop the batterer from violent behavior, society expects battered women to leave in order for the violence to end.

A woman's culture or cultural belief systems also influence her decision to stay or leave an abusive relationship.[42] In some cultures the emphasis on family unity and the woman's role as caregiver make leaving a violent relationship even more challenging. Male authority, and a woman's deference to that authority, may be culturally imposed, thereby making a challenge to such beliefs through leaving a relationship increasingly difficult. Some cultural traditions (eg, female genital mutilation in parts of Africa, former Taliban rule in Afghanistan that prohibited women from leaving the home for school or work) may be perceived by outsiders as abusive toward women, but have a level of acceptance within that culture.[28] A full exploration of these cultural issues is beyond the scope of this chapter; however, a person's culture should be recognized as a potentially powerful barrier to a battered woman's leaving an abusive relationship.

Immobilization and Psychological Impact of Abuse

Women may not be able to leave a violent relationship, because they feel immobilized by psychological trauma or fear. Studies show that battered women have lower self-esteem levels than nonbattered women.[43,44] Years of verbal, emotional, or physical abuse often lower a woman's self-esteem to the point of feeling powerless to control or change her situation. If a woman has listened to her batterer's consistently berating comments, insults, or accusations (eg, accusing her of being unfaithful or crazy) while threatening violence, her self-esteem may be destroyed. Wuest and Merritt-Gray describe a process by which an abused woman's survival strategy is to attempt to counteract the abuse by relinquishing psychological or emotional parts of herself.[45] As a result, the abused woman becomes vulnerable to believing her batterer's comments, which repeatedly tell her that she is worthless, so she feels helpless. For example, a woman with a good job may give it up because her abuser constantly tells her that she is stupid, which makes her believe that she is too stupid to be good at her job. If one aspect of the woman's abuse is imposed isolation, then the batterer's words may be the victim's only source of information.[46] This misinformation provided by the batterer through insults (eg, telling her that she is crazy, accusing her of having an affair, taunting her by saying that no one else would want her) may become truth in the eyes of the victim since she does not hear any other perspectives. Such verbal abuse may make a victim unable to think for herself, thereby maintaining the batterer's control over her.[19] In addition, the lack of power and control she has in the relationship may make her feel even more helpless and powerless to change her situation. A woman who suffers from such low self-esteem may believe that she could never attain the necessary strength and faith in herself needed to overcome the numerous obstacles that prevent her from leaving the violent relationship. For example, she may be unable to interview for a job to become financially independent, look for new housing, apply for assistance, tell her health care provider about the violence, or phone the police department or domestic violence hotline.

In addition, the high levels of trauma to which an IPV victim may be exposed can lead to the development of defense mechanisms that may challenge her ability to leave the relationship (eg, minimization of the degree of danger, denial of the abuse, numbing to or dissociation from the abuse). A victim may turn to drug or alcohol abuse in an effort to numb the pain of living in a violent relationship. Although these strategies do enable a woman living with violence to survive her situation, they may impair her ability to judge the degree of danger in which she finds herself.[18] If she is unable to appreciate the risks she is taking by remaining in the relationship, she may not be able to consider the risks involved in leaving.

As previously mentioned, one trauma theory that has been applied to battered women is *learned helplessness*. This trauma theory suggests that a battered woman will remain in her violent relationship, because she has learned that escape is impossible.[26,47,48] In applying this theory to battered women, an IPV victim experiences 3 types of deficits:

1. *Motivational deficit.* The woman believes her responses will not affect the outcome (ie, she believes that there is nothing she can do to change her situation). As a result, she does not try to change the situation.

2. *Cognitive deficit.* This follows a motivational deficit and includes poor problem solving capabilities. As a result, the abused woman cannot learn that her response affects the outcomes.

3. *Affective deficit.* This deficit includes emotional trauma and a depressive state that contributes to the woman's increased feelings of helplessness.[26,28,47-50] In fact, 38% to 83% of battered women experience depression.[51] Women who experience the severe depression that often accompanies abuse can feel immobilized.[52]

In addition to depression, studies have found high rates of posttraumatic stress disorder (PTSD) among battered women. In fact, studies estimate the prevalence of PTSD among battered women as between 33% to 84%.[44,51] PTSD is an anxiety disorder occurring in response to an extremely stressful event. This disorder is characterized by the following[28,53]:

— Re-experiencing trauma with intrusive thoughts or recurrent dreams

— Numbing or diminished responsiveness accompanied by feelings of detachment

— Disruption in sleep, memory, and concentration

— Avoidance of anything that recalls the stressful or traumatic event

Although experiencing physical violence can certainly cause PTSD, for IPV victims the experience of psychological abuse is also a significant factor in PTSD. Psychological abuse may actually be more damaging to women than physical abuse. Women may be experiencing psychological abuse more frequently than physical abuse and, rather than discrete episodes of physical violence that have a beginning and end, psychological abuse may be ongoing or prolonged.[44] A woman may hear insults, threats, and accusations from her batterer on a daily basis but may only experience violence occasionally. This constant verbal and emotional abuse may have a greater impact than physical abuse on a woman's psychological well-being and degree of functioning, thereby crippling her with low self-esteem and depression that tend to accompany such constant insults, threats, and fear.[44,51,54] Studies show that women who experience more severe or more frequent violence may have a greater likelihood of PTSD, possibly related to an increased fear and lack of a sense of safety.[51] Even when controlling for the effects of physical abuse, Arias and Pape found that greater levels of psychological abuse directly correlate to greater levels of PTSD. This study also found that women with higher levels of psychological abuse had greater intentions to end their relationship; however, in women who experience high levels of PTSD symptomatology, neither physical nor psychological abuse were associated with a high likelihood of leaving the abusive situation. In contrast, with women who experience low levels of PTSD, both physical and psychological abuse did predict their intentions to terminate the relationship. Perhaps resulting from the stress of the symptoms themselves and the association of PTSD with inadequate coping skills, PTSD interferes with a battered woman's ability to leave the relationship as well as her ability to function after leaving.[44] Therefore, PTSD may be both an effect of IPV and a barrier to ending the violence.[18]

A history of previous violence or victimization in a woman's life may contribute to her psychological immobilization and difficulty in ending an abusive relationship. Grigsby and Hartman contend that childhood neglect or abuse serve as barriers faced by victims of IPV.[18] Substantial evidence exists that indicates an intergenerational transmission of violence. That means that when a person's family of origin teaches him or her that violence is a common or acceptable behavior in relationships, then that person will use violent behavior in his or her adult relationships.[55-58] Since children learn communication and relationship skills from their families, those children who are abused by their families may learn that they cannot trust anyone and cannot escape abusive situations. They may also believe that abuse is a normal part of adult relationships, so violence from a partner only confirms this viewpoint. In addition, the effects of childhood trauma may include depression, anxiety, PTSD, and substance abuse. Any of these factors may make a woman more vulnerable to abuse in her adult relationships.[18] An early study by Gelles found that 1 of the 3 main reasons women stayed in abusive relationships was the experience of violence in her childhood home.[59] More recent data, however, are not as supportive of this idea. In fact, some studies have found that a history of abuse in childhood is no more prevalent in battered women than in the general population.[28,60-63]

Fear is another aspect of the psychological impact of abuse on a woman's ability to leave a violent relationship. Such fear stems from a batterer's threats of violence (eg, toward the victim, the children, or other loved ones) if the woman leaves him; sometimes the batterer will even threaten to kill the woman if she leaves. Fear of further abuse or an escalation of violence based upon such threats, fear of retribution for calling the police or seeking help, and fear of being killed if she does leave are all powerful reasons women remain in abusive relationships.[28,33,64]

Anderson and colleagues found that fear of a partner and fear of being alone were some of the reasons reported for staying in or returning to an abusive relationship. Women in this study felt safer staying with the abusive partner, because they would "know what he was doing"; such a statement certainly demonstrates the women's fears about what their batterers might do otherwise. According to this study, other reasons given for remaining in an abusive relationship include the fear of not being able to survive without their partner and the fear of losing their children.[19] Since a battered woman's self-esteem may be tied in with her success as a partner or may be so low as a result of years of abuse, she may believe that she could not function independently of her batterer, which accounts for her fear of being on her own. She may also fear that she would never have another partner or could not find a better partner. In addition, she may have very practical fears about her ability to acquire money, shelter, childcare, and supportive help, all of which are essential to a woman successfully leaving an abusive situation.[20,21]

HOME

Several factors within a woman's home life can also present barriers to leaving a violent relationship. These include the woman's children, social network (ie, family members and friends), and the batterer.

Children

For a number of reasons the presence of children in an abusive relationship can greatly compromise a woman's ability to end that relationship. As previously mentioned, a woman may believe that her children need a father or an intact family.[20,21] This may be more important to her than her own emotional or physical safety. Even if she believes that her children would be better off away from their father and not being exposed to the violence, she may determine that leaving is impossible. She may fear leaving her children with their violent father if she leaves the situation on her own. This fear may be well founded, since the likelihood is high that the children will be abused, too. In fact, between 50% and 70% of men who beat their wives also frequently abuse their children.[15,65] The woman may also fear the batterer's threats that he will hurt or kill the children in order to punish her if she leaves.

If the woman is able to leave the relationship with her children, she faces increased demands for food, clothing, shelter, and childcare. This may place a financial burden on her that she is unable to overcome, so she returns to her abuser. A study by Bell found that few women who had children with their batterer were able to end their relationships because of the ongoing need for emotional and financial support required to care for children.[24] Even if an abused woman successfully leaves with her children, she may face continued contact with her abuser regarding custody and visitation. Such continued contact may place her in danger.[64] In addition, she may need to rely on the batterer for ongoing childcare or child support, thereby making a true escape from the relationship difficult.[24] If she seeks separation or divorce from her batterer, she may risk losing custody of her children or being reported to Child Protective Services (CPS) for failure to protect her children.[20,21]

In spite of the potential consequences to children who grow up in a violent home, when a woman considers all of these factors, remaining in the abusive relationship may seem safer to the victim to retain custody of her children and keep them safe. When a woman does decide to leave, freeing her children from a violent home can be a major motivator.

Social Network

A woman's social network of family members and friends may also impact her decision to remain in an abusive relationship. Though family members and friends can certainly be sources of support for helping a woman to leave, oftentimes the batterer's actions may have increasingly isolated relatives and friends from the abused woman. Given this physical or psychological distance, relatives and friends may not fully understand the situation, especially if the victim has hidden the abuse because of feelings of shame and humiliation. In addition, they might only see the batterer's public persona, which may be kind or charismatic, and may not believe the woman about the abuse.[18] Support from family members and friends could also be lost if the victim were forced to move away during the leaving process. Also, they may not know exactly how to help or could be afraid to help. Remember, the batterer may have threatened family members or friends, so they may not want to get involved for fear of potential danger to themselves.[20,21]

Family members may also discourage a victim from leaving. They may encourage the woman to keep the couple together or preserve her family. If she leaves, people in her social network may criticize her for a failed marriage.[20,21,26,45] The belief system of a woman's family of origin and the rules she has learned as a child may make ending an abusive relationship difficult for her. By ending her relationship, even a violent one, she may be violating the very rules, ethics, and values of her family, which could lead to consequences within her family of origin such that her relatives may not help or support her if she leaves.[18] Family members may also tell the woman that her children need a father and that an abusive father is better than no father at all. In addition, if violence has been experienced or witnessed by the victim in her family of origin, the acceptance of violence in relationships may have been transmitted across generations.[55-58] Her family may, therefore, view the violence as normal or acceptable behavior. If there are strong religious values regarding the sanctity of marriage or family sexual roles, or if divorce is prohibited by the family's religion, then family members may encourage the woman to uphold these beliefs. Family and friends may also be unwilling or unable to provide shelter, childcare, or financial support, all of which a woman needs to leave successfully. An abused woman may feel quite discouraged by such responses. She may wonder why others such as health care providers or IPV advocates would help her leave her situation if her own relatives and friends cannot or will not provide support her.

The Batterer
The batterer's behavior toward the IPV victim creates an atmosphere of tension and fear from which the woman may find escape difficult. For example, batterers may minimize the severity of abuse or blame the victim for the abuse.[20,21,38] In such a setting, a battered woman may begin to believe that the abuse is not really that bad or that if she stopped nagging and just did things "right," then the violence would stop. However, all of this serves to remove the blame from the perpetrator of the violence. In fact, the batterer chooses to use violent behavior to maintain control over his partner and nothing, not the victim's behavior or alcohol or drug use, can excuse these violent outbursts. In addition, the batterer may make promises to change. Given the victim's previously mentioned emotional attachment issues and personal and social values, the victim may be all too willing to believe the batterer's promises and hope for a change to occur.[28,33] The combined effects of the batterer's behaviors and promises, which create learned hopefulness in a setting of fear from emotional or physical abuse, may immobilize a woman and make her incapable of terminating the relationship.[28,35]

Threatening Behaviors
Threats and threatening behaviors from the batterer may be significant barriers to leaving a violent relationship. Specifically, the abuser may threaten to kill her if she leaves him or threaten that if he cannot have her, no one can. In addition, he may threaten to kill himself if she leaves him or is with anyone else. The batterer may also

threaten the children and other family members with abuse or death. Another powerful threat is that the batterer will take away the children, kidnap them, or fight for custody if she leaves him. Threatening behaviors include the destruction of property, waving a knife or gun with threats to use the weapon, stalking the woman, harassing her with phone calls, and hurting the pets.[15,20,21] When accompanied by violence or the promise of further violence, these threats become very real to women living in abusive relationships. These women are intimidated by the batterer and may have come to believe that their abuser is capable of anything; they certainly believe that he would carry out his threats. To avoid the possibility of these threats being carried out, women stay in the abusive relationship.

Isolating Behaviors

Another powerful aspect of IPV is the isolation of the woman from her family members and friends by the batterer. He may restrict visits or insist on being present during visits. He may not allow her to remain in touch with her social contacts and sometimes even moves the family away to increase the woman's isolation. He may not allow her to leave the house without him and may even lock her inside the home. He may not allow her to use the telephone or might record or listen to any phone calls. Any Internet activity could easily be monitored. A woman's access to basic resources like food, clothing, and shelter may be restricted or controlled by her batterer. He may prevent her access to health care by not taking her to physician visits or by accompanying her and controlling the interaction. The batterer may not allow the woman to take necessary medications or comply with treatment plans. He may not allow her to work or, if she does work, he may impose economic abuse by controlling all of the household finances.[15] At work, he may threaten her with frequent, harassing phone calls or visits. For some women, keeping a job may be difficult because of the abuser's behaviors.[24]

One thought-provoking paper by Avni compared women living in the isolation of a violent relationship to inmates in prison. As with inmates, battered women lose their autonomy when their abusers control connections to the outside world, activities, use of time, and use of personal space.[46] In addition to the isolation imposed by a batterer, an IPV victim may experience a self-imposed isolation; that is, she may experience so much shame about the abuse that she defends the privacy of the home and, therefore, her violent relationship remains private.[46] In essence, she imprisons herself within the myth of a happy family, because she is too embarrassed to tell others the truth and, therefore, is incapable of asking for help.

Alcohol and Drug Use

Another batterer behavior that may hinder an IPV victim from leaving the relationship is that a batterer may blame the violence on alcohol or drug use. Alcohol use can certainly contribute to IPV. Studies show that alcohol abuse may be involved in 25% to 50% of IPV cases, and men seeking alcohol treatment show higher rates of IPV than the general population.[66-71] Some data show that alcohol use increases the occurrence of violence.[66,72,73] In such cases, when the batterer is not drinking, there may be violence-free periods, so women are hopeful that if their partner remains sober, the violence will stop. In fact, studies by O'Farrell and colleagues of men in treatment for alcoholism and marital therapy did show a reduction in violence 1 and 2 years after treatment.[69-71] Therefore, victims may be correct in hoping that alcohol treatment will reduce or even end the violence. Although alcohol is associated with an increase in frequency and severity of violence, alcohol use is only found in a few episodes of IPV, and the intoxication of a batterer does not excuse his violence.[66]

Types of Batterers

There is a growing body of evidence that suggests that not all batterers are the same. In their study, Holtzworth-Munroe and Stuart indicate that different types of batterers and different etiologies for the perpetration of relationship violence may exist; therefore, leaving a violent relationship or the treatment provided for a batterer may depend on the type of batterer initiating the violence or on the possible causes of his violence. Though a complete review of batterers and the etiology of violence in intimate relationships are beyond the scope of this chapter (see Dixon and Browne[74] and Holtzworth-Munroe and Stuart[75] for more information), 3 batterer types have been identified[75]:

1. Family-only batterer

2. Dysphoric or borderline batterer

3. Generally violent or antisocial batterer

Batterer treatment may be more effective if tailored to the type of batterer. The ineffectiveness of batterer treatment may result from interventions not matching the right batterer types.[74,76]

The family-only batterer restricts his violence to the family and tends to be the least severe of the 3 types of batterers. Few family-only batterers exhibit psychopathology or personality disorders. This group accounts for 50% of all batterers.

The dysphoric/borderline type makes up 20% of batterers. Such batterers tend to perpetrate moderate to severe abuse, which is primarily directed only toward the family, but they may also have some extra-familial violence or criminal behavior. These batterers tend to be dysphoric, psychologically distressed, and emotionally volatile. Evidence of borderline or schizoid personality disorders may exist. Also, some drug or alcohol abuse issues may exist.

The batterers in the generally violent/antisocial group engage in the most severe violence in their relationships but also exhibit the most aggressive behaviors outside the family. They tend to have extensive histories of criminal behavior and legal problems. In addition, they are the most likely group to exhibit antisocial personality disorder or be psychopathic and have the highest rates of alcohol and drug abuse. They represent 30% of batterers.[75]

Other researchers, like Gottman and colleagues, who study the physiology of violent couples have placed batterers into 2 categories:

— *Type 1 batterers.* Their heart rates drop below the baseline during interactions with their spouses; this indicates low physiological reactivity, which is associated with criminality.[77,78] When interacting with their wives, type 1 batterers rapidly escalate the aggression but act deliberately and physiologically relaxed. Type 1 batterers are more severely violent, more emotionally abusive, use more drugs and alcohol, engage in more violence outside the home, and show more antisocial behaviors. These batterers are most similar to the generally violent or antisocial type described by Holtzworth-Munroe and Stuart.[74,75] Based on several studies of the motivation for battering, it appears that type 1 batterers are motivated to violence as a way of gaining control and power over their wives.[78]

— *Type 2 batterers.* They have higher heart rates during interactions with their wives. They are comparable to the family-only batterer type proposed by Holtzworth-Munroe and Stuart.[74,75] Aggression shown by type 2 batterers seems associated with a lack of emotional control, rather than the deliberate actions of type 1 batterers. This may be related to the batterer's fear of abandonment as a motivator for abuse by a type 2 batterer.[78]

Leaving different types of batterers requires different strategies. A woman facing the more severe violence of the type 1 or generally violent or antisocial batterer may require more extensive safety planning with the help of law enforcement officers, because she will likely be at greater risk for danger when she attempts to leave. In addition, she will require extensive counseling and possible treatment for PTSD considering the severe emotional and physical abuse she has suffered.

The cessation of violence is least likely in the most severely aggressive men.[74,79,80] An understanding of the different types of batterers faced by victims as well as an understanding of the batterers' motivations may help people better understand the risk factors and causes for IPV; such knowledge can help direct the care and treatment of both victims and batterers.[75]

Danger
Although the best advice to give a battered woman may seem to be to tell her "just leave" to end her abusive relationship and remain safe, leaving can actually be the most dangerous time for IPV victims.[14,81,82] Despite the misconception that ending the relationship will end the violence, many abusers continue or escalate the violence once the relationship has ended.[64] The Department of Justice's 1994 National Crime Victimization Survey (NCVS) reported that 70% of reported battering incidents occurred after separation.[83] One study that looked at NCS data over a 10-year period found that most IPV victims were divorced, separated, or otherwise living apart from their partner at the time of assault.[84] In addition, the abusive partner is more likely to kill the battered woman if the woman has left or is trying to leave the relationship.[28,64,85] This reality of separation assault and separation homicide may be an extension of the power and control issues inherent in violent relationships.[14,64,81] Leaving the relationship threatens the batterer's control, so he continues using violence to exert control over his partner or ex-partner. If the batterer assaults the woman because she has threatened or tried to leave, then this may create enough fear of future assaults or possibly death that this fear prevents the woman from ending the abusive relationship. Women living in the midst of a violent relationship know that leaving is dangerous, therefore, only the victim should decide whether staying or leaving the relationship is safest for her.[15,64]

COMMUNITY
The community and institutions within the community in which a battered woman lives may also present barriers to ending her violent relationship.

Institutional Obstacles
Within the institutional systems that are available to a woman who leaves a violent relationship, many barriers exist that actually hinder her leaving. First, community resources are organized so that the victim must initiate contact, make changes, and leave her home and relationship.[20,21] As a result, the responsibility for ending the abuse falls on the victim, rather than the batterer, who causes the problem and ultimately controls whether he abuses his partner.[1] In addition, a woman may find accessing these resources difficult because of her isolation, depression, and low self-esteem. Yet another challenge to the woman's ability to end the relationship lies with the responsiveness of the resources to the woman's expressed need, or lack thereof.

Police

Police officers are often the battered woman's first point of contact with any community resource when she tries to leave her abusive relationship. Though police officers can provide support to an IPV victim by arresting the batterer, initiating a restraining order, providing help in finding alternate shelter, or providing advocacy group information, the police may inadvertently provide significant barriers.[18]

When called to the scene of a domestic assault or a violation of protection order, a police officer's response can significantly impact a woman's perception of her ability to leave her situation. For example, if police officers do not respond strongly to the batterer, both the batterer and victim learn that the police officers will not hold the abuser accountable for the violence and that they will not stop the violence.[18] Research shows that police officers typically avoid arresting batterers, even in jurisdictions with pro-arrest policies.[14] Studies also show that if police officers do arrest a batterer, he is unlikely to serve jail time.[20,21] In addition, police officers may also arrest victims for injuries inflicted on the batterer in self-defense.[18,20,21] Also, police officers may inadequately refer perpetrators and victims to social agencies.[14] As a result, if women perceive police response as negative, these women are more likely to report feelings of self-blame, which can impede their ability to end the relationship.[14,86]

An estimated 61% of IPV incidents go unreported because the victims fear that police officers will not believe them; 73% of incidents remain unreported because women lack faith in the system.[87,88] Victims of IPV report a lack of support from police officers and legal professionals as reasons for returning to abusive relationships.[19] Ironically, victims of IPV also identify police encouragement and explanation of victims' legal rights as factors that motivate these victims to request a restraining order or warrant for arrest of their batterers.[14]

One study surveyed victims' experiences with the criminal justice system in 2 Ohio counties and found that victims described insensitive comments made by police officers, a general lack of understanding of the IPV victim's situation, and instances of police officers blaming the victim for the violence or violent situation. Most of the women surveyed (66%) stated that police officers did not collect evidence. Half of the victims felt that police officers minimized the extent of the victims' injuries. In addition, 71% of the women reported that a criminal processing agent encouraged them to drop the complaint.[14]

Legal System

Within the court system, many IPV cases are dismissed either because the victim drops the case or does not show up in court. In the previously mentioned Ohio study, 48% of victims dropped their complaints because they feared for their safety, that is, they did not believe that the courts could protect them from their abusers.[14] Other reasons cited by victims for noncompliance with the attorneys prosecuting the batterer include the justice system's ineffectiveness, the victim's distrust of or difficult experiences with the criminal justice system, the victim's concern for her children, and the victim's emotional or financial dependence upon the batterer. In addition, IPV victims may face sexist, victim-blaming attitudes of professions working within the criminal justice system. In fact, most victims who participated in this study reported that prosecutors asked them whether they had provoked their abusers.[14] These attitudes, when coupled with the low number of arrests and prosecutions of batterers, lead victims to believe that the criminal justice system is colluding with the abuser.[19] As a result, though the criminal justice system can certainly help IPV victims, the system may simultaneously serve as a major barrier.

Domestic Violence Shelters and Advocacy Groups

Victims may find the difficulty in accessing domestic violence shelters and advocacy groups to be yet another obstacle to leaving their violent relationship. As previously mentioned, a victim's access to such shelters or groups may be limited by the physical isolation imposed by the batterer (ie, she may be unable to leave the house or use the telephone) or her own mental illness, physical disability, substance abuse, immigration status, and language or cultural barriers.[18,20,21,89]

In addition, the shelters may restrict access in several ways. For example, they may not provide bilingual services or be equipped for disabled victims. Admission policies may not allow prostitutes, women who have tested positive for human immunodeficiency virus (HIV), women with mental health or substance abuse issues, or victims who have been arrested. The shelter may also prohibit re-admittance to the shelter if the victim has previously returned to her batterer. In addition, shelters are frequently full, have long waiting lists, and may allow only limited stays (eg, 30 to 90 days).[18,20,21] Domestic violence shelters are certainly lifelines for battered women who are trying to escape; however, their limitations, which may result from underfunding and a lack of available shelters, also create institutional barriers to women trying to leave an abusive situation.

Experiencing IPV in a same-sex couple can serve as a significant obstacle to ending the violent relationship. As well as facing the same barriers to leaving as battered women in heterosexual relationships, victims of same-sex relationship violence may experience an increased sense of isolation or may have to "come out" to his or her social network to obtain support, which may not feel safe either. In addition, fewer resources are available to victims of same-sex violence, especially male victims.[28]

Child Protective Services

Child Protective Services presents another institutional barrier, in that the woman risks having her children removed from the home if she reports the violence. If the victim seeks help, whether from agencies or within the criminal justice system, she may risk being reported to CPS for exposing her children to violence, and thereby putting them in harm's way, failing to protect them, or neglecting them.[15,20,21]

Religion

As previously mentioned, the institution of religion may hinder a woman's decision to leave her abusive relationship. For example, a woman's religion may prohibit divorce, or religious leaders to whom a battered woman may turn for advice might encourage her to keep her family together. Such religious leaders may also erroneously tell the woman that the abuse is her fault, that the abuse could be prevented if she were more obedient to her husband, or that the abusive situation is God's will. Battered women rarely report that a religious leader advised her that her personal safety was the most important issue.[18] One third of clergy members felt that the abuse would have to be severe to justify a woman leaving her abusive husband; 21% of clergy members felt that no amount of abuse would justify ending the relationship.[28,90]

Health Care System

Battered women frequently see health care providers for annual examinations or with complaints that may result from the abuse (eg, depression, chronic pelvic pain, physical injuries)[15,91]; however, IPV often remains undetected by health care providers. In fact, approximately 95% of IPV cases are incorrectly identified.[38,92-95] This is usually because health care providers do not ask victims about IPV.[94] Health care providers may not ask women about abuse because they lack the knowledge and skills regarding intervention for battered women, feel that they do not have the time to deal with the issue, believe that IPV is a personal matter, or fear offending the patient.[96,97] Although health care providers can greatly assist women who try to leave a violent relationship, more education is needed to improve the response of health care providers to battered women.

Socioeconomic

Though the societal values imposed on IPV victims as barriers to leaving and how victims internalize those values have already been discussed, victims of abuse must also overcome the socioeconomic realities of leaving an abusive relationship and reestablishing their lives. A major impediment to women who attempt to leave their violent relationship is their inability to access the economic resources necessary to live independently.[4] Many studies show that women who have limited economic resources are more likely to stay with or return to their abusers.[14,19,23,24,31-33,59]

As previously mentioned, part of the batterer's means of controlling the victim may be his control of the resources, which includes money.[19] An IPV victim may be economically abused and, therefore, completely economically dependent upon the batterer. The batterer may prohibit the woman from working or, if she does work, he may not allow her to have any money of her own. All household assets may be in the batterer's name alone, including bank accounts, home loans or deeds, car loans or titles, and credit card accounts, thereby eliminating the victim's access to money or assets.

Leaving a violent relationship can be an expensive process that requires money for housing, childcare, attorney fees, transportation, and the creation of a new home if the victim must leave everything behind.[18,28] Although domestic violence agencies can supply access to some of these items, they have limited resources. Such agencies may provide free legal help and housing in a shelter, but if a woman cannot pay for childcare or food, she may need to return to her abusive relationship. As previously mentioned, a shelter may only allow women to remain for a limited time (ie, 30 to 90 days). For a woman who has not been allowed to work or who possesses few job skills, finding a job that will adequately pay her so that she can afford alternate housing within the allotted time may pose a challenge; she may feel that she must return to her abusive situation. In addition, a lack of affordable housing and long waiting lists for subsidized housing may present still more barriers to her leaving or staying away from the abusive relationship. As a result, an IPV victim may not have any place to go. In fact, 50% of homeless women and children in the United States are leaving violent relationships. Intimate partner violence ranks as the number one cause of homelessness in 44% of surveyed cities within the United States.[15,28,87]

If a victim of abuse does find a job, that job may not pay enough to cover all of her expenses, so she often returns to the abusive relationship. If a victim of abuse already has a job, she may fear losing that job if she leaves her abuser because of absenteeism, a need to relocate, or an inability to access the tools or services that enable her to work (eg, transportation, childcare).[20,21]

Poverty certainly contributes to women remaining with or returning to abusive partners.[89] If an IPV victim can obtain public assistance, the welfare program may require her to work. The woman may have difficulty maintaining a job without formal child support or childcare or if her abuser harasses her in the workplace. As a result, the cycle between low-wage work and welfare may be directly related to IPV.[24] After all, without adequate economic resources, an IPV victim may find herself returning to or unable to leave her abuser.

LEARNING THEORIES

Several theoretical models are utilized to explain battered women's decision-making process for staying or leaving. Constructs that explore the psychology of remaining in an abusive relationship as well as the process of deciding to leave that relationship include the following models:

— Learned helplessness

— Traumatic bonding

— Psychological entrapment

— Investment

— Social-learning

— Reasoned action or planned behavior

— Transtheoretical or stages of change

Understanding these models can have implications for helping and caring for battered women who choose to remain in the relationship, are in the process of leaving the relationship, or have already left the relationship. Though the following sections summarize these models, the cited references provide more in-depth information.

LEARNED HELPLESSNESS

The theory of learned helplessness was initially identified during animal testing. When animals were given shocks that could be avoided or escaped, the animals learned a new task (ie, pressing a food bar or jumping over a barrier) to avoid the shock. When given inescapable shocks, however, the animals did not learn the new behavior and exhibited a sense of helplessness.[28,49,50]

In learned helplessness, the victim loses the ability to initiate avoidance behavior of a painful situation and will not attempt escape from a noxious or painful situation after having learned from previous, similar situations that escape is impossible.[28] As previously discussed, for women in violent relationships this is often expressed as depression or PTSD, both of which can contribute significantly to their remaining in the abusive relationship because of their psychological immobilization.

TRAUMATIC BONDING

With traumatic bonding, strong emotional attachments develop from the imbalance of power and intermittent good-bad treatment, which are features of violent relationships. According to this theory, the woman's combined hope for change and fear entraps her in the violent relationship.[28,30,98] Honeymoon periods, during which the batterer may act more lovingly toward the victim, often follow episodes of violence. Such intermittent abuse is thought to strengthen the victim's emotional attachment.[30,36,98] Honeymoon periods may serve to highlight the desirable aspects of the relationship and abusive partner for the victim, which makes recalling past abuse or perceiving the possibility of future abuse more difficult for her.

In addition, the power imbalance present in abusive relationships serves to lower the victim's self-esteem and increase her dependence upon the batterer. Both factors may make leaving the relationship more difficult. After the woman does leave an abusive relationship, her attachment may actually increase as her fear subsides. Also, the needs previously filled by her partner increase the longer she remains away from her abuser, which may contribute to the reasons a woman may return to an abusive partner.[30,98]

PSYCHOLOGICAL ENTRAPMENT

Psychological entrapment is another theory that asserts that a battered woman's commitment to the relationship increases to justify her previous investments (eg, time, energy, emotional involvement) in the relationship.[22,26,99] While the violent situation she is in remains intolerable the psychological entrapment model makes clear that the thought of leaving is seen as less and less an appropriate solution.

INVESTMENT

In Rusbult's investment model, a battered woman decides whether to remain in or leave her relationship by weighing the costs and benefits of both options. This theory especially examines the benefits of relationship satisfaction versus the costs of the quality of alternatives to the relationship, as well as how these impact the investments that have bound a woman to her partner.[22,26,100]

SOCIAL-LEARNING THEORY

The social-learning theory model, similar to the investment model, predicts that a battered woman will stay in an abusive relationship because investments with previous, positive outcomes (eg, children, a home) have increased her expectations for future happiness. On the other hand, an abused woman would be more likely to leave if investments had a prior negative outcome (eg, increasing physical violence), thereby decreasing her expectations for happiness.[22]

REASONED ACTION/PLANNED BEHAVIOR

The reasoned-action and/or planned-behavior model assumes that people will make rational decisions based on the information available to them. For battered women, this theory suggests that a woman will be more likely to leave if she views leaving as a positive outcome that is under her control and supported by significant others such as friends or family members.[26,101]

TRANSTHEORETICAL/STAGES OF CHANGE

Another model used to understand the process of ending an abusive relationship is the transtheoretical or stages-of-change model. In this model, behavior change requires 5 stages of change before that change can be achieved. These stages include the following:

1. *Precontemplation.* No interest in changing behavior, because the situation is not considered problematic

2. *Contemplation.* Recognition of the need for change

3. *Preparation.* Intent to change in the future

4. *Action.* Actively involved in making changes

5. *Maintenance.* Taking steps to prevent relapse

A study by Burke and colleagues investigated this model in the context of IPV and found this theory consistent with the experience of battered women trying to end their relationships.[102]

CONCLUSION

For many victims of IPV the decision to leave an abusive relationship is clearly difficult and complex. Victims may be unable to even consider leaving their situation, because they feel immobilized by psychological abuse, fear, or isolation. The personal, family, and social values imposed on an abuse victim, whether externally or internally, may encourage her to keep her relationship and family together even at the cost of her own safety. The process of actually leaving the situation may be quite difficult as well. A victim may lack outside support; have a limited access to resources; and may have little or no access to money, housing, transportation, or childcare. Facing these challenges, a battered woman may experience some doubts, setbacks, or ongoing emotional attachment that lead her to return to her abuser.[30,98,104] Additionally, the victim may find that escape from her violent relationship may be more dangerous for her than staying, because she is more likely to be killed when she has attempted or is attempting to leave; therefore, asking "why doesn't she just leave" fails to account for the complexity of an abused woman's situation. In addition, such a question inaccurately places the responsibility for ending the abuse on the victim, rather than the batterer, who ultimately controls abuse.[1]

Rather than ask "why doesn't she just leave?," more research and intervention needs to be conducted to focus on batterers rather than on victims' decisions to remain in or leave the situation, since the batterer's abusive behavior ultimately determines a victim's experience with violence.[64] In fact, many women do leave, though doing so may take an average of 7 tries for the victim to accomplish this goal; between 40% and 70% of battered women eventually do end their violent relationships.[15,17,52] The safer the leaving process and the more extensive safety planning and support from IPV agencies, police officers, legal professionals, therapists, and health care providers, the more effective the victim's leaving will be. Furthermore, sustaining separation after the victim leaves may require even more support than her leaving.[45]

Understanding the barriers women face can help providers of victim services empower battered women to live more safely, whether that means remaining in or leaving the abusive relationship. As caregivers to IPV victims and as part of the broader community, providers must support women who attempt to leave their abusive relationships to maintain a violence-free life; this will help end IPV.

REFERENCES

1. Follingstad DR, Runge MM, Ace A, Buzan R, Helff C. Justifiability, sympathy level, and internal/external locus of the reasons battered women remain in abusive relationships. *Violence Vict.* 2001;16:621-644.

2. Nicolaidis C, Curry M, Gerrity M. Health care workers' expectations and empathy toward patients in abusive relationships. *J Am Board Fam Pract.* 2005;18:159-165.

3. Bachman R. *Violence Against Women: A National Crime Victimization Survey Report.* Washington, DC: US Dept of Justice, Bureau of Justice Statistics; 1994. NCJ 145325.

4. Alpert EJ. Violence in intimate relationships and the practicing internist: new "disease" or new agenda? *Ann Intern Med.* 1995;123:774-781.

5. Ganley AL. Understanding domestic violence. In: Warshaw C, Ganley AL, eds. *Improving the Health Care Response to Domestic Violence: A Resource Manual for Healthcare Providers.* San Francisco, CA. Family Violence Prevention Fund:1995;14-45.

6. Cascardi M, Langhinrichsen J, Vivian D. Marital aggression: impact, injury, and health correlates for husbands and wives. *Arch Intern Med.* 1992;152:1178-1184.

7. Vivian D, Langhinrichsen-Rohling J. Are bi-directionally violent couples mutually victimized? A gender-sensitive comparison. *Violence Vict.* 1994;9:107-124.

8. Phelan MB, Hamberger LK, Guse CE, Edwards S, Walczak S, Zosel A. Domestic violence among male and female patients seeking emergency medical services. *Violence Vict.* 2005;20:18/-206.

9. Hamberger LK, Guse CE. Men's and women's use of intimate partner violence in clinical samples. *Violence Against Women.* 2002;8:1301-1331.

10. Saunders DG. When battered women use violence: husband-abuse or self-defense. *Violence Vict.* 1986;1:47-60.

11. Hamberger LK, Lohr JM, Bonge D, Tolin DF. An empirical classification of motivations for domestic violence. *Violence Against Women.* 1997;3:401-423.

12. Barnett OW, Lee CY, Thelen RE. Gender differences in attributions of self-defense and control in interpartner aggression. *Violence Against Women.* 1997;3:462-481.

13. Cascardi M, Vivian D. Themes and context for specific episodes of marital aggression. Paper presented at: Hartford Conference on Family Violence; June of 1993; New London, CT.

14. Erez E, Belknap J. In their own words: battered women's assessment of the criminal processing system's responses. *Violence Vict.* 1998;13:251-268.

15. Philadelphia Family Violence Working Group. *RADAR: A Domestic Violence Intervention for Health Care Providers.* Philadelphia, Pa: Philadelphia Family Violence Working Group; 1998.

16. Adams D. Treatment programs for batterers. *Clin Fam Pract.* 2003;5:159-176.

17. Schecter S, Edelson J. In the best interest of women and children: a call for collaboration between child welfare and domestic welfare constituencies. Paper presented at: Domestic Violence and Child Welfare: Integrating Policy and Practice for Families; June 8-10, 1994; Racine, Wis.

18. Grigsby N, Hartman B. The barriers model: an integrated strategy for intervention with battered women. *Psychotherapy.* 1997;34:485-497.

19. Anderson MA, Gillig PM, Sitaker M, McCloskey K, Malloy K, Grigsby N. "Why doesn't she just leave?" A descriptive study of victim reported impediments to her safety. *J Fam Violence.* 2003;18:151-155.

20. Hamby S. Domestic violence in sociocultural context [training package]. Eastport, ME: Possible Equalities; 1999. Quoted by: Liebshutz JM, Frayne SM, Saxe GN, eds. *Violence Against Women: A Physician's Guide to Identification and Management.* Philadelphia, PA: American College of Physicians. 2003; 18-19.

21. Hamby SL, Koss MP. Violence against women: risk factors, consequences, and prevalence. Quoted by: Liebschutz JM, Frayne SM, Saxe GN, eds. *Violence Against Women: A Physician's Guide to Identification and Management.* Philadelphia, PA: American College of Physicians; 2003:3-38.

22. Bauserman SA, Arias I. Relationships among marital investment, marital satisfaction, and marital commitment in domestically victimized and nonvictimized wives. *Violence Vict.* 1992;7:287-296.

23. Strube MJ. The decision to leave an abusive relationship: empirical evidence and theoretical issues. *Psychol Bull.* 1988;104:236-250.

24. Bell H. Cycles within cycles: domestic violence, welfare, and low-wage work. *Violence Against Women.* 2003;9:1245-1262.

25. Straus M. Sexual inequality and wife beating. In: Straus MA, Hotaling GT, eds. *The Social Causes of Husband-Wife Violence.* Minneapolis, MN: University of Minnesota Press; 1980:86-93.

26. Choice P, Lamke LK. A conceptual approach to understanding abused women's stay/leave decisions. *J Fam Issues.* 1997;18: 290-314.

27. Towns A, Adams P. "If I really loved him enough he would be okay": women's accounts of male partner violence. *Violence Against Women.* 2000:6:558-585.

28. LaViolette AD, Barnett OW. *It Could Happen to Anyone: Why Battered Women Stay.* 2nd ed. Thousand Oaks, CA: Sage Publications; 2000.

29. Langhinrichsen-Rohling J. Top 10 greatest "hits": important findings and future directions for intimate partner violence research. *J Interpers Violence.* 2005;20: 108-118.

30. Dutton DG, Painter S. Emotional attachments in abusive relationships: a test of traumatic bonding theory. *Violence Vict.* 1993;8:105-120.

31. Strube MJ, Barbour LS. The decision to leave an abusive relationship: economic dependence and psychological commitment. *J Marriage Fam.* 1983; 45:785-793.

32. Griffing S, Ragin DF, Sage RE, Madry L, Bingham LE, Primm BJ. Domestic violence survivors' self-identified reasons for returning to abusive relationships. *J Interpers Violence.* 2002;17: 306-319.

33. Barnett O, Lopez-Real D. Women's reactions to battering and why they stay. Paper presented at: American Society of Criminology; November, 1985; San Diego, CA.

34. Gordon KC, Burton S, Porter L. Predicting the intentions of women in domestic violence shelters to return to partners: does forgiveness play a role? *J Fam Psychol.* 2004;18:331-338.

35. Muldary PS. Attribution of causality of spouse assault. *Dis Abstrs Int.* 1983; 44:1249B.

36. Walker L. *The Battered Woman Syndrome.* New York, NY: Harper and Row; 1979.

37. Langhinrichsen-Rohling J, Schlee K, Monson C, Ehrensaft M, Heyman R. What's love got to do with it? Perceptions of marital positivity in h-to-w aggressive, distressed, and happy marriages. *J Fam Violence.* 1998;13: 197-212.

38. Salber P, Taliaferro E. *The Physician's Guide to Domestic Violence: How to Ask the Right Questions and Recognize Abuse.* Volcano, CA: Volcano Press; 1995.

39. Gilligan C, Rogers AG, Tolman DL. *Women, Girls, and Psychotherapy: Reframing Resistance.* New York, NY: Harrington Park Press; 1992.

40. Ferguson KE. *Self, Society, and Womankind: The Dialectic of Liberation.* Westport, CT: Greenwood; 1980.

41. Debold E, Wilson MC, Malave I. *Mother-Daughter Revolution: From Good Girls to Great Women.* New York, NY: Bantam; 1993.

42. Sokoloff NJ, Dupont I. Domestic violence at the intersections of race, class, and gender: challenges and contributions to understanding violence against marginalized women in diverse communities. *Violence Against Women*. 2005; 11:38-64.

43. Aguilar RJ, Nunez Nightingale N. The impact of specific battering experiences on the self-esteem of abused women. *J Fam Violence*. 1994;9:35-45.

44. Arias I, Pape KT. Psychological abuse: implications for adjustment and commitment to leave violent partners. *Violence Vict*. 1999:14:55-67.

45. Wuest J, Merritt-Gray M. Not going back: sustaining the separation in the process of leaving abusive relationships. *Violence Against Women*. 1999; 5:110-133.

46. Avni N. Battered wives: the home as a total institution. *Violence Vict*. 1991; 6: 137-149.

47. Walker L. Battered women and learned helplessness. *Victimology*. 1978; 2: 525-534.

48. Walker L. Victimology and the psychological perspective of battered women. *Victimology*. 1983; 8: 82-104.

49. Seligman MEP. *Helplessness: On Depression, Development, and Death*. San Francisco, CA: WH Freeman; 1975.

50. Maier S, Seligman M. Learned helplessness: theory and evidence. *J Exp Psychol*. 1976;105:3-46.

51. Cascardi M, O'Leary KD, Schlee KA. Co-occurrence and correlates of posttraumatic stress disorder and major depression in physically abused women. *J Fam Violence*. 1999; 14: 227-249.

52. Sheehan Berlinger J. Domestic violence: how you can make a difference. *Nursing*. 2001; 31: 58-63.

53. American Psychiatric Association. *Diagnostic and Statistical Manual of Mental Disorders*. 4th ed. Washington, DC: American Psychiatric Association Press; 1994.

54. Murphy CM, Cascardi M. Psychological aggression and abuse in marriage. In: Hampton RL, ed. *Family Violence: Prevention and Treatment*. 2nd ed. Newbury Park, CT: Sage Publications; 1999:198-226.

55. Widom CS. The cycle of violence. *Science*. 1989; 244: 160-166.

56. Crick NR, Dodge KA. A review and reformation of social-information processing mechanisms in children's social adjustment. *Psychol Bull*. 1994; 115: 74-101.

57. Lochman JE, Dodge KA. Social-cognitive processes of severely violent, moderately aggressive, and nonaggressive boys. *J Consult Clin Psychol*. 1994; 62: 366-374.

58. Langhinrichsen-Rohling J, Hankla M, Stormberg CD. The relationship behavior networks of young adults: a test of the intergenerational transmission of violence hypothesis. *J Fam Violence*. 2004;19:139-151.

59. Gelles RJ. Abused wives: why do they stay. *J Marriage Fam*. 1976;38:659-668.

60. Astin MC, Lawrence KJ, Foy DW. Posttraumatic stress disorder among battered women: risk and resiliency factors. *Violence Vict*. 1993;8:17-28.

61. Bergman B, Larsson G, Brismar B, Klang M. Aetiological and precipitating factors in wife battering. *Acta Psychiatr Scand*. 1988; 77: 338-345.

62. Hamberger L. Research concerning wife abuse: implications for training physicians and criminal justice personnel. Paper presented paper at: American Psychological Association; August, 1991.

63. Hotaling GT, Sugarman DB. A risk marker analysis of assaulted wives. *J Fam Violence*. 1990; 5: 1-13.

64. Fleury RE, Sullivan CM, Bybee DI. When ending the relationship does not end the violence: women's experience of violence by former partners. *Violence Against Women*. 2000;6:1363-1383.

65. Straus MH, Gelles RJ. *Physical Violence in American Families*. New Brunswick, NJ: Transaction Publishers; 1991.

66. Leonard K. Domestic violence and alcohol: what is known and what do we need to know to encourage environmental interventions? *J Substance Use*. 2001; 6: 235-247.

67. Bureau of Justice Statistics. *Alcohol and Crime: An Analysis of National Data on the Prevalence of Alcohol Involvement in Crime*. Washington, DC: US Dept of Justice, Office of Justice Programs; 1998. NCJ 168632.

68. Kaufman Kantor G, Straus MA. The "drunken bum" theory of wife beating. In: Straus MA, Gelles RJ, eds. *Physical Violence in American Families*. New Brunswick, NJ: Transaction Publishers; 1990:203-224.

69. O'Farrell TJ, Choquette KA. Marital violence in the year before and after spouse-involved alcoholism. *Fam Dyn Addict Q*. 1991;1:32-40.

70. O'Farrell TJ, Murphy CM. Marital violence before and after alcoholism treatment. *J Consult Clin Psychol*. 1995; 63: 256-262.

71. O'Farrell TJ, Van Hutton V, Murphy CM. Domestic violence before and after alcoholism treatment: a two-year longitudinal study. *J Stud Alcohol*. 1999; 60: 317-321.

72. Leonard KE, Roberts LJ. The effects of alcohol on the marital interactions of aggressive and non-aggressive husbands and their wives. *J Abnorm Psychol*. 1998; 107: 602-615.

73. Fals-Stewart W. The occurrence of partner physical aggression on days of alcohol consumption: a longitudinal study. *J Consult Clin Psychol*. 2003; 71: 41-52.

74. Dixon L, Browne K. The heterogeneity of spouse abuse: a review. *Aggress Violent Behav*. 2003; 8: 107-130.

75. Holtzworth-Munroe A, Stuart GL. Typologies of male batterers: three subtypes and the differences among them. *Psychol Bull*. 1994; 116: 476-497.

76. Holtzworth-Munroe A, Meehan JC, Herron K, Rehman U, Stuart GL. Testing the Holtzworth-Munroe and Stuart (1994) batterer typology. *J Consult Clin Psychol*. 2000; 68: 1000-1019.

77. Gottman JM, Jacobson NS, Rusher RH, et al. The relationship between heart rate reactivity, emotionally aggressive behavior, and general violence in batterers. *J Fam Psychol*. 1995; 9: 227-248.

78. Coan J, Gottman JM, Babcock J, Jacobson N. Battering and the male rejection of influence from women. *Aggress Behav.* 1997; 23: 375-388.

79. Jacobson NS, Gottman JM, Gortner E, Berns S, Shortt JW. Psychological factors in the longitudinal course of battering: when do the couples split up? when does the abuse decrease? *Violence Vict.* 1996; 11: 371-392.

80. Quigley BM, Leonard KE. Resistance of husband aggression in the early years of marriage. *Violence Vict.* 1996; 11: 355-370.

81. Mahoney MR. Legal images of battered women: redefining the issue of separation. *Mich Law Rev.* 1991;90:1-94.

82. Campbell JC. "If I can't have you, no one can": power and control in homicide of female partners. In: Radford J, Russel DEH, eds. *Femicide: The Politics of Woman Killing.* New York, NY: Twayne Publishers; 1992:99-113.

83. Department of Justice. *National Crime Victimization Survey.* Washington, DC: US Dept of Justice; 1994.

84. Schwartz MD. Marital status and woman abuse theory. *J Fam Violence.* 1988; 3: 239-248.

85. Wilson M, Daly M. Spousal homicide risk and estrangement. *Violence Vict.* 1993;8:3-16.

86. Brown SE. Police responses to wife beating: neglect of a crime of violence. *J Crim Justice.* 1984;12:277-288.

87. Catania S. The counselor. *Mother Jones.* 2005;30:45-49.

88. Gonnerman J. The unforgiven. *Mother Jones.* 2005; 30: 38-43.

89. Zweig JM, Schlicter KA, Burt MR. Assisting women victims of violence who experience multiple barriers to services. *Violence Against Women.* 2002; 8: 162-180.

90. Alsdurf JM. Wife abuse and the church: the response of pastors. *Response.*1985; 8: 9-11.

91. Sutherland C, Bybee D, Sullivan C. The long term effects of battering on women's health. *Womens Health.* 1998; 4: 41-70.

92. Abbott J, Johnson R, Koziol-McLain J, Lowenstein SR. Domestic violence against women: incidence and prevalence in an emergency department population. *JAMA.* 1995; 273: 1763-1767.

93. Stark E, Flitcraft A, Zuckerman D, Grey A, Robison J, Frazier W. *Wife Abuse in the Medical Setting: An Introduction for Health Personnel.* Washington, DC: National Clearinghouse on Domestic Violence; 1981. Monograph Series, No. 7.

94. Liebschutz J, Paranjape A. How can a clinician identify violence in a woman's life? Quoted by: Liebschutz J, Frayne S, Saxe G, eds. *Violence Against Women, A Physician's Guide to Identification and Management.* Philadelphia, PA: American College of Physicians; 2003:39-69.

95. Goldberg WG, Tomlanovich MC. Domestic violence victims in the emergency department. New findings. *JAMA.* 1984; 251: 3259-3264.

96. Rodriguez MA, Bauer HM, McLoughlin E, Grumbach K. Screening and intervention for intimate partner abuse: practices and attitudes of primary care physicians. *JAMA*.1999; 282: 468-474.

97. Gerbert B, Caspers N, Milliken N, Berlin M, Bronstone A, Moe J. Interventions that help victims of domestic violence: a qualitative analysis of physicians' experiences. *J Fam Pract*. 2000; 49: 889-895.

98. Dutton DG, Painter SL. Traumatic bonding: the development of emotional attachments in battered women and other relationships of intermittent abuse. *Victimology*. 1981; 1: 139-155.

99. Brockner J, Rubin JZ. *Entrapment in Escalating Conflicts: A social Psychological Analysis*. New York, NY: Springer-Verlag; 1985.

100. Rusbult CE. Commentary on Johnson's "Commitment to personal relationships": what's interesting, and what's new? In: Jones WH, Perlman DW, eds. *Advances in Personal Relationships*. Vol. 2. London, England: Jessica Kingsley; 1991: 151-169.

101. Ajzen I. From intentions to actions: a theory of planned behavior. In: Kuhl J, Beckman J, eds. *Action Control: From Cognition to Behavior*. Heidelberg, Germany: Springer; 1985: 11-39.

102. Burke JG, Gielen AC, McDonnell KA, O'Campo P, Maman S. The process of ending abuse in intimate relationships: a qualitative exploration of the transtheoretical model. *Violence Against Women*. 2001; 7: 1144-1163.

103. Martin AJ, Berenson KR, Griffing S, et al. The process of leaving an abusive relationship: the role of risk assessments and decision-certainty. *J Fam Violence*. 2000; 15: 109-122.

Chapter 6

THE ABUSED PATIENT: A CLINICAL RESPONSE USING THE STAGES OF CHANGE MODEL

Janice B. Asher, MD

Angelo P. Giardino, MD, PhD, MPH, FAAP

Health care providers cite many reasons for not assessing their patients for intimate partner violence (IPV) during the clinical encounter. The stages of change (SOC), more broadly the transtheoretical, model offers a perspective to health care providers who seek to screen for and respond to the risk of IPV to their patients. One of the most common reasons given for not assessing IPV is health care providers do not feel confident that they will know how to respond affirmatively to a question about a patient's exposure to violence.[1,2] In other words, health care providers do not know what they should do when a patient says, "Yes, I'm being abused." This concern was likened to "opening Pandora's box." The difficult issues raised by primary care providers about exploring IPV included their[3]:

— Lack of comfort with the topic

— Fear of offending the patient

— Powerless feelings in the face of such an overwhelming problem

— Time pressures in the busy office, which often prevent delving into complex psychosocial issues such as IPV

It is difficult for health care providers to appropriately respond to a patient disclosing abuse because of the potential awkwardness of the situation. Few health care providers have any training in the subject of IPV.[4,5] Further, public health issues in general, and IPV in particular, do not lend themselves to the traditional medical model of a solo practitioner. Treating such problems cannot be achieved in a linear fashion.[6,7]

In addition, health care providers may instinctively respond in ways that may place an IPV patient in even greater jeopardy. For example, a well-intentioned physician may tell a patient that the abusive relationship is dangerous and she should leave immediately, but this may prompt a highly dangerous response. Evidence shows that serious injuries and homicide increase when a victim makes clear her intentions of leaving the relationship or after she has left.[8]

A more practical and successful way for health care providers to help their patients is to know what methods and advice help patients change their behavior. When viewed from this perspective, health care providers tend to respond more appropriately, thereby making the interaction more effective, satisfying, and time-efficient.[9] This chapter examines practical approaches to responding to IPV in the clinical setting while exploring the underpinnings of a SOC model, especially when used to help victims of abuse move toward safety and independence.

HEALTH CARE SCREENING FOR INTIMATE PARTNER VIOLENCE

Even a decade after the Pandora's box analogy was published, health care providers continue to voice these concerns to some extent, and primary care physicians are reported to routinely screen for IPV in their female patients at a rate as low as 10%.[2] Obstetrics and gynecology specialists screen at the highest rate; emergency medicine specialists screen at the lowest rate. Despite increased training efforts directed at health care providers, misperceptions continue about IPV and the role of the physician during screening and intervention.[2,10-12]

Screening for various health risks related to social issues remains an evolving field. Until the second half of the 20th Century, health care providers did not routinely ask patients about their alcohol consumption, sexual practices, or smoking habits.[13] These behaviors were considered social rather than medical issues. Presently, health care providers view these practices from a public health perspective and know that these issues have enormous medical ramifications.

In 1998, the Centers for Disease Control and Prevention (CDC) described IPV as a "public health emergency."[14] In addition, the American Medical Association (AMA), American College of Obstetricians and Gynecologists (ACOG), and American Pediatric Association (APA) recognized that assessing IPV is a mandatory standard of medical care practice.[15-17] Simply put, assessment of IPV is indeed "part of the job" for health care providers from all disciplines, including physicians.

The American Academy of Nurse Practitioners (AANP) also challenges their members (eg, participants in primary care, women's health care, specialty care, and emergency medical services) to identify and respond to IPV victims. In fact, the AANP's Statement on Violence, issued in 2000, includes IPV as a form of violence that requires assessment, identification, and referral.[18]

Despite the increasing number of calls from professional organizations to include assessment for IPV in the health care setting, rates for domestic violence screening continue to lag other risk behaviors (eg, behaviors associated with tobacco use, alcohol use, human immunodeficiency virus [HIV], sexually transmitted infections [STI]).[13] Reasons given for these lower IPV screening rates, when compared to the other situations typically seen as private and socially related, include[13]:

— Physicians believe that they do not know how to accurately screen for IPV.

— Physicians do not know how to appropriately intervene.

— Interventions for IPV are less successful than those for the other risk situations.

Chang and colleagues conducted a qualitative study regarding the consequences experienced by women after a screening by a health care provider. Their analysis supports the claim that sensitivity is needed when raising the issue of possible IPV in patients' lives.[19] In fact, these screenings helped abused women acknowledge the existence and seriousness of IPV in their lives, and also affirmed their concerns, distress, and fears about the violence in their lives.[19] In following up with these women, researchers asked them whether they perceived that a difference had been made by having the issue of IPV raised with them. One woman responded that, "It helps us to believe in ourselves. People respect doctors, and when a doctor says something, you know it [reflects] better on you that somebody that's professional would actually believe in you."[19] Intimate partner violence survivors clearly indicate that health care providers' screenings about the violence in their lives provided an opportunity to build their awareness about IPV, experience compassion regarding their difficult situation, and acquire needed information that went beyond a simple screening exercise.[19]

BACKGROUND OF THE STAGES OF CHANGE MODEL

The transtheoretical model of behavioral change, as formulated by James O. Prochaska, addresses the process by which people change problematic behaviors and uses the construct of moving from stage to stage as an organizing principle.[20,21] This model is called *trans*theoretical because the model emerged from a scholarly process that sought to systematically integrate what was known about the behavior change process and the principles from various schools of thought, which were fragmented into more than 300 theories of psychotherapy.[22] Important to health care clinicians, the transtheoretical model provides a framework for assessing readiness to change; therefore, it facilitates an appropriate response that respects where the patient is psychologically while setting the health care provider's expectations at the appropriate level for the given situation. The transtheoretical model, which contains a number of component parts, is often referred to by its most recognized component, the stages of change, and was initially developed within the context of tobacco smoking. Since its development, this model has been applied to many issues, which include alcohol and substance abuse, anxiety and panic disorders, delinquency, eating disorders and obesity management, promotion of low carbohydrate diets, HIV and AIDS prevention, mammography screening, medication compliance, unplanned pregnancy prevention, sun exposure reduction, and IPV.[22]

The SOC model consists of the following 5 stages:

1. ***Precontemplation.*** No intention to take action toward change within the next 6 months.

2. ***Contemplation.*** Intention to take action toward change within the next 6 months.

3. ***Preparation.*** Intention to take action within the next 30 days, and some initial behavioral steps taken.

4. ***Action.*** Overt behavior has changed for fewer than 6 months.

5. ***Maintenance.*** Overt behavior has changed for more than 6 months.

The following sections briefly describe each stage of change within this model as it applies to victims of IPV. Bear in mind that these descriptions are generic in nature.

PRECONTEMPLATION

In this stage, the victim of violence does not see the violence as a problem, does not recognize the partner's behavior as abusive, or feels hopeless about any possibility for change. As a result, she does not think about making changes regarding her response to the violence and abuse. A victim in the precontemplation stage tends to blame herself for inducing the abuse.

CONTEMPLATION

The victim is aware of the problem, but tends to minimize it while in the contemplation stage. She may perceive that her partner is abusive and that his behavior negatively affects her children, even if the children are not in immediate physical danger. She may think of ways to avoid situations in which violence could occur. Though the victim is not ready to take action, the situation does concern her.

PREPARATION

During the preparation stage, the victim prepares to make changes regarding the abusive behavior or abuser. She may consider ways to de-escalate potentially explosive situations; seek a support group; or develop a temporary, emergency exit strategy, potentially including ending the relationship. At this stage, the victim does recognize the potential danger of her situation.

ACTION

During the action stage, the victim carries out the plan she has prepared. It should be noted that no one plan is appropriate for all IPV victims. Instead, each situation and each individual person needs to make a plan that makes sense for her and her family and will end their exposure to the abusive situation.

MAINTENANCE

The victim either takes steps to decrease her physical and emotional vulnerability to the violence or has left the relationship. According to Prochaska's original model that applied to smoking cessation, the maintenance stage begins after approximately 6 months of action. For IPV victims, the 6-month time frame is useful as well because it serves as a time or transition milestone for monitoring the victim's movement from action to maintenance.

THE PROCESS OF CHANGE

Prochaska and DiClemente described in 1984 how 10 processes of change facilitate a person's progression through the 5 stages of change.[23] In addition, they sought to develop a theoretically cohesive and inclusive answer to the question, "How does a person move from one stage to the next?". What is radical about their answer, and the concept this answer espouses, is that several of these processes are not based on any action or change in the person's behavior at all; rather, the changes are internal. That is, people gain awareness and understanding that they then use to move themselves through the later action-oriented stages of change.[24] In other words, attitudinal changes precede behavioral changes. People outside of the situation looking in (eg, health care providers, family members, friends) find understanding the reasons victims do not exchange their unhealthy situations for healthier ones difficult to comprehend. The SOC model is described as "spiral-shaped" because a person typically moves back to a previous stage, but such a move is not a sign of failure (or "noncompliance," in medical terms). For example, most people who successfully quit smoking experienced prior unsuccessful attempts. Although few patients stop smoking immediately after a discussion with their physicians, most people who do quit smoking indicate that their doctors' advice was a key motivating factor. The SOC model recognizes that a person's modifications in attitude and behavior that occur over time actually move that person from one stage to the next. Using an empirical analysis that compared people who independently stopped smoking and smokers involved in professional smoking cessation programs, researchers identified the following 10 processes[25]:

1. Consciousness raising

2. Dramatic relief

3. Self-reevaluation

4. Environmental reevaluation

5. Social liberation

6. Helping relationships

7. Self-liberation

8. Counter conditioning

9. Contingency management

10. Stimulus control

Burke and colleagues found that women use these processes of change when dealing with IPV and ending the abusive relationships.[26] Different processes of change appear more prominently and are used during different stages. In the earlier stages of change (eg, precontemplation, contemplation) the victim tends to rely upon the more cognitive-affective processes rather than using the processes that are seen as behavioral tools, which victims tend to use during the preparation, action, and maintenance stages. Burke and colleagues also found that consciousness raising and social liberation appeared in both early and late stages, while helping relationships became critical to the woman's change process throughout each stage. **Table 6-1** provides a graphic representation of the process.

Table 6-1. Processes of Change that Mediate Progression Between the Stages of Change

PRECONTEMPLATION	CONTEMPLATION	PREPARATION	ACTION	MAINTENANCE

Processes   Consciousness Raising
Dramatic Relief
Environmental Reevaluation
Self-reevaluation
Self-liberation
Counterconditioning
Helping relationships
Reinforcement
management
Stimulus control

Note: Social liberation was omitted because of its unclear relationship to the stages.

Adapted with permission from: Prochaska JO, Redding CA, Evers KE. The transtheoretical model of stages of change. In: Glanz K, Rimer BK, Lewis RM, eds. Health Behavior and Health Education: Theory, Research and Practice. 3rd ed. San Francisco, CA: Jossey-Bass; 2002:99-120.

When trying to help an abused patient, health care providers may easily become frustrated and fail to realize that attitudinal changes precede behavioral changes; therefore, they must remember that, especially in the beginning of the process, the abused woman may have acquired positive effects but not yet show any visible signs of improvement or growth. Thus, tenacity in caring for patients may be of great value, especially as applied to the process of changing behaviors and reducing exposure to the risks associated with IPV.

The following are descriptions of each of the 10 processes as they apply to IPV victims. Understanding these processes on the part of the health care provider working with the IPV victim may help illuminate for the clinicians the underlying processes of change that may facilitate the patient's progression through the 5 stages of change.

CONSCIOUSNESS RAISING

The process of consciousness raising increases the victim's awareness and understanding of the abuse. The victim begins to understand that her partner's behavior is actually abusive. The woman also sees that the abuse does not occur because of what the victim does, but because of who the perpetrator is. Perhaps most importantly, the victim realizes that no one deserves to be abused under any circumstances.

DRAMATIC RELIEF

Dramatic relief is an emotional process by which the victim begins to anticipate and experience the potential benefits, affectively, of taking effective action to reduce the risk of and exposure to IPV. According to Prochaska et al,[22] psychodrama, role playing, personal testimonies, and public service announcements may be particularly effective at stimulating this emotional process and motivating change.

SELF-REEVALUATION

As with consciousness raising, the process of self-reevaluation is both cognitive and emotional. The reevaluation process encompasses the victim's assessment of her relationship, her realization of what she herself can change, and the determination of her goals.

ENVIRONMENTAL REEVALUATION

It is critical to assess the way an abusive behavior affects the environment of its victim. In doing so, she comes to understand the devastating effects the violence has on her children, even if they are not actually being abused themselves. Such reevaluation often helps victims to move from the contemplation to the preparation stage. A victim can also use this process to consider her available options for change. For example, she may consider moving temporarily or permanently, or consider staying with friends, relatives, or in shelter facilities. She may also consider strategies for saving money, getting a job, or going to school.

SOCIAL LIBERATION

Also a cognitive process, a victim uses social liberation to progress from the stage of action to maintenance. With this process, the victim increasingly accepts and becomes comfortable with her life, which is free from the abuser, or at least free from the abuse.

HELPING RELATIONSHIPS

In every stage of change, the victim requires support from others. Actually receiving and experiencing this help is essential for change to occur. For example, health care providers may overlook the importance of being supportive and nonjudgmental in their approach to an abused patient who is not yet ready to move toward an action-oriented stage of change.

SELF-LIBERATION

The victim commits to changing the problem behavior during the process of self-liberation. An abused woman uses this process to free herself from her feelings of self-worth as defined by the abusive partner. She may become free of the false hope that the violence will end or free from the notion that she cannot live without her abuser.

COUNTER CONDITIONING

This is an experiential process by which the IPV victim substitutes healthy behaviors for the counterproductive and problematic behaviors that may keep them in the abusive situation. Techniques such as assertiveness training, self-esteem building exercises, and desensitization sessions may be useful in assisting victims to make progress in making the healthier substitutes.

CONTINGENCY MANAGEMENT

Contingency management is another experiential process, similar to the counter conditioning, by which the IPV victim receives reinforcement for the choices made. With regard to the movement toward effective action that gets the victim away from the abuse, positive reinforcers would be preferable to negative or punishing reinforcers. Techniques to help the victims experience positive reinforcement for good choices might include group work that recognizes good choices, consistent action, and the implementation of one's plans.

STIMULUS CONTROL

During the process of stimulus control, the victim can control stimuli that may precipitate the problem behavior. For example, a woman may develop an exit strategy for herself and her children for a situation when her partner becomes drunk and is likely to be violent. During the maintenance stage, she may avoid his telephone calls.

Remember that in the original SOC model, as applied to smoking, the concept was that the individual's behavior is the problem (ie, their own smoking). This is not the case in IPV, where the perpetrator's behavior is the problem, not that of the victim. Thus, this change process is one part of the model that tends to be less applicable to IPV as opposed to quitting smoking. The use of this process is limited in the case of IPV and is often not useful over time while the victim remains in the relationship.

ADDITIONAL CONSTRUCTS OF CHANGE CONSIDERATION AS APPLIED TO IPV

In addition to the 5 stages and the 10 processes of change, the transtheoretical model also uses other constructs to help health care providers further understand how a person moves from one stage to another stage.

DECISIONAL BALANCE

A decisional-balance construct exists in which the individual weighs the pros and cons of changing behavior and seeks to balance the perceived benefits with the perceived costs of change.[22] When applied throughout the stages of change, this process typically begins with the contemplation stage. For most IPV victims, decisional balance applies most strongly to issues regarding the victim's safety and the safety of her children.[26,27] Other acute concerns include the emotional welfare of her children, as well as financial and cultural considerations.

SELF-EFFICACY

This construct delineates the balance between the person's confidence to make a change against the temptation to continue in the current health risk. Within this construct, *confidence* is described as the perceived assurance that the person can engage in the changed health behavior throughout different, challenging situations; whereas, *temptation* is described as the pull felt by the person to continue engaging in the unhealthy behavior throughout those challenging situations.[22]

THE STAGES OF CHANGE MODEL IN CLINICAL PRACTICE

The application of the stages of change model is particularly useful insofar as the model addresses 2 primary concerns for health care providers. These concerns include addressing the issue of IPV in a time-efficient manner and responding appropriately when a patient discloses IPV.

Haggerty and Goodman synthesized recent research regarding IPV and the stages of change that support the ways women demonstrate typical behaviors for the various stages of change.[28] They reviewed the literature and incorporated findings from various studies that supported the idea that women who are exposed to violence show behaviors that are similar to the movement through the stages of change seen with other health issues. The Haggerty and Goodman article is important because the synthesis provided by the authors provides a clinically relevant application of the SOC model to the experience of the IPV victim.

Burke and colleagues also make an important contribution in their examination of the application of the SOC model to the experiences of women dealing with IPV issues.[26] They found clear evidence that women ending IPV relationships use the processes and constructs of change described in the traditional transtheoretical model. This supports the development and implementation of practices based on interventions that use the stages of change approach.

In most IPV cases, health care providers encounter a patient who is either in the precontemplation or contemplation stage. By using the SOC model, health care providers can respond to the patient in an appropriate and helpful manner.

Before applying the SOC model to IPV, first consider the issue of tobacco smoking, which was the first behavior on which Prochaska applied this model. Most health care providers feel experienced and comfortable discussing smoking with their patients. The patient who smokes and is in the precontemplation stage states that she will be able to stop smoking any time she likes. Obviously, there is no point in providing the patient with the telephone number for a smoking-cessation clinic or a prescription for medication to decrease nicotine craving. On the other hand, the health care provider should address smoking regardless of the patient's current stage; ample evidence shows that people who quit smoking successfully cite their health care provider's recommendation as one of the factors that encouraged them to quit. In this case, the provider may remind the patient that at some point all tobacco addicts think they will be able to stop smoking any time they like. Since many precontemplative smokers are young, health care providers may find appealing to their personal vanity worthwhile (eg, yellow teeth, bad breath, wrinkles).

As with smoking cessation, most women who have left abusive relationships cite physician support and encouragement as a key factor to their leaving the relationship. When applying this model to the abuse victim, health care providers remember that a patient may be in the precontemplation stage. Perhaps she does not perceive that her partner's behavior is his fault or that he is significantly different from other men. Perhaps she feels utterly hopeless and believes that she cannot do anything about the abuse or her life. A health care provider who only responds to an abused patient by telling her that she should immediately leave the relationship is wasting time as well as making the patient feel even more guilty for staying and hopeless for change. The provider's appropriate goal, regardless of the patient's stage, is to be non-judgmental and help the patient maximize her safety.

Even the abused patient in the precontemplation stage can be reminded that no one deserves to be abused, that help is available, and that she may wish to consider what she might do to protect herself in the future. Even in the precontemplative stage, abuse victims find abuse-related materials that include safety planning information and local resources useful. Evidence shows that one factor that helps move abused victims toward the preparation stage is their recognition of the deleterious effects the abuse has on their children.[26]

Implicit in this discussion is the concept that behavioral change is a process rather than an event. In other words, health care professionals will not be able to "cure" a patient, but through compassion, support, and information, health care providers can help abuse patients engage in the process of changing their behavior.

CLINICAL EXAMPLES OF USING THE STAGES OF CHANGE MODEL

The previously described 10 processes of change prove useful in helping women leave IPV relationships.[29] Theory and practice point out that these 10 processes are essentially strategies that help support the woman as she progresses through the 5 stages of change. As a result, health care providers should continue to use these processes in helping women, and should also connect each process with the stages in which that process most supports the change.

Ongoing research conducted with IPV survivors gives health care providers information regarding the best ways to sensitively ask abused women about their situations. Those women who have survived IPV generally advise the following[30]:

1. Health care providers should explain their reasons for asking the woman about IPV-related issues during the health assessment. This reduces a woman's suspicions and may minimize any sense of stigma she may feel.

2. Health care providers should maintain a supportive, safe atmosphere during the interaction.

3. Regardless of whether the woman discloses abuse or not, health care providers should make information and resources available.

From the specific perspective of informing practice based on an SOC method approach to working with women who may be experiencing IPV, Zink and colleagues studied women dealing with IPV issues and asked about their interactions with health care providers, particularly during the precontemplation and contemplation stages.[24] These women believed that health care providers should screen both routinely and in high-risk situations when symptoms suggesting violence are present.[24] These women advised that though screening is acceptable during the precontemplative stage when the abuse victim does not recognize the abuse, going beyond sensitively asking about abuse may actually alienate the woman. In addition, during a woman's early stages of recognition, health care providers should explore the clues provided by the woman. As an abused woman recognizes the abuse as victimization, she will be more willing to disclose her abuse situation and explore options. The women in this study further advise physicians to affirm the existence of abuse, know the local resources and support systems available to IPV victims, assist with referrals for services and support systems, educate victims about the health effects of IPV, and document the abuse.[24] **Table 6-2** provides a stage of change, informed, clinical approach developed from this study for the precontemplation and contemplation stages.

Health care providers encounter women who are IPV victims during all stages of change. **Table 6-3** also lists responses for the precontemplation and contemplation stages. Additionally, **Table 6-3** provides examples of what patients might say during the later stages of preparation, action, and maintenance. It also gives possible responses that the health care provider may use in these situations.

In addition to the verbal cues and responses listed in **Table 6-3**, other responses may be useful as well. For example, Frasier and colleagues suggest a number of possibly effective

Table 6-2. Stages of Change (Precontemplation and Contemplation) for Intimate Partner Violence with Matched Physician Interventions From Study Data and Published Guidelines

STAGE OF CHANGE	PHYSICIAN STAGE-MATCHED INTERVENTIONS FROM STUDY DATA AND RATIONALE	ADDITIONAL INTERVENTIONS FROM PUBLISHED GUIDELINES INTERPRETED FOR APPROPRIATE STAGE MANAGEMENT
Precontemplation: the patient-victim does not see the relationship as abusive	Ask about IPV when there is an injury; ask how injury occurred Ask during pregnancy Ask routinely (annual examination) and when warning symptoms and illnesses are present* Have and make pamphlets available. Do not spend time reviewing them in detail Educate about the impact of IPV on the physical and mental health of the victim and her children Document suspicions about IPV	Ask about IPV at the annual examination Ask during each trimester of pregnancy Ask when warning symptoms and illnesses are present* Ask at well-child examination and if abuse is suspected (child abuse, failure to thrive, behavior problems, school problems, ADHD/hyperactivity, depression, teen risk-taking behaviors, worried parent) Make pamphlets with safety plan information available in the office Assess safety.† If any risk factors are present, share concerns with the patient-victim or follow mandated reporting guidelines
Early contemplation: the patient-victim sees the relationship as abusive, but may choose not to share this with the physician	Ask about IPV as above despite nondisclosure–women want to be screened Listen and watch for clues (hints or evidence of abuse). Victims are observing whether physician is willing to discuss abuse Discuss observations about the abuser's controlling behavior–if physicians observe abuse, discuss concerns in private with the patient-victim Have and make pamphlets available. Do not spend time reviewing them in detail	Ask as above Assess safety.† If any risk factors are present share concerns with the patient-victim or follow mandated reporting guidelines Make pamphlets with safety plan information available in the office

(continued)

Table 6-2. *(continued)*		
Early contemplation *(continued)*	Educate about the impact of IPV on the physical and mental health of the victim and her children	
	Document suspicions about IPV	
	Document subjective and objective findings	
Late contemplation: the patient-victim sees the relationship as abusive and is weighing the pros and cons of making a change	Ask as above	Ask as above
	Affirm abuse is occurring and that no one deserves to be abused	Assess safety.[†] If any risk factors are present share concerns with the patient-victim or follow mandated reporting guidelines
	Educate about the impact of IPV on the physical and mental health of the victim and her children	Consider reviewing safety plan[‡] with the patient-victim, educate staff about IPV and have them review safety plan, or refer the patient to IPV agency
	Review local IPV crisis numbers with the patient-victim	
	Offer to have the patient telephone the crisis number from a private room in the office	
	Make referrals for counseling to a counselor knowledgeable about IPV for the patient or her children	
	Document subjective and objective findings	

IPV = intimate partner violence; ADHD = attention deficit hyperactivity disorder.

* Warning symptoms and conditions: injuries (ask about the mechanism of the inquiry, if mechanism does not make sense, consider probing further in a nonjudgmental manner); chronic pain (headache, abdominal pain, including irritable bowel syndrome, pelvic pain, back pain, etc); vague somatic complaints (fatigue, dizziness); mental health issues (depression, anxiety, post-traumatic stress disorder, substance abuse); abuser's inappropriate behavior in the office.

† Safety assessment: evaluate suicide or homicide risk (victim and abuser), weapons or threat to use weapons (victim and abuser), drug and alcohol use (victim and abuser), abuse of children, abuse of pets, escalating severity of abuse, threats to life.

‡ Safety plan: where to go, important documents and items to have ready to take with such as keys, medications, children's immunizations, money.

Adapted with permission from: Zink T, Elder Z, Jacobson N, Klosterman B. Annals of Family Medicine. American Academy of Family Physicians. June 2004;2(3):231-239.

interventions for patients in various stages of change.[31] **Table 6-4** lists these interventions and matches them with the appropriate stage of change.

RELAPSE

Understanding the likely "relapse" is integral to the application of the SOC model. As previously mentioned, Prochaska describes his model as a spiral, in that returning to a previous stage is common. Thus, people do not only move forward, they may move back and forth between stages. Such relapse is often temporary and not a sign of failure or "non-compliance." Rather, relapse signals that maintenance strategies may not have

Table 6-3. What Patients and Providers Might Say at Different Stages of Change Around IPV

STAGE OF CHANGE	POSSIBLE PATIENT COMMENTS	POSSIBLE PROVIDER RESPONSES
Precontemplation	"It's not a problem."	"I'm glad you told me about this."
	"I know my husband loves me."	"I am concerned for your safety and the safety of your children."
	"My husband is under a lot of stress."	
	"My boyfriend hits me only when he's drunk."	"The behavior you described is abusive."
	"It's better now. He says it won't happen again."	"Violence usually gets worse, not better."
	"All men are like this."	"Even if he never hits your children, they are being hurt, too."
	"I've given up. This will never change."	
Contemplation	"I'm afraid of my husband."	"No one deserves to be hit or threatened."
	"I don't deserve this."	
	"I'm afraid to ask my boyfriend to use a condom."	"Do you want safety information?"
	"My kids are scared."	"Do you want information about resources for support, assistance and/or shelter?"
Preparation	"I'm moving next week."	"I am glad you told me about this."
	"I'm going to get a job so that I can support my children if I need to."	"You have come a long way to have reached this point."
	"I'm going to open my own savings account."	"Be careful. You are potentially in the greatest danger when you leave and even after you leave."
Action	"I moved into a shelter."	
	"I'm back in school."	
	"I changed the locks."	"Sometimes people decide not to leave or they decide to return, but that doesn't mean they have failed."
	"I don't answer his telephone calls anymore."	
	"I have a new boyfriend who treats me with respect."	
	"The kids and I leave the house whenever he drinks."	

Adapted with permission from: Glanz K, Rimer BK, Lewis FM. Health Behavior & Health Education, Theory, Research, and Practice. 3rd ed. Hoboken, NJ: Jossey-Bass;2002:107.

Table 6-4. Effective Intervention Matched with Stages of Change*

STAGE OF CHANGE	CHARACTERISTICS	INTERVENTION
Precontemplation	Denial of need to change situation	Acknowledge that victim is not ready to make changes
	Avoidance in discussing problem	Emphasize that you do not plan to 'pressure' victim to make changes
	Refusal of information	
	Minimization of situation's seriousness	Affirm that no person deserves to be hit or abused
	Defending batterer	Focus on provision of information about abuse
	Scapegoating	Indicate that other victims have started where the patient is now
	Hopelessness	Urge the patient to think seriously about the situation
	Belief that abuse is victim's fate	Ask the patient to think about reasons she might consider a change
		Reaffirm you are there to help
		Help patient develop a safety plan
Contemplation	Awareness of problem, seeking information, asking questions	Ask "Have you ever tried to make a change in the past?" "What happened?"
	Planning to take action within 6 months	Ask "What problems do you anticipate?"
	Struggling to understand why ("What can I do differently?")	Solicit 'pros' and 'cons' using a worksheet kept in patient's chart
	Wishful thinking ("I wish I knew what to do differently.")	Discuss options to overcome barriers
	Procrastination	Offer support: "I know you'll do the best you can to make the right decision."
	'Fence sitter'	Report your experiences with other patients, information from reading, television, etc. that may encourage the victim
	Anxiety ("What if…")	

(continued)

Table 6-4. *(continued)*		
Preparation	Planning to take action within the month	Ask the patient how you can help
	Publicly acknowledges plans to safe individuals/organizations	Mutually set a definite date to prevent premature or prolonged planning
	Some ambivalence, with last-name resolution	Offer information on community resources, referrals
	Careful detailed planning	Review safety plan
Action	Very busy	Schedule follow-up visits to reinforce patient's behavior
	High commitment level for specific change	Referrals to group support if necessary and mutually agreeable
		Check for symptoms of 'return'
Maintenance	Strong commitment to activities to prevent return	Be alert to danger signs that patient may be contemplating return
Termination	Confident	
	Problem no longer present or a threat	

* Characteristics are applications from Prochaska and DiClemente [8-10]. Interventions were developed by two of the authors (PF and PG) based on their experiences with abuse victims.

Adapted with permission from: Frasier PY, Slatt L, Kowlowitz V, Glowa PT. Patient Education and Counseling. Elsevier. May 2001;43(2):7.

been as successful as hoped.[32] Both the health care provider and patient need to recognize this phenomenon and its inevitability, otherwise they may both feel a sense of frustration, failure, and even anger.

Though relapse to precontemplation is highly unusual, the health care provider who displays ignorance or a judgmental attitude toward patients who feel unable to leave abusive relationships may contribute to a patient's sense of lack of self-worth and increasing hopelessness. In such a case, a patient may revert to precontemplation and assume there is no way out of her abusive relationship.

LIMITATION OF THIS MODEL

The SOC model was originally designed to address a person's process of changing his/her own problematic behavior (eg, smoking). In the case of IPV, the perpetrator's behavior is unacceptable, not the victim's behavior.

Women face many obstacles when changing their violent situations and these obstacles may be well beyond their control. For example, women are limited in some situations if they lack the financial, educational, or social support needed to implement the change. Though the SOC model does not fully address the social and economic contexts in which the abuse may occur, these factors do impact the victim's readiness for change and her success in maintaining it within the realm of IPV.[32] Despite these obstacles, a victim of abuse may successfully adapt this model and develop strategies for safety within an abusive relationship and, perhaps ultimately, safely end the abusive relationship.

CONCLUSION

Although the SOC model was developed initially in relationship to cigarette smoking, it has proved highly useful to health care professionals to describe the process by which people change a problematic behavior. With IPV, understanding the 5 stages of change and the behavioral and cognitive modification processes required in making change allows health care professionals to know how to effectively and appropriately reach out to abuse victims. Because victims often cite their health care provider's reaching out to them as being an eye-opening experience, the SOC model as applied to IPV will prove useful far into the future as the health care provider screens for, and seeks to respond to, IPV.

REFERENCES

1.   Rodriquez MA, Bauer HM, McLoughlin E, Grumbach K. Screening and intervention for intimate partner abuse: practices and attitudes of primary care physicians. *JAMA*. 1999;282:468-474.

2.   Elliott L, Nerney M, Jones T, Friedmann PD. Barriers to screening for domestic violence. *J Gen Intern Med*. 2002;17:112-116.

3.   Sugg NK, Inui T. Primary care physicians' response to domestic violence. Opening Pandora's box. *JAMA*. 1992;267:3157-3160.

4.   Bair-Merritt MH, Giardino AP, Turner M, Ganetsky M, Christian CW. Pediatric residency training on domestic violence: a national survey. *Ambul Pediatr*. 2004;4:24-27.

5.   Varjavand N, Cohen DG, Gracely EJ, Novack DH. A survey of residents' attitudes and practices in screening for, managing, and documenting domestic violence. *J Am Med Womens Assoc*. 2004;59:48-53.

6.   Alpert EJ, Sege RD, Bradshaw YS. Interpersonal violence and the education of physicians. *Acad Med*. 1997;72(suppl 1):41-50.

7.   Warshaw C. Domestic violence: changing theory, changing practice. *J Am Med Womens Assoc*; 1996;51:87-91.

8.   Koziol-McLain J, Coates CJ, Lowenstein SR. Predictive validity of a screen for partner violence against women. *Am J Prev Med*. 2001 Aug;21:93-100.

9.   Zimmerman GL, Olsen CG, Bosworth MF. A "stages of change" approach to helping patients change behavior. *Am Fam Physician*. 2000;61:1406-1416.

10.   Berger RP, Bogen D, Dulani T, Broussard E. Implementation of a program to teach pediatric residents and faculty about domestic violence. *Arch Pediatr Adolesc Med*. 2002;156:804-810.

11.   Chez RA, Horan DL. Response of obstetrics and gynecology program directors to a domestic violence lecture module. *Am J Obstet Gynecol*. 1999;180(pt 1):496-498.

12.   Ernst AA, Weiss SJ, Cham E, Hall L, Nick TG. Detecting ongoing intimate partner violence in the emergency department using a simple 4-question screen:

the OVAT. *Violence Vict.* 2004;19:375-384.

13. Gerbert B, Gansky SA, Tang JW, et al. Domestic violence compared to other health risks: a survey of physicians' beliefs and behaviors. *Am J Prev Med.* 2002;23:82-90.

14. Centers for Disease Control and Prevention. *Youth Risk Behavior Surveillance— United States, 1997. MMWR.* 1998;47:1-28.

15. Violence against women. Relevance for medical practitioners. Council on Scientific Affairs, American Medical Association. *JAMA.* 1992;267:3184-3189.

16. The American College of Obstetricians and Gynecologists. Violence Against Women: Screening Tools—Domestic Violence. 2008. *http://www.acog.org/ departments/dept_notice.cfm?recno= 17&bulletin=585.* Accessed June 13, 2008.

17. American Academy of Pediatrics Committee on Child Abuse and Neglect. The Role of the Pediatrician in Recognizing and Intervening on Behalf of Abused Women. *Pediatrics.* 1998;101(6):1091-1092.

18. American Academy of Nurse Practitioners. 2000. Statement on Violence. Washington, DC. *http://www.aanp.org/Publications/AANP+Position+Statements/ Position+Statements+and+Papers.asp.* Accessed June 13, 2008.

19. Chang JC, Decker M, Moracco KE, Martin SL, Petersen R, Frasier PY. What happens when health care providers ask about intimate partner violence? A description of consequences from the perspectives of female survivors. *J Am Med Womens Assoc.* 2003;58:76-81.

20. Prochaska JO, DiClemente CC. Stages and processes of self-change of smoking: toward an integrative model of change. *J Consult Clin Psychol.* 1983;51:390-395.

21. Prochaska, JO. *Systems of Psychotherapy: A Transtheoretical Analysis.* Pacific Grove, Calif: Brooks-Cole; 1979.

22. Prochaska, JO, Redding, CA, Evers KE. The transtheoretical model of stages of change. In: Glanz K, Rimer BK, Lewis RM, eds. *Health Behavior and Health Education: Theory, Research and Practice.* 3rd ed. San Francisco, Calif: Jossey-Bass; 2002:99-120.

23. Prochaska JO, DiClemente CC. Self change processes, self efficacy and decisional balance across five stages of smoking cessation. *Prog Clin Biol Res.* 1984;156:131-140.

24. Zink T, Elder N, Jacobson J, Klostermann B. Medical management of intimate partner violence considering the stages of change: precontemplation and contemplation. *Ann Fam Med.* 2004;2:231-239.

25. DiClemente CC, Proschaska JO. Self-change and therapy change of smoking behavior: a comparison of processes of change in cessation and maintenance. *Addict Behav.* 1982;7:133-142.

26. Burke JG, Denison JA, Gielen AC, McDonnell KA, O'Campo P. Ending intimate partner violence: an application of the transtheoretical model. *Am J Health Behav.* 2004;28:122-133.

27. Zink T, Elder N, Jacobson J. How children affect the mother/victim's process in intimate partner violence. *Arch Pediatr Adolesc Med.* 2003;157:587-592.

28. Haggerty LA, Goodman, LA. Stages of change-based nursing interventions for victims of interpersonal violence. *J Obstet Gynecol Neonatal Nurs*. 2003;32:68-75.

29. Anderson C. Evolving out of violence: an application of the Transtheoretical Model of Behavior Change. *Res Theory Nurs Pract*. 2003;17:225-240.

30. Chang JC, Cluss PA, Ranieri L, et al. Health care interventions for intimate partner violence: what women want. *Wom Health Iss*. 2005;15:21-30.

31. Frasier PY, Slatt L, Kowlowitz V, Glowa PT. Using the stages of change model to counsel victims of intimate partner violence. *Patient Educ Couns*. 2001;43:211-217.

32. Littell JH, Girvin H. Ready or not: uses of the stages of change model in child welfare. *Child Welfare*. 2004;83:341-366.

Chapter 7

CHILDREN WHO WITNESS VIOLENCE: THE SPECIFIC PROBLEM OF CHILDREN WHO ARE EXPOSED TO INTIMATE PARTNER VIOLENCE

Kathleen Franchek-Roa, MD
Marcy Witherspoon, MSW
Angelo Giardino, MD, PhD, MPH, FAAP

Our understanding of children as witnesses, observers, or "silent victims" of various forms of violence has been slow to develop over time.[1] Only over the past 40 years has the medical community recognized that children may be physically injured by severe, intentional trauma (ie, child abuse/child maltreatment).[2] Therefore, it comes as no surprise that the recognition of potentially detrimental effects of witnessing violence, either in the home or from others outside of the home, has an even shorter history. As professional attention has turned to issues related to children's exposure to violence, the potentially damaging effects of witnessing all forms of violence—particularly intimate partner violence (IPV)—are becoming more apparent.[3,4] Betsy McAllister Groves, a pioneer in the study of children who have witnessed violence, highlights the unique character of IPV for children as she states[5]:

Domestic violence, violence that occurs between adult caregivers in the home, seems to be the most toxic form of violence for children… For many children, the first lessons they learn about violence are not from television or from the streets, but from their parents. These lessons are generally the wrong lessons: that it is acceptable to use threats or force to get one's way, that violence has a place in an intimate relationship, that adults can hurt one another and not apologize or take some responsibility for their actions.

This chapter addresses our current understanding of children's exposure to violence—particularly IPV. The field is evolving and, as the following excerpt documents, even its terminology is still developing[6]:

Several different terms have been used by researchers and others to refer to children in households with domestic violence. Early researchers spoke of these children as either "witnesses" or "observers" of the violence… these terms have been replaced by "exposure" to the violence, which is more inclusive and does not make assumptions about the specific nature of the children's experiences with the violence. Exposure to domestic violence can include watching or hearing the violent events, direct involvement (for example, trying to intervene or calling the police), or experiencing the aftermath (for example, seeing bruises or observing maternal depression).

This chapter, while recognizing the wide range of forms of violence to which children may be exposed worldwide, focuses primarily on children who are exposed to violence in their own homes—specifically, those who witness their caregiver threatened, victimized, or harmed by a current or former partner.

CHILDREN'S EXPOSURE TO INTIMATE PARTNER VIOLENCE

An expanding body of literature supports the fact that IPV is a common, frequent, and persistent form of violence throughout the world, including in American society. Surveys indicate that one quarter to one half of women throughout the world have suffered violence at the hands of an intimate partner at some point in their lives.[7,8] While horrible for the women affected, what may be even more detrimental is the fact that many women who are victims are also mothers who have children living with them; thus, the children are inevitably exposed to the violence as well. Indeed, at least 50% of female victims of IPV in the United States have children less than 12 years of age in the household.[9] It is estimated that 3 to 10 million children annually witness acts of family violence.[10] Dr. Straus suggests that "at least a third of American children have witnessed violence between their parents, and most have endured repeated instances of these painful and distressing events."[11] The report, entitled "In Harm's Way: Domestic Violence and Child Maltreatment,"[12] draws attention to the overlap between IPV and child maltreatment in the United States. **Figure 7-1** graphically represents this overlap and should encourage health care providers to screen caregivers who bring children in for care for the presence of IPV to permit early identification or prevention of child maltreatment. The following report complements this idea[12]:

Research studies clearly document that children are affected by domestic violence and that, not infrequently, child maltreatment and spouse abuse occur in the same families. Children in abusive families may be seriously affected by the violence found in their homes. Studies show that the effect of both experiencing maltreatment and witnessing family violence may produce greater negative effects than either factor alone..."

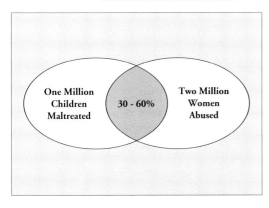

Figure 7-1.
Overlap of Child Maltreatment and Domestic Violence

CHILDREN'S INVOLVEMENT IN INTIMATE PARTNER VIOLENCE

In 2006, the United Nations issued a report entitled "Behind Closed Doors: The Impact of Domestic Violence on Children,"[13] and made the following observations about the risk of ever-increasing harm to the child's physical, emotional, and social development from exposure to IPV[13]:

Infants and small children who are exposed to violence in the home experience so much added emotional stress that it can harm the development of their brains and impair cognitive and sensory growth. Behaviour changes can include excessive irritability, sleep problems, emotional distress, fear of being alone, immature behaviour, and problems with toilet training and language development.[14] At an early age, a child's brain is becoming 'hard-wired' for later physical and emotional functioning. Exposure to domestic violence threatens that development."

The 1998 policy statement of the American Academy of Pediatrics (AAP) that "the abuse of women is a pediatric issue" highlights the overarching need to explore the effect of IPV on children and their development.[14] Over the years, the realization that children are intimately involved in the violence in their homes has become clearer. In the 1970s, there was an increasing awareness that many women were victims of abuse by their intimate partners, and, soon after that, researchers began evaluating how witnessing violence in the home could affect children—this area of research has been growing ever since.[3] What has become clear is that children become involved in IPV in a number of ways, including by sustaining physical injuries, trying to stop the violence, affecting the mother's decision-making process, and witnessing the violence or its aftermath. Dr. Jeffrey Edleson, a prolific investigator of how IPV impacts children and families, summarizes our growing understanding of how children are exposed to IPV[16]:

In their national curriculum for child protection workers, Ganley and Schechter (1996)[15] highlight several additional ways that children experience adult domestic violence. These include hitting or threatening a child while in its mother's arms, taking the child hostage in order to force the mother's return to the home, using a child as a physical weapon against the victim, forcing the child to watch assaults against the mother or to participate in the abuse, and using the child as a spy or interrogating him or her about the mother's activities. Children are also frequently told by abusive fathers that their families would be together were it not for their mother's behavior, thus attempting to put pressure on the mother through the children to return to him or risk driving a wedge between the mother and her children.

The Overlap between Child Maltreatment and Intimate Partner Violence

Living in violent homes not only places children at risk of witnessing violence but also of becoming victims of violence themselves. **Figures 7-2 to 7-10** are pictures created by children who have witnessed violence. Edleson reported that in 30%–60% of families where domestic violence or child maltreatment occurs, the other form of violence is also present.[17] Appel and Holden, in a comprehensive review examining the co-occurrence of IPV and child physical abuse, have drawn attention to the wide variation in reported prevalence figures of the overlap between IPV and child injury.[18] Specifically, they reviewed 42 different studies that provided data on the co-occurrence of IPV and child physical abuse, and 31 of these studies had sufficient detail to be included in their analysis. They found that in studies done on clinical populations, namely settings where victims of either IPV or child abuse were the populations studied, the prevalence of co-occurrence or overlap between the two problems was relatively high, ranging from 20% to 100%. In

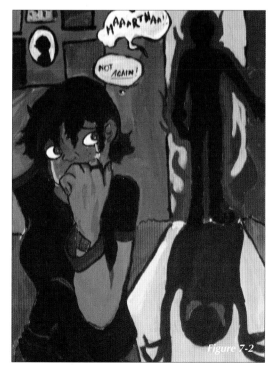

Figure 7-2

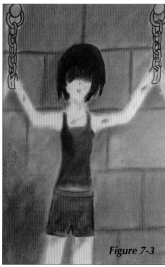

Figure 7-3

Figure 7-2. *A 9th grader's drawing of a girl crying and looking over her shoulder as a figure stands at the door.*

Figure 7-3. *A bruised girl bound by chains, as portrayed by a 16-year-old.*

studies of the overall community, however, where randomly selected populations were examined, the prevalence of overlap was much lower than in the "clinical studies," ranging from 6% to 11%. This variation would be expected from an epidemiological perspective, in that the clinical samples are the people most at risk and not randomly selected; therefore, they would be the most likely to have overlap between IPV and child physical abuse (thus overestimating the overlap) while the community-based samples selected by random would likely have fewer cases of IPV and child physical abuse and would find less overlap as a result (thus potentially underestimating the overlap). These researchers concluded that, using a conservative definition of child physical abuse, a reasonable estimate of the co-occurrence of IPV and child physical abuse would be 40%.

Sustaining Injuries

Children may sustain injuries during violent episodes between adults in the home in a number of ways. Among the more commonly described injury scenarios are being unintentionally injured by an object, being thrown or kicked, being in their mother's arms when their mother is assaulted, being injured as they directly intervene during an assault, or being intentionally injured by the perpetrator to further intimidate or gain control over the adult victim. Appel and Holden have developed a list of models drawn from their extensive review of the co-occurrence of IPV and child physical abuse, which describes the various ways that the child may come to be abused in the setting of IPV.[18] **Table 7-1** displays these models and offers a brief description of each.

Pediatricians, family medicine practitioners, and emergency medicine physicians may be called upon to evaluate children who are harmed as a result of the various IPV related scenarios. Christian and colleagues, in their case series of 139 children between the ages of 2 weeks and 17 years who were harmed during IPV, found that the most common mechanism of injury sustained by children during an IPV altercation was a direct hit (36%), followed by being hit by an object (27%), being thrown or pushed (15%), and being dropped (11%).[19] Of the 67 children who were fewer than 2 years old, 59% were injured while being held by a parent. Eighty-three percent of the cases identified the person who injured the child, and the child's father was responsible for the injury in 50% of cases, the mother's boyfriend in 10%, and the mother herself in 13%. Fifty-seven percent of the injuries were minor, not requiring additional treatment after the evaluation, and 9% required hospitalization. The child's head, face, and eyes were most commonly injured. Seventy-three percent of children returned to their homes, while the other 27% went to other, alternative homes.[19]

Trying to Stop the Violence

Many children living in homes where intimate partner violence occurs are victimized on multiple occasions. Studies have supported the finding that 30%–60% of children who live in violent homes are likely to be victims of child abuse.[20,21] Many of these episodes of violence in the home are chronic, featuring multiple events that are repeated over

Figure 7-4. This split image shows two houses: one in which abuse occurs and one in which a happy family resides.

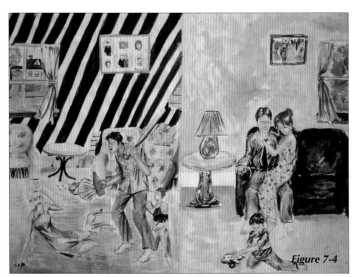

Figure 7-4

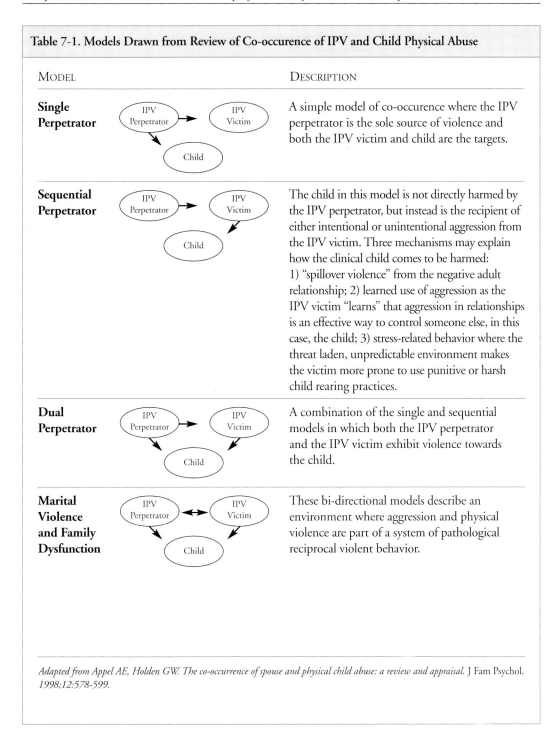

Table 7-1. Models Drawn from Review of Co-occurence of IPV and Child Physical Abuse

MODEL		DESCRIPTION
Single Perpetrator		A simple model of co-occurence where the IPV perpetrator is the sole source of violence and both the IPV victim and child are the targets.
Sequential Perpetrator		The child in this model is not directly harmed by the IPV perpetrator, but instead is the recipient of either intentional or unintentional aggression from the IPV victim. Three mechanisms may explain how the clinical child comes to be harmed: 1) "spillover violence" from the negative adult relationship; 2) learned use of aggression as the IPV victim "learns" that aggression in relationships is an effective way to control someone else, in this case, the child; 3) stress-related behavior where the threat laden, unpredictable environment makes the victim more prone to use punitive or harsh child rearing practices.
Dual Perpetrator		A combination of the single and sequential models in which both the IPV perpetrator and the IPV victim exhibit violence towards the child.
Marital Violence and Family Dysfunction		These bi-directional models describe an environment where aggression and physical violence are part of a system of pathological reciprocal violent behavior.

Adapted from Appel AE, Holden GW. The co-occurrence of spouse and physical child abuse: a review and appraisal. J Fam Psychol. *1998;12:578-599.*

time. Children are held captive by these situations because they do not have the coping mechanisms or resources to escape their abusive homes. Edleson and colleagues found that 23% of mothers reported that their children became physically involved during an abusive incident.[22] Children may also verbally try to stop the abuse. Edleson and colleagues found that 52% of the mothers reported that their children, at least occasionally, yelled from another room during an abusive incident; 53% reported that

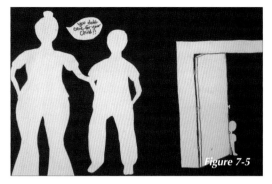

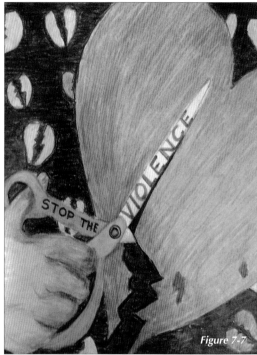

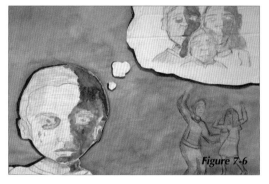

Figure 7-5. A 15-year-old's drawing of a child who watches from afar as his parents argue and shout, "You don't care for your child!!".

Figure 7-6. A 6th grader's wish while a violent scene occurs.

Figure 7-7. An 11-year-old child's drawing of scissors that read, "stop the violence" as they cut through a heart.

their children, at least occasionally, yelled while in the same room during an abusive incident; and 21% of their children sought help from someone else during the abuse.[22] This study highlights the potential risk for physical injury to children during these abusive episodes, in which many children are taking an active role in attempting to stop the abuse.

Affecting the Mother's Decision-Making Process

In working with mothers who are victims of IPV, a common theme emerges regarding children: children are often the reason why many women *leave* their abuser, *stay* with their abuser, or *return* to their abuser. Zink and colleagues found that more than half of the mothers they interviewed reported that something related to the child (eg, the child was injured, the child was mimicking the perpetrator's behavior, the child commented on the abuse) motivated them to take action against the abuse.[23] Some of the women in this study delayed seeking help because of the children's attachment to the abuser. Also, financial concerns, threats of injury to the children if she left, and fear of losing her children all play important roles in a woman's decision to stay.[24] In cases where victims and their children have to leave their home, the children are often removed from their support systems (eg, their friends, neighborhoods, schools) and this can further magnify the problems that these children face in dealing with the trauma. These women are often confronted with the challenge of making painful decisions that may affect their children adversely in the short-term but will benefit them in the long-term. Bancroft and Silverman have examined the mother-child bond in the face of IPV and have drawn attention to the strength of this relationship and its potential to contribute positively to the child's resilience and ability to cope with exposure to violence.[25] They also explored the potential damage that the perpetrator can do to the mother-child relationship by undermining the mother's authority with the child. **Table 7-2** displays Bancroft and Silverman's inventory of potential negative impacts that a perpetrator may have on the exposed children, which includes damaging the mother-child bond.[25]

Table 7-2. Bancroft and Silverman's "Risk to Children from Batterers" Framework

Component	Description
Exposure to threats or acts of violence	After separation, especially when restraining orders are involved, children are at high risk of witnessing or becoming deliberately or accidentally involved in new assaults, the retraumatization or exposure, all of which are likely to impede a child's emotional recovery. During visitation, threats or revictimizations often occur, the likelihood of which is increased if the mother begins a new relationship. Evidenced more by the batterer's attempt to address causes of past behavior than his violent record alone, he is likely to repeat behavior in subsequent relationships, especially because the new partner is unlikely to disclose, because of fear, the belief that he has changed or an influenced opinion of his former partner.
Undermining mother's relationship	The most important factor in the emotional recovery of child victims of abuse is the relationship with the nonbattering parent. This relationship can be weakened by abuse, the deterioration possibly intensifying even after separation, and is therefore one of the most serious risks to children's recovery.
Physical, sexual, or emotional abuse	Batterers may display verbally abusive parenting, increasing after separation with visitation as the only means to control the mother, emotionally abuse children, or risk parentification of children by instilling guilt. Furthermore, higher rates of child physical and sexual abuse exist among batterers, likely to increase after separation when the mother is unable to oversee the batterer's behavior. Though a batterer may not have abused his children while the family was together, there is still the possibility that the batterer will seek revenge on the mother through their children, or that children will become insubordinate with their father, placing them at a higher risk of physical abuse.
Modeling violent or threatening behavior	As adults, sons and daughters of batterers have increased chances of becoming perpetrators or victims. Additionally, systemic decisions, such as granting custody to a battering parent, might be perceived by the child as supporting the father's behavior and placing blame on the mother. Therefore, the batterer's effect on his children's value system needs to be addressed and his relationship with them should require limitation of his power as a role model.
Rigid parenting	Nurturing and structured environments ease the recovery of child victims of abuse; however, the common authoritative parenting styles used by batterers impede healing. The achievement of a sense of security is crucial for recovery, but a parent's intimidation reminds the child of violence, slowing progress for a child trying to regain self-esteem while aggression is sustained.

(continued)

135

Table 7-2. *(continued)*

COMPONENT	DESCRIPTION
Neglect or irresponsible parenting	Batterers typically focus more on themselves and are less likely to focus on their children's needs or to provide consistency, which often increases after separation. With typically more time to care for children during visitation than they have done previously, batterers are often more lenient to increase favor with the children, hindering the mother's ability to provide structure in her own home, a necessary element in children's recovery. Neglect by the visiting father can sometimes escalate to leaving children unattended or exposing them to entertainment that is frightening or inappropriate, an experience highly disturbing and influential to children who have been exposed to domestic violence.
Abduction	Many abductions take place under the circumstances of domestic violence, usually fulfilled by the father or a representative, and often have traumatizing effects on children. Abductions, are most commonly accomplished by failing to return a child from visitation and occur either before separation or years after the separation, instances varying little by race. Family abductions are much more likely than stranger abductions, and half of these have been threatened in some way prior to the abduction.

Adapted with permission from Sage Publications Inc.[25]

PSYCHOLOGICAL AND DEVELOPMENTAL EFFECTS OF WITNESSING VIOLENCE

Literature on the effects of violence on children has expanded significantly over the past two decades. In 1998, Holden identified 56 published articles over a 20-year period between 1975 to 1995 that addressed children exposed to marital violence.[3] A major theme that emerged from this extensive literature review is that children of all ages can be affected by the violence in their homes, even if they are not the direct recipients of that violence. The adverse effects on children of witnessing violence in the home are generally considered to be internalizing behaviors (eg, anxiety, depression, social withdrawal), externalizing behaviors (eg, aggressiveness, hyperactivity, conduct problems, truancy, bullying), poor academic performance, stress-related physical symptoms, and post-traumatic stress disorder (PTSD). The chronological and developmental age of the child, the gender of the child, the severity of the violence, the chronicity of the violence, and the child's social supports all play a role in the child's response to the violence. In a more recent meta-analysis, Kitzmann and colleagues examined 118 studies on psychosocial outcomes of children exposed to IPV and confirmed that exposure to IPV is associated with significant disruption in children's psychosocial functioning.[26] The researchers make clear in their meta-analysis, however, that, like others in the field, they find gaps and inadequacies in the available literature—especially concerning the differences in gender response to exposure to IPV, age of child at time of exposure, length of exposure, severity of violence to which they are exposed, and the child's inherent resilience. Each of these factors requires further study.[26]

Table 7-3. Examples of Programs Addressing the Needs of Children Who Witness Violence

PROGRAM	DESCRIPTION	WEBSITE

Child Development-Community Policing Program in New Haven, CT.
 	
The evaluation component of this program occurs in the Childhood Violent Trauma Center (a collaboration of the CD-CP program at the Yale Child Study Center, the Northeast Program Evaluation Center at the Yale School of Medicine Dept of Psychiatry, and the Department of Psychiatry Center at the University of Connecticut Health Center.
	Collaborative alliance among law enforcement, juvenile justice, domestic violence, medical and mental health professionals, child welfare, schools and other community agencies.
	— provides opportunities to understand
	   — the relationship between a child's exposure to violence
	   — the traumatic stress symptoms that can develop
	   — effective ways to assist children exposed to violence
	— The primary emphasis is on the child's perspective; therefore, it is a nontraditional service delivery model. This model has been replicated and now exists in eleven other cities in the country, in addition to New Haven, and is explicitly focused on the effects of violence on children.
		Office of Juvenile Justice and Delinquency Prevention http://ojjdp.ncjrs.org/pubs/gun_violence/profile48.html. Accessed March 27, 2008.

Preschool Witness to Violence Program-Child Trauma Research Project This is a collaboration of San Francisco General Hospital, Department of Psychiatry, the San Francisco Department of Community Mental Health and the San Francisco Department of Human Services.	This project addresses children's exposure to abuse and neglect and their exposure to domestic violence to: — "ensure that the most vulnerable infants and toddlers are identified early and linked to intensive services." The program serves children from birth to 6: — ages 3 to 6 are served through a randomized clinical research project funded by the NIMH, and — those from birth to 3 are seen through a treatment-focused evaluation outcome research program for infants and toddlers and their families.	http://psych.ucsf.edu/research.aspx?id=1554 Accessed March 27, 2008
Miller Children's Abuse and Violence Intervention Center Miller Children's Hospital in Long Beach, California.	Coordinates investigative, medical and mental health services to children, adolescents and families who have experienced child abuse, family violence, child abduction and parental substance abuse conducted at a child-oriented facility located near the hospital provides: — immediate interventions, — longer-term services, and — advocacy for children and families.	http://www.memorialcare.org/miller/services/abuse.cfm Accessed March 27, 2008.

(continued)

Table 7-3. *(continued)*

PROGRAM	DESCRIPTION	WEBSITE
Violence Intervention Program in Los Angeles, California Began as the Center for the Vulnerable Child (CVC) in 1984 at the Los Angeles County and USC Medical Center.	Comprehensive medical and mental health services for victims of sexual assault, domestic violence, and elder or dependent adult abuse and provides: — medical, forensic, mental health, social and legal services for all victims of violence, regardless of gender or age (although children continue to be the focus) — emphasizes community-based prevention efforts to end the cycle of family violence.	http://www.violence interventionprogram.org/ Accessed June 23, 2008.
Cognitive-Behavioral Intervention for Trauma in Schools (CBITS). RAND Corporation, the University of California at LA (UCLA) and the Los Angeles Unified School District (LAUSD).	Intervention designed to help children cope with the many forms of violence to which they are exposed. — Implemented by school-based mental health clinicians — Deals with all kinds of violence and exposure to violence — Students are eligible to participate if they: — have experienced substantial direct exposure to violence — exhibit PTSD symptoms in the clinical range, and — are willing to discuss their symptoms in a group setting	http://www.hsrcenter.ucla. edu/research/cbits.shtml Accessed March 27, 2008.

A number of programs have been developed to address the psychological impact witnessing violence has on children. **Table 7-3** arrays the similarities among these programs while **Table 7-4** lists several model programs along with a brief description of each.

A thorough review from Knapp sheds light on how children of different ages may potentially respond in different ways to their exposure to violence.[27] Many symptoms of violence exposure exhibited by children are common pediatric complaints. Infants have been noted to suffer disrupted sleep patterns and disruptive feeding routines. These infants may present with failure to thrive or developmental delays. Infants may present with the complaint of excessive screaming and these infants may be misdiagnosed with colic.

Preschoolers can exhibit regression of developmental behaviors, such as thumb-sucking or nocturnal enuresis. These children can become needier or more anxious. They also show decreased willingness to explore their environment and exert their independence.

School-aged children can exhibit behavioral problems or poor academic performance. McFarlane and colleagues found that children exposed to domestic violence had significantly higher incidences of internalizing behaviors, externalizing behaviors, and other behavioral problems than children not exposed to violence in the home.[28]

Table 7-4. Similarities Among Programs Serving Children Who Witness Violence

COMPONENT	DESCRIPTION
Providing Information and Building Group Cohesion	Common ground rules address issues such as use of violent words or actions, the ability to not speak or "pass" your turn to speak, interrupting others when they are speaking, and confidentiality (and the limitations of confidentiality in cases of child abuse).
"Breaking the Silence"	A primary goal of many therapeutic interventions is to promote open discussion of the children's experiences.
Dealing with Feelings of Responsibility for Violence in the Family	Children should be helped to understand that parental actions are adult issues, and not the responsibility of the children. Children should be dissuaded from the belief that they can change their parents' violent behavior.
Identifying Feelings	Learning to identify and label feelings helps children to not only express themselves to others, but also better understand their reaction to fighting between their parents. Group facilitators will commonly ask children to identify different feelings, and describe situations when they might feel that way.
Dealing with One's Own Anger	Teaching children to effectively manage anger is an important step in breaking the intergenerational cycle of violence. Developing relaxation skills is a common anger control strategy. Another strategy is to have groups of children brainstorm healthy and unhealthy ways of dealing with anger.
Identifying/Using Social Supports	Social support interventions often focus on the positive aspects of the children's current social support system and provide them with resources for maintaining or enlarging this network.
Self-Concept and Self-Confidence	Exploring children's self-concept and boosting their self-confidence.
Learning about the Cycle of Violence and the Dynamics of Family Violence	Children's concerns that violence is inevitable in their own lives. Misconceptions around spouse abuse, for example, that all batterers are mentally ill, can be discussed and accurate information provided.

(continued)

Table 7-4. *(continued)*	
COMPONENT	DESCRIPTION
Conflict Resolution/Problem Solving/Communication Skills	Children from violent homes often lack healthy models of adult relationships. Teaching and modeling assertive (as opposed to aggressive) communication skills, problem solving skills, and other healthy relationship skills are an important step in the process of breaking the cycle of violence
Symptom Reduction	In addition to needing emotional support, increased coping and safety skills, and preventive interventions, many children exposed to domestic violence will also need relief from specific symptoms that result from exposure to violence such as insomnia, nightmares, depression, anxiety, and other post-traumatic stress (PTSD) symptoms.
Increasing Safety and Stability	Typical small group interventions with children include problem solving various ways to handle "unsafe" situations and identifying or role-playing ways to stay safe while parents are fighting (ie, going to neighbors, calling the police)
Dealing with Repeated Separations	Discussing how the children have dealt with other separations and stresses in their lives and encouraging them to focus on the positive aspects of their experiences and relationships helps terminate the group on a positive note

Adapted from http://www.uic.edu/orgs. Permission granted from author: Schewe PA. Interventions for children exposed to domestic violence. The Community Psychologist. 2004;37(4)31-34.

[a] *Peled E, Jaffe PG, Edleson JL. Ending the Cycle of Violence: Community Responses to Children of Battered Women. Thousand Oaks, CA: Sage Publications; 1994.*

[b] *Grusznski RJ, Brink JC, Edleson JL. Support and education groups for children of battered women. Child Welfare. 1998;67:431-444.*

[c] *Wilson SK, Cameron S, Jaffe P, et al. Children exposed to wife abuse: an intervention model. Soc Casework: J Contemp Soc Work. 1989;70(3):180-184.*

Poor academic performance can be a result of school absenteeism or school suspension or expulsion caused by behavioral problems. Kernic and colleagues found that children exposed to domestic violence or child abuse were more likely to have significant school absenteeism and were twice as likely to have been suspended from school for disruptive, delinquent, or aggressive behaviors.[29] This study also found that speech delay, as manifested by speech pathology referrals, was seven times more likely in IPV-exposed children than in those not exposed to IPV. Huth-Bocks and colleagues also found that children who witnessed domestic violence had poorer verbal abilities than nonwitnesses.[30] This difference was thought to be caused in part by maternal depression and a poorer intellectual environment in these homes. Children exposed to domestic violence also exhibit problems with their ability to concentrate, stay on task, and complete their work.[6] All of these behaviors interfere with academic success. Children may also present with common pediatric complaints (eg, chronic headache, chronic abdominal pain, sleep disturbances, vomiting), which may actually be a somatic manifestation of their stress from exposure to violence.

Adolescents experience a wide range of responses to the violence. They may experience extreme guilt from their perceived inability to protect their mother. They may experience shame and betrayal. Adolescents may become aggressive, and may exhibit high-risk behaviors such as drug use, sexual promiscuity, truancy, or running away from home. They may also lose impulse control, which can be deadly if there are lethal weapons available in the home.

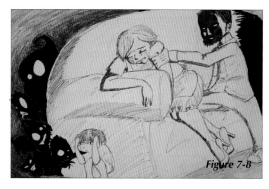

One of the most debilitating mental health disorders that occur with exposure to violence is PTSD. The symptoms of PTSD in children include recurring intrusive recollection of the traumatic event, persistent avoidance of stimuli that recreate the traumatic event, a numbing of the general normal physiological response to trauma, and hyperarousal. These physiological conditions are expressed in children as anxiety, social withdrawal, depression, sleep problems, and impulsivity. Many children who may be suffering from PTSD are misdiagnosed with attention deficit hyperactivity disorder (ADHD), conduct disorders, mood disorders, or anxiety disorders.[31] Studies demonstrate that 19%-50% of children who witnessed abuse of their mothers had clinical criteria consistent with PTSD.[32,33]

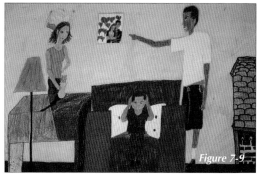

The ongoing Adverse Childhood Experiences (ACE) Study provides a powerful link between exposure to violence during childhood (either child abuse or IPV) and long-term health consequences experienced in adulthood. Felitti and colleagues showed an association between adverse childhood experiences, defined as experiences during childhood of personal abuse (ie, psychological, physical, sexual abuse) or household dysfunction (ie, adult in home abused drugs/alcohol, had mental illness, was a victim of IPV, was incarcerated), to many of the leading causes of illness and death in adulthood, including obesity, diabetes, pulmonary disease and cardiac disease.[34] Felitti and colleagues concluded that these adverse experiences in childhood had a strong and cumulative effect on adult health.[34] This impact on adult health is believed to be caused by the adoption of poor health habits (eg, smoking, drinking, drug use, overeating, sexual promiscuity). Felitti and colleagues found that adults used these behaviors as ways to cope with these stressful events that had occurred, in most cases, half a century ago.[34] **Figure 7-11** graphically represents the interrelationship between the exposure to adverse childhood experiences such as child abuse or exposure to IPV and subsequent poor adult health recognized in the ACE studies.

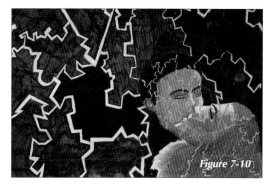

Figure 7-8. *A high school freshman's drawing of monsters that lurk around the corner of the couch behind which a child hides to escape an abusive scene.*

Figure 7-9. *A high school sophomore's drawing of a child covering his ears during a fight.*

Figure 7-10. *A 13-year-old child's drawing of a man and woman kissing in front of a shattered background.*

Figure 7-11. *The ACE Pyramid shows how negative experiences in childhood lead to social, emotional, and cognitive impairments.*

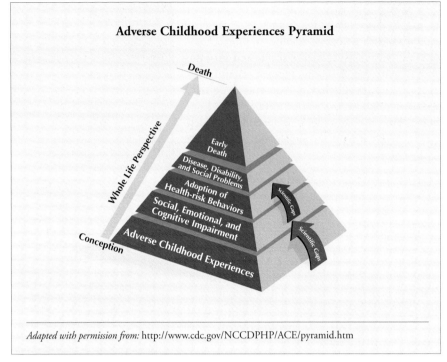

Adapted with permission from: http://www.cdc.gov/NCCDPHP/ACE/pyramid.htm

The ACE Pyramid represents the conceptual framework for the Study. During the time period of the 1980s and early 1990s information about risk factors for disease had been widely researched and merged into public education and prevention programs. However, it was also clear that risk factors, such as smoking, alcohol abuse, and sexual behaviors for many common diseases were not randomly distributed in the population. In fact, it was known that risk factors for many chronic diseases tended to cluster, that is, persons who had one risk factor tended to have one or more others.

EMERGING GLOBAL PERSPECTIVES OF CHILDREN'S EXPOSURE TO ALL FORMS OF VIOLENCE

In the past decade, medical professionals have begun to understand that children are not just unaffected observers of the violence around them but are "silent victims" of the violence they witness.[2] Described as forgotten, unacknowledged, hidden, and unintended victims, these children exposed to violence may suffer significant negative impact on their physical, developmental, and emotional health.[3] **Figures 7-12 to 7-14** are representations of violence witnessed by children.

Throughout the world, children are exposed to all forms of violence (eg, war, media, community, school, home). All levels of violence can create trauma that children need to cope with—there is much debate as to what kinds of violence are more troubling—but clearly, some of the violence that children are exposed to is within our control to end. The UN Secretary General in August of 2006 received an in-depth global study of violence against children by an independent expert, Paolo Sergio Pinheiro.[36] It begins with the observation that no violence against children can be justified and that all violence is preventable. Specifically, Mr. Pinheiro states[36]:

The study should mark a turning point—an end to adult justification of violence against children, whether accepted as 'tradition' or disguised as 'discipline'. There can be no compromise in challenging violence against children. Children's uniqueness—their potential and vulnerability, their dependence on adults—makes it imperative that they have more, not less, protection from violence."

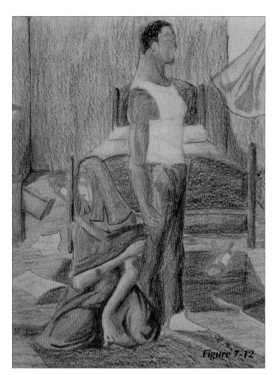

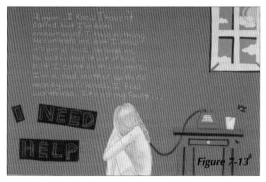

Figure 7-12. *A 14-year-old child's depiction of a man standing over an injured women in a room in disarray.*

Figure 7-13. *Created by a 17-year-old artist, this image displays a woman calling for help.*

Figure 7-14. *A woman grabbed by the hair with smeared, red handprints. The 15-year-old artist included text, some of which reads, "Hello, my name is [censored], but you can call me 'whore,' 'wench,' 'tramp,' 'skank'…"*

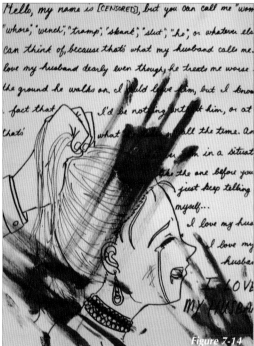

Regretfully, violence in many forms is part of everyday life for many families in all parts of the world, and many children experience that violence daily. Children in troubled areas experience war violence either directly from injury, victimization, or loss of loved ones or indirectly from starvation, homelessness, and disease. In more developed nations where overall social turmoil may be less prevalent, children are nonetheless exposed to both actual and vicarious violence, graphically displayed in various forms of media such as news and entertainment programs, video games, and most recently via the Internet and the World Wide Web.[3,*] Because violence in modern life is increasingly seen as pervasive, children are at risk for witnessing community violence in the many places they frequent. In addition, as discussed throughout this chapter, children are exposed to violence in their homes either as direct recipients of abusive assaults from family members, from witnessing or hearing assaults on their siblings or caregivers, or from observing the aftermath of any of these types of violence. Professionals concerned with the safety, well being, and optimal development of children find themselves concerned with how this exposure to violence affects those they serve.

---

* AAP, 2001, http://aappolicy.aap publica-tions.org/cgi/reprint/pediatrics;108/5/1222.pdf

Table 7-5. Summarizes the UN Report, Taking a Global Perspective, Identifies the Following Range of Violence-Related Issues Facing the World's Children Today

COMPONENT	DESCRIPTION
Homicide	WHO has estimated, through the use of limited country-level data, that almost 53,000 children died worldwide in 2002 as a result of homicide.
Physical Punishment	Studies from many countries worldwide suggest that 80% to 98% of children suffer physical punishment in their homes, with a third or more experiencing severe physical punishment resulting from the use of implements.
Bullying	Reporting on a wide range of developing countries, the Global School-based Health Survey recently found that between 20% and 65% of school-aged children reported having been verbally or physically bullied in the past 30 days. Bullying is also frequent in industrialized countries.
Sexual Violence	WHO estimates that 150 million girls and 73 million boys under 18 experienced forced sexual intercourse or other forms of sexual violence during 2002.
Genital Mutilation	According to a WHO estimate, between 100 and 140 million girls and women in the world have undergone some form of female genital mutilation/cutting. Estimates from UNICEF published in 2005 suggest that in sub-Saharan Africa, Egypt, and Sudan, 3 million girls and women are subjected to genital mutilation/cutting every year.
Child Labor	Recent ILO estimates indicate that, in 2004, 218 million children were involved in child labor, 126 million of whom were subjected to hazardous work. Estimates from 2000 suggest that 5.7 million were in forced or bonded labor, 1.8 million in prostitution and pornography, and 1.2 million were victims of trafficking. Compared with estimates published in 2002, however, the incidence of child labor has diminished by 11%, and 25% fewer children were found working in hazardous occupations.

Adapted from United Nations Report of the Independent Expert for the United Nations Study on Violence Against Children. 2006. Available at: http://www.violencestudy.org/IMG/pdf/English-2-2.pdf. Accessed March 27, 2008.

Table 7-5 summarizes the UN report with a global perspective, identifying the following range of violence-related issues facing the world's children today.[36] Many of the psychiatric and psychological disturbances found in children who witness violence are similar across the different forms of violence to which they are exposed. The common theme emerging from studies of child witnesses to violence shows that the occurrence of anxiety disorders, depression, use of aggression, PTSD, poor academic performance, and symptoms of ADHD are similar among children exposed to violence whether from war trauma[38,39,40]; media exposure[37,41,42]; community violence[43,44,45]; or school violence, including bullying.[46,47,48,49]

THE HEALTH CARE RESPONSE

As we learn more and more about children and violence, the implication for primary care providers who care for children is clear—these issues have to be addressed. The medical community must begin routinely asking patients and their families about their exposure to violence as well as examining and understanding the critical role health professionals play in the response to the issue of IPV. If the cycle of violence is interrupted, then children and families may begin to heal. If we have healthy families, then we will have healthy children.

With so many families impacted by violence, many professional medical, nursing, and social worker organizations and associations have set forth policy statements and guidelines outlining intervention and prevention recommendations (please see **Table 7-6** for a summary of the position statements). The AAP has taken a very active advocacy role in violence detection and prevention because family violence issues are relevant to pediatric medicine. As this chapter has illustrated, violence exposure significantly impacts a child's health and well being, and the symptoms manifested by violence-exposed children overlap with many common pediatric complaints (eg, sleep disturbances, school performance issues, chronic somatic complaints). It has been argued that one of the most effective means of preventing child abuse may be identifying maternal IPV victims.[50]

Pediatricians have a long history of advocating for preventive measures such as the use of car seats and bike helmets and screening for lead, anemia, and tuberculosis. Issues such as disciplinary methods, television viewing, and access to lethal weapons in the home[51] are topics that many pediatricians discuss routinely at well-child visits. Screening for family violence should also be part of the preventive screening discussed with families.

The AAP's Task Force on Violence has set forth recommendations to make children's homes and communities safer.[51] These recommendations include identifying high-risk families, providing violence intervention and prevention counseling, advocating for nonviolent disciplinary methods, reducing exposure of children to media violence, stricter hand-gun laws, increasing funding for prevention programs such as home-visitation programs,[51] and teaching pediatric residents about domestic violence.[14] Martin and colleagues showed that abused women bring their children in for well-child care as often as nonabused women[52]; therefore, the pediatric setting may be an important health care setting to identify IPV victims.

Specifically, regarding pediatrician's response to IPV, the AAP's Committee on Child Abuse and Neglect, has issued guidelines that could guide the response for most health care professionals, including[14]:

— Recognizing that intervention is crucial as children are likely to be victims;

— Attempting to identify evidence of family or IPV in the clinical setting;

— Intervening in a sensitive and skillful manner that prioritizes the safety of women and children who are victimized; and

— Supporting local and national multidisciplinary efforts to identify, treat, and ultimately to prevent family violence and IPV.

Table 7-6 lists a variety of national professional organizations along with IPV guidelines or recommendations.

Table 7-6. Selected Health Care Professional Organizations Positions Regarding Family Violence

GROUP	GUIDELINES AND RECOMMENDATIONS	SOURCE
American Academy of Family Physicians	These guidelines include education, screening, recognition, intervention, and advocacy for victims of IPV and their families	American Academy of Family Physicians. Policy and Advocacy. *Violence Position Paper.* Available at: www.aafp.org. Accessed December 24, 2007
American Academy of Pediatrics (AAP)	The AAP advocates educating residents and pediatricians to identify, intervene, and advocate for victims of family violence and their children.	American Academy of Pediatrics Committee on Child Abuse and Neglect. The role of the pediatrician in recognizing and intervening on behalf of abused women. *Pediatrics.* 1998;101:1091-1092.
American Association of the Colleges of Nursing (AACN)	The AACN recognizes that IPV requires health care interventions. Therefore, the AACN recommends education of nursing students in identifying IPV victims; intervening with violence victims to enhance their safety; and developing cultural competency skills in dealing with violence as a health problem.	www.aacn.org. Accessed February 8, 2008)
American College of Emergency Physicians (ACEP)	Recommends screening patients for IPV because "… The identification and assessment for domestic violence is an important, specialized part of the evaluation of the emergency patient…" The ACEP also recommends educating residents and physicians in the recognition of and intervention and referral for IPV victims.	American College of Emergency Physicians. Policy Compendium 2007. Available at: www.acep.org. Accessed February 9, 2008.

(continued)

Table 7-6. *(continued)*

Group	Guidelines and Recommendations	Source
American College of Obstetrics and Gynecology (ACOG)	ACOG recommends that physicians screen all patients for intimate partner violence.	Available at: www.acog.org. Accessed February 8, 2008.
American Medical Association (AMA)	The AMA asserts that future physicians need to be competent in identifying and appropriately intervening with IPV victims and assessing the safety of violence victims and their families	American Medical Association. *H-515.965 - Family and Intimate Partner Violence - Policy Statement.* Available at: www.ama-assn.org. Accessed December 24, 2007.
American Psychiatric Association (APA)	The APA recommends that its members learn about the prevention of domestic violence; participate in the development and implementation of protocols for identifying and assessing victims of family violence; and advocate on the behalf of violence victims at the state, local, and national levels.	American Psychiatric Association. *Domestic Violence Position Statement.* APA Document Reference No. 200111. 2001. Available at: www.psych.org. Accessed February 8, 2008.
National Association of Social Workers (NASW)	NASW supports the education of social workers in addressing and advocating for victims of family violence.	Available at: www.socialworkers.org. Accessed February 8, 2008.

Conclusion

The message is clear —children's exposure to IPV places their normal development and well being at significant risk. The prevention of violence will require enhanced awareness, committed effort, and education at all levels—the education of families, communities, and the society at large as well as professionals who are best positioned to identify and assist IPV victims. Education of health care professionals includes making family violence curriculum part of the core curriculum taught in the various professional schools, teaching entry level as well as advanced practitioners by example about how to recognize victims of violence and how to intervene on their behalf, and the development of advocacy courses in professional schools and advanced training programs to provide the skills and tools that will enable health care providers to be effective in dealing with this pervasive problem. Health care professionals have to convey the message that "violence is not okay." The various health care disciplines need to join forces with community advocates to change the way that society views violence within the family and clearly establish that violence is unacceptable.

REFERENCES

1. Groves BM, Zuckerman B, Marans G, Cohen DJ. Silent victims. Children who witness violence. *JAMA*. 1993; 269:262-264.

2. Kempe CH, Silverman FN, Steele BF, Droegemueller W, Silver HK. The battered-child syndrome. *JAMA*. 1962; 181:17-24.

3. Holden GW, Geffner RA, Jouriles EN, eds. *Children Exposed to Marital Violence: Theory, Research and Applied Issues*. Washington, DC: American Psychological Association; 1998.

4. Carlson BE. Children exposed to intimate partner violence: Research findings and implications for intervention. *Trauma, Violence, and Abuse*. 2000; 1:321-340.

5. Groves BM. *Children Who See Too Much: Lessons from the Child Witness to Violence Project*. Boston, MA: Beacon Press; 2002.

6. Fantuzzo F, Mohr W. (1999). Prevalence and effects of child exposure to domestic violence. *Dom Viol Child* [serial online]. 1999; 9:21-31. Available at: www.futureofchildren.org. Accessed June 4, 2008.

7. The Commonwealth Fund. *Health Concerns Across a Woman's Lifespan: 1998 Survey of Women's Health*. New York, NY: The Commonwealth Fund. May 1999.

8. *State of the World's Children 2000*. New York, NY: UNICEF; 2000.

9. US Dept of Justice. *Violence by Intimates: Analysis of Data on Crimes by Current of Former Spouses, Boyfriends, and Girlfriends*. Washington, DC; U.S.Dept. of Justice, Bureau of Justice Statistics. March 1998.

10. Carlson BE. Children's observations of interparental violence. In: Roberts AR, ed. *Battered Women and Their Families*. New York, NY: Springer; 1984:147-167.

11. Straus M. Children as witnesses to marital violence: a risk factor for lifelong problems among a nationally representative sample of American men and women. In: Schwartz DF, ed. *Children and Violence: Report of the Twenty-third Ross Roundtable on Critical Approaches to Common Pediatric Problems*. Columbus, OH: Ross Laboratories; 1992:98-104.

12. US Dept of Health and Human Services. Children's Bureau, Administration on Children, Youth Families. Administration for Children and Families. National Clearing House on Child Abuse and Neglect Information. *In Harm's Way: Domestic Violence and Child Maltreatment*. Available at: http://www.calib.com/dvcps/facts/harmway.doc. Accessed March 27, 2008.

13. Child Protection Section. Stop the Violence Campaign. *Behind Closed Doors: The Impact of Domestic Violence on Children*. New York, NY: UNICEF, Child Protection Section; 2006.

14. American Academy of Pediatrics. Committee on Child Abuse and Neglect. The role of the pediatrician in recognizing and intervening on the behalf of abused women. *Pediatrics*. 1998; 101:1091-1092. (Reaffirmed 2004; 114:1126.)

15. Ganley AL, Schechter S. *Domestic Violence: A National Curriculum for Children's Protective Services*. San Francisco, CA: Family Violence Prevention Fund; 1996.

16. Edelson JL. Children's witnessing of adult domestic violence. *J Interpers Violence*. 1999;14(8):839-870.

17. Edleson JL. The overlap between child maltreatment and woman battering. *Violence Against Women*. 1999; 5:135-154.

18. Appel AE, Holden GW. The co-occurrence of spouse and physical child abuse: a review and appraisal. *J Fam Psychol*. 1998; 12:578-599.

19. Christian CW, Scribano P, Seidl T, Pinto-Martin JA. Pediatric injury resulting from family violence. *Pediatrics*. 1997; 99:E8.

20. English DJ, Marshall DB, Stewart AJ. Effects of family violence on child behavior and health during early childhood. *J Fam Violence*. 2003; 18:43-57.

21. Edleson JL. The Overlap Between Child Maltreatment and Woman Abuse: National Electronic Network on Violence Against Women; 1999. http://new.vawnet.org/category/Main_Doc.php?docid=389. Accessed June 22, 2008.

22. Edelson JL, Mbilinyi LF, Beeman SK, Hagemeister AK. How children are involved in adult domestic violence—results from a four-city telephone survey. *J Interpers Violence*. 2003; 18:18-32.

23. Zink T, Elder N, Jacobson J. How children affect the mother/victim's process in intimate partner violence. *Arch Pediatr Adolesc Med*. 2003; 157:587-592.

24. Schecter S, Edleson JL. In the best interest of women and children: a call for collaboration between child welfare and domestic violence constituencies. *Prevention Report*; 1995. Available at: http://www.mincava.umn.edu/papers/wingsp.htm. Accessed October 2005.

25. Bancroft L, Silverman JG. Risks to children from batterers. In: Bancroft L, Silverman JG, eds. *The Batterer as Parent*. Thousand Oaks, CA: Sage Publications Inc. Books; 2002:29-83.

26. Kitzmann K, Gaylord N, Holt A, Kenny E. Child witness to domestic violence: a meta-analytic review. *J Consult Clin Psychol*. 2003; 71:339-352.

27. Knapp JF. Violence among children and adolescents—the impact of children witnessing violence. *Pedia Clin N Am*. 1998; 45:355-364.

28. McFarlane JM, Groff JY, O'Brien JA, Watson K. Behaviors of children who are exposed and not exposed to intimate partner violence: an analysis of 330 Black, White, and Hispanic children. *Pediatrics*. 2003; 112:e202-e207.

29. Kernic MA, Holt VL, Wolf ME, McKnight B, Huebner CE, Rivara FP. Academic and school health issues among children exposed to maternal intimate partner abuse. *Arch Pediat Adolesc*. 2002; 156:549-555.

30. Huth-Bocks AC, Levendosky AA, Semel MA. The direct and indirect effects of domestic violence on young children's intellectual functioning. *J Fam Violence*. 2001; 16: 269-290.

31. LaCerva V. Teaching violence prevention: A critical role for medication education. In: Hamberger LK, Burge SK, Grahma AV, Costa AJ, eds. *Violence Issues for Health Care Educators and Providers*. New York, NY: The Haworth Press; 1997:11-31.

32. McCloskey LA, Walker M. Posttraumatic stress in children exposed to family violence and single-event trauma. *J Am Acad Child Adolesc Psychiatry*. 2000; 39:108-115.

33. Lehmann P. The development of posttraumatic stress disorder (PTSD) in a sample of child witnesses to mother assault. *J Fam Violence*. 1997; 12:241-257.

34. Felitti VJ, Anda RF, Nordenberg D, Williamson DF, Spitz AM, Edwards V, Koss MP, Marks JS. Relationship of childhood abuse and household dysfunction to many of the leading causes of death in adults—the Adverse Childhood Experiences (ACE) Study. *Am J Prev Med*. 1998 ;14:245-258.

35. US Dept of Health and Human Services, Center for Disease Control and Prevention. *Ace Childhood Experiences Study*. Available at: http://www.cdc.gov/NCCDPHP/ACE/Pyramid.HTM. Accessed April 2, 2008.

36. United Nations. *United Nations Report of the Independent Expert for the United Nations Study on Violence Against Children*. 2006. Available at: http://www.violencestudy.org/IMG/pdf/English-2-2.pdf. Accessed March 27, 2008.

37. American Academy of Pediatrics. Committee on Public Education. Media violence. *Pediatrics*. 2001;108:1222-1226. Available at: http://aappolicy.aappublications.org/cgi/reprint/pediatrics;108/5/1222.pdf. Accessed April 2, 2008.

38. Kinzie JD, Sack WH, Angell RH, Manson S, Rath B. The psychiatric effects of massive trauma on Cambodian children. I. The children. *J Am Acad Child Adolesc Psychiatry*. 1986; 25:370-376.

39. Goldstein RD, Wampler NS, Wise PH. War experiences and distress symptoms of Bosnian children. *Pediatrics*. 1997; 100:873-878.

40. Allwood MA, Bell-Dolan D, Husain SA. Children's trauma and adjustment reactions to violent and nonviolent war experiences. *J Am Acad Child Adolesc Psychiatry*. 2002; 41:450-457.

41. Robinson TN, Wilde ML, Navracruz LC, Haydel F, Varady A. Effects of reducing children's television and video game use on aggressive behavior: a randomized controlled trial. *Arch Pediatr Adolesc Med*. 2001; 155:17-23.

42. American Psychological Association. I*s Youth Violence Just Another Fact of Life?* Available at: http://www.apa.org/ppo/issues/pbviolence.html. Accessed October 2005.

43. Hurt H, Malmud E, Brodsyy NL, Giannetta J. Exposure to violence—psychological and academic correlates in child witnesses. *Arch Pediatr Adolesc Med*. 2001; 155:1351-1356.

44. Schwab-Stone ME, Ayers TS, Kasprow W, Voyce C, Barone C, Shiver T, Weissberg RP. No safe haven: a study of violence exposure in an urban community. *J Am Acad Child Adolesc Psychiatry*. 1995 ;34:1343-1352.

45. Delaney-Black V, Covington C, Ondersma SJ, Nordstrom-Klee B, Templin T, Ager J, Janisee J, Sokol RJ. Violence exposure, trauma and IQ and/or reading deficits among urban children. *Arch Pediatr Adolesc Med*. 2002; 156:280-285.

46. Nansel TR, Overpeck MD, Haynie DL, Ruan WJ, Scheidt PC. Relationships between bullying and violence among US youth. *Arch Pediatr Adolesc Med*. 2003;157:348-353.

47. Saluja G, Iachan R, Scheidt PC, Overpeck MD, Sun W, Giedd JN. Prevalence of and risk factors for depressive symptoms among young adolescents. *Arch Pediatr Adolesc Med*. 2004; 158:760-765.

48. Nansel TR, Craig W, Overpeck MD, Saluja G, Ruan WJ, Health Behaviour in School-aged Children Bullying Analyses Working Group. Cross-national consistency in the relationship between bullying behaviors and psychosocial adjustment. *Arch Pediatr Adolesc Med*. 2004; 158:730-736.

49. Nansel TR, Overpeck M, Pilla RS, Ruan WJ, Simons-Morton B, Scheidt P. Bullying behaviors among US youth: prevalence and association with psychosocial adjustment. *JAMA*. 2001; 285:2094-2100.

50. Wright RJ, Wright RO, Isaac NE. Response to battered mothers in the emergency department: A call for an interdisciplinary approach to family violence. *Pediatrics*. 1997; 99:186-192.

51. American Academy of Pediatrics. Task Force on Violence. The role of the pediatrician in youth violence prevention in clinical practice and at the community level. *Pediatrics*. 1999; 103:173-181.

52. Martin SL, Mackie L, Kupper L, Buescher PA, Moracco KE. Physical abuse of women before, during and after pregnancy. *JAMA*. 2001; 285:1581-1584

Chapter 8

THE SEXUAL ASSAULT NURSE EXAMINER RESPONSE TO NON-STRANGER SEXUAL ASSAULT

Linda Ledray, PhD, SANE

Sexual assault is rarely a stranger attacking an unknown victim. Rape victims are far more likely to be assaulted by someone they know and trust, that is, someone with whom they feel comfortable and safe. Oftentimes, victims are attacked by a significant other (eg, husband, boyfriend, or partner). Until 1980, states did not recognize rape by a marital partner as a crime. Previously, sex was considered the "right" of a husband and the "obligation" of a wife. During the early 1980s, states began to eliminate the marital exceptions to their rape laws and included marital rape as a crime against the state. It wasn't until 1993, however, that every state included marital rape as a crime under all circumstances.[1]

The first sexual assault nurse examiner (SANE) programs were developed in Memphis, Tennessee in 1976[2]; in Minneapolis, Minnesota in 1977[3]; and in Amarillo, Texas in 1979.[4] The success of these initial programs provided better care to victims, which resulted in the development of additional SANE programs throughout the United States. Before the development of SANE programs, sexual assault victims waited in emergency department waiting rooms for as many as 12 hours while other patients with "more serious" wounds received priority treatment. Nurses frustrated by the long delays in treatment for sexual assault victims developed many of the early SANE programs.

At this time, medical staff members were often hesitant to collect evidence of sexual assault, because they did not want to be called to testify if the case went to trial. In addition, victims were often assessed by health care providers who were not trained in forensic evidence collection or in addressing the specialized needs of these victims. Evidence collected was often inadequate, the chain-of-custody was not maintained, and the victims often received incomplete medical care. For example, health care providers did not tend to offer rape victims emergency contraception or antibiotics to prevent sexually transmitted diseases (STDs).[5]

Much as the acknowledgement of marital rape and acquaintance rape as a crime has changed laws in the United States and the response to victims of intimate partner violence (IPV), so too has the development of SANE programs and sexual assault response teams (SARTs) improved forensic evidence collection and clinical care for victims of rape. While the team members that make up a SART may vary depending upon community resources, most teams include the SANE or specially trained medical professional, law enforcement officer, prosecutor, rape crisis center advocate, and crime laboratory specialist. Some SARTs also include a domestic violence advocate, chaplain, social worker, or mental health professional.

As the benefits of the SANE-SART model became more clearly demonstrated, rape crisis centers, law enforcement departments, and community groups became more active in SART program development. Since 2000, these community groups have been a driving force in SANE-SART program development.[6]

Today an estimated 1 in 5 adult victims report rape to law enforcement officers. Though the rate of reported rapes remains relatively low, those who do report are 9 times more likely to receive medical care than those who do not report the rape.[7] In the mid 1980s, after rape crisis centers across the United States made a concerted effort to educate women that non-stranger rape was a reportable crime, acquaintance rape was reported more often than stranger rape for the first time. This trend continues today as between 70% and 80% of reported rapes occur with a non-stranger.[8] Despite this continued trend, the better the victim knows her assailant, the less likely she is to report the rape, which suggests that non-stranger rape, especially intimate partner rape, is still likely to be significantly under reported.[9-11] Datner, Asher, and Rubin indicate reported rates of intimate partner sexual assault vary from a low of 7.7% in a national survey of women to a high of 55% of a smaller sample of women seeking help for IPV.[1]

This chapter focuses on non-stranger sexual assault and IPV. Thus, an obvious question is, "Does the relationship of the offender to the victim change the response of the SANE?" (Or perhaps, "should it change the response?") This chapter will discuss these questions and make recommendations for the SANE response.

ADEQUACY OF THE CURRENT RESPONSE TO SEXUAL ASSAULT

In the emergency department, there are two distinct and interconnected overall focuses in the care of sexual assault victims: 1) the clinical or medical evaluation and treatment of the victim and 2) forensic evidence collection. In order to adequately meet the needs of sexual assault victims, health care providers must effectively address both aspects. Before the development of the SART model, health care providers focused on the clinical needs of victims, while law enforcement officers and prosecutors focused on evidence collection. These groups worked independently and did not recognize that, by collaborating, they could better meet their own goals, as well as the needs of the rape victims.[12,13]

Unfortunately, with fewer than 500 identified SANE programs across the United States, most sexual assault examinations are still completed by untrained medical personnel. All too often, they work in isolation and read the directions for evidence collection while actually collecting the evidence.[14,15]

With the current advances in DNA recovery, it is no longer possible to collect all the evidence available on the victims body by simply reading and following the directions on the sexual assault evidentiary examination kit. With the implementation of the Combined DNA Index System (CODIS) established by the Federal Bureau of Investigation (FBI) used to identify repeat offenders throughout the United States through recovered biological samples, the collection of all possible evidence has become even more crucial. Every day, SANE nurses literally "think outside the box" and collect evidence that would have been missed had they simply followed the evidence collection kit's directions. Time and time again such additional evidence has played a key role in identifying serial rapists who otherwise would have gone undetected.

SANE-SART PROGRAM IMPACT

Researchers are only beginning to scientifically evaluate the effectiveness of the SANE programs. Initial studies indicate that SANE programs do a significantly better job of collecting the proper evidence and maintaining chain of custody of that evidence once the evidence is collected,[16] of providing immediate crisis intervention and emotional support for victims, and of increasing police reporting rates.[5,17] In addition, SANE programs effectively increased the rate of guilty pleas[2,18] and increased community prosecution rates.[17] Many people had initially feared that either clinical care of victims (ie, medical and psychological care) or the collection of forensic evidence and ability to prosecute would suffer if the other aspect improved, yet research shows that both aspects have improved.[12,17,19,20] By working as a team, the SART members, SANEs, victim's advocates, law enforcement officers, prosecutors, and crime laboratory specialists have better met both the forensic and clinical needs of victims and the systems.

The SANE model has supported advances in prosecution in 2 ways:

1. Better evidence collection

2. The ability to effectively testify in court

Though certainly important, better collection of evidence is not the most important role that the SANE plays. In fact, evidence collection involves much more than merely obtaining the evidence. Proper evidence collection includes knowing the following:

— What evidence to collect

— How to properly collect the evidence

— How to properly document the evidence collected in terms understood by law enforcement officers, prosecutors, and jury members

— How to maintain proper chain-of-custody to ensure that the evidence will be admissible in court

— How to either effectively testify about the significance of the evidence collected or explain why evidence was not found

In order to do all of this, the SANE needs to know when and what evidence will likely be available for collection. The case presented later about anal sperm evidence underscores the importance of a SANE's ability to relate the time when evidence is available and explain when evidence is not available.

Unfortunately, even with the implementation of SANE-SART programs, few examiners systematically track the results of the evidence they collect. Feedback from the crime laboratory about the evidence collection results is essential for SANEs to improve their evidence collection skills and more effectively testify in court regarding the evidence collected or not found.

Understanding the importance of the SANE's role the Sexual Assault Resource Service (SARS) in Minneapolis obtained funding to develop a national database for SANEs. This database encourages SANEs to collect and share vital information.[14] In November 2005, the West Virginia State Police worked closely with the West Virginia Foundation for Rape Information and Service to initiate the first statewide data-tracking and feedback system for sexual assault evidence.[21,22] Within the West Virginian system, each sexual assault evidence collection kit is coded. The SANE enters this code into the computer with the basic victim information. Once the evidence is processed, the SANE who collected the evidence can log onto the secure computer site and see the results of the collected evidence. Soon, SANEs will be able to track the case's progress through the court system with this tracking system, too.

PROTOCOL STANDARDIZATION

Significant advances continue to be made in standardizing the sexual assault protocols for evidence collection. In 1987, California was the first state to standardize these protocols.[23] Though other states have followed California's example, significant variation remains regarding the type of evidence collected and the way in which evidence is collected even within the same state. Nationally, the first attempt to standardize the protocols came from the American College of Emergency Physicians,[24] the Association of Genitourinary Medicine, and the Medical Society for the Study of Venereal Diseases when they established guidelines for the management of sexual assault survivors. In September 2004, the Office on Violence Against Women released *A National Protocol for Sexual Assault Medical Forensic Examinations*.[25] While the development of this protocol was a monumental task and has added substantially to the sexual assault field, the protocol remains only a guide for suggested practice rather than a requirement and does not supersede existing protocols. In addition, this protocol was met with immediate, harsh criticism from experts, organizations, and the media for the way it addressed sexually transmitted infections (STI) and for the lack of information provided regarding emergency contraception.

Institutional, state, and national protocols vary considerably regarding the specifics of what evidence to collect, the way to collect the evidence, and even the time frame for evidence collection. Most protocols recommend the completion of an evidentiary examination for up to 72 hours or 96 hours after a sexual assault occurs.[5,24,25] Examinations occurring after this 72 or 96 hour deadline are also recommended in cases that include documentable injuries, or when a survivor has not changed clothes or showered, which means that evidence may still be available for collection.

Though SANE-SART programs have advanced the care of sexual assault victims and helped prosecute offenders, health care professionals without proper evidence collection training still care for most rape victims. This means that though the model of care has been advanced, sufficient progress has not been made in making the model accessible to victims across the United States. The US Joint Armed Services is in the process of rapidly changing this for military personnel. As a result of recommendations from the Joint Armed Service Task Force, military rape victims are now cared for by SARTs.[26] As a result of this effort, the military community will likely rapidly surpass civilian medical facilities in providing widespread access to state-of-the-art care for rape victims.

USE OF EVIDENCE

When assessing how the victim's relationship to the offender may impact the importance of the collected evidence, understanding what evidence the SANE collects and how the evidence is used becomes essential. Evidentiary examination of the sexual assault survivor includes evidence collected for the following 4 purposes[5,27]:

1. Evidence to identify the assailant

2. Evidence to confirm recent sexual contact

3. Evidence to show force, coercion, or lack of consent

4. Evidence to corroborate or refute the survivor's history of the assault

EVIDENCE TO IDENTIFY THE ASSAILANT

In cases of intimate partner sexual assault the identity of the assailant is clearly not the issue. An exception may be drug-facilitated sexual assault (DFSA), because the victim is unsure whether and by whom she has been assaulted. Today the primary evidence used to identify an unknown assailant is DNA, which can also help link a known assailant to other sexual crimes when that DNA evidence is entered into the Combined DNA Index System (CODIS). States that do not run DNA in known cases miss this opportunity, however.

The Importance of DNA Evidence

Arguably the typing of DNA from biological specimens may be the most important advance in forensic science in the 20th Century. The evidence from DNA samples can be used to identify an unknown assailant, corroborate the identity of a suspect, and exonerate the falsely accused.

In 1987, the first man was convicted of sexual assault with the help of DNA evidence. The case was upheld upon appeal the following year.[28] In 1991, the Minnesota Bureau of Criminal Apprehension Laboratory became the first state crime laboratory to identify a suspect on the basis of DNA evidence alone. As a result of this valuable investigative resource, an otherwise unidentified rapist was found and convicted.[29] More recently, in West Virginia, a suspect was arrested after a positive eyewitness identification, but later released when his DNA did not match the biological evidence collected from the victim. Despite a positive eyewitness identification, West Virginia judicial policy mandates that DNA evidence must always be entered into the CODIS system. In this case, when the DNA evidence was entered into the CODIS system, the DNA matched a man serving a prison term in an out-of-state prison. While out of prison briefly, this man visited a relative who lived blocks away from the victim's residence. He also looked nearly identical to the man initially arrested for the crime.[19]

The Combined DNA Index System

The recognition of DNA as a valuable investigative tool and the knowledge that many rapists are repeat offenders led to the development of CODIS by the FBI. This system serves as a national DNA database used to identify assailants who move from state to state.[30] In fact, every state participates in CODIS and, as of 2007, CODIS has matched 45 400 forensic, biological specimens obtained from victims to offender profiles (referred to as ***forensic hits***) and has aided 46 300 investigations.[31]

The Expansion of DNA Testing

The federal DNA Identification Act, included in the 1994 Crime Bill, allocated $40 million to expand DNA testing capabilities nationally. Since that time, millions of additional dollars have been allocated to assist crime laboratories with DNA analysis of backlogged cases. These databases are used for "DNA fingerprinting" in much the same way as conventional fingerprint databases were once used, but with much greater specificity. As previously mentioned, genetic profiles found in body fluids and other biological evidence are used to link serial cases, identify offenders of multiple assaults, and exonerate falsely accused suspects.[29]

Initially only nuclear DNA markers were used for comparison of forensic evidence collected to suspect data; however, since 1996, mitochondrial DNA (mtDNA) also provides valuable additional information. Mitochondrial DNA helps in cases in which the biological evidence may be degraded or in a very small quantity. The technology based upon the polymerase chain reaction (PCR) can create many copies of the DNA for additional analysis so that very small samples of biological evidence can help solve crimes.

An assailant's DNA can be obtained from any cell with a nucleus (eg, hair, blood, saliva, perspiration, semen). Such evidence may have remained on the survivor's body or clothing. Since the newer, PCR-based technology can test much smaller samples, specimens are more easily susceptible to contamination, making it even more important that the SANE use impeccable care in evidence collection to avoid specimen contamination.

Very impressive and convincing population frequency estimates are also available for nuclear DNA. These estimates suggest the likelihood that an offender is someone other than the person identified through the DNA analysis is, in some cases, one in more than 200 million.[32]

The once primarily relied upon restriction fragment length polymorphism (RFLP) method of DNA analysis requires a comparatively large quantity of good-quality DNA. In fact, this method requires approximately 100 000 or more cells that have not been degraded. The RFLP method isolates DNA fragments by using a protein called a restriction enzyme. The DNA fragments are then separated by their relative length, which varies distinctly from person to person. The result is visualized as a series of bands on film. A suspect's DNA pattern is then compared to evidence collected from the survivor. Because of the large sample size required, small samples are unsuitable for RFLP testing procedures, but now these can be tested using the PCR technique.

In contrast, PCR testing of nuclear DNA can be completed on samples as small as 50 cells (ie, the size of a dot of blood or a single hair root). This method can also be used effectively with degraded or damaged samples. With PCR testing, specific regions of the DNA sample are copied using an enzyme. Both RFLP and PCR testing procedures are generally accepted as valid in the scientific community; that is, they meet the Frye test and are admissible in a court of law.[33]

Evidence Collection

The SANE can obtain potential DNA evidence by collecting any possible biological specimen from the survivor's skin that could be from the assailant (eg, saliva from a bite mark or any other area of oral contact, perspiration, hair, or blood). To best collect skin specimens, slightly moisten a cotton swab with a couple of drops of sterile water and then firmly swab the suspected area in a circular motion. The SANE should also collect any clothing that could contain these specimens. Each specimen should be properly labeled and described (eg, "saliva") in order to assist the laboratory technicians as they fully analyze the specimen. The forensic examiner should always err on the side of collecting skin specimens wherever the survivor reports oral contact or possible semen deposits, even if the alternate light source reading is negative. While an alternate light source can help identify skin specimens, history is the most accurate guide.[5] If the location of the specimen is wet when the clothing is collected, the SANE should circle the wet spot with a marker, being careful to stay outside the specimen area. This will help the crime laboratory technicians locate the specimen.

If the survivor reports that she scratched the assailant, the SANE should also collect fingernail swabs in hopes of obtaining the assailant's blood or cells. Samples of DNA can also be obtained by swabbing the involved orifices with a standard-size, cotton-tip swab to collect sperm and seminal fluid.[29] In addition, when the SANE completes the evidentiary examination, DNA evidence must be collected from the survivor to distinguish her DNA from that of her assailant. Most states now request buccal swabs of the inside of the victim's mouth, except in cases of oral assault. In cases in which the assailant's DNA may contaminate the victim's oral specimen, the SANE should still collect the victim's blood.

EVIDENCE TO CONFIRM RECENT SEXUAL CONTACT

Important evidence used to verify that recent sexual contact has occurred includes the identification of trauma to an orifice that the victim indicates was involved in the assault, and by semen obtained from that orifice or from the victim's skin or clothing. In non-stranger sexual assault cases, proof of recent sexual contact is usually not helpful, because even if the known assailant initially claims that sexual contact did not occur with the victim, if proof of recent sexual contact is obtained, the assailant may then change his defense to "consent."

In addition to helping identify or confirm an assailant's identity through the recovery of DNA, semen can also help prove that recent sexual contact occurred; however, the absence of positive sperm or seminal fluid findings does not prove that sexual intercourse did not recently occur.[34] Evidence suggests that at least 34% of rapists are sexually dysfunctional,[35] and 40% or more wear condoms.[36] Seminal fluid evidence may be analyzed for sperm, motile (ie, live sperm that moves when observed under a microscope) or non-motile sperm, and acid-phosphatase (AP). This enzyme is present in large quantities in seminal fluid and in minimal concentrations in vaginal fluids, so if a high level of AP is collected in a sexual assault survivor, this indicates that recent sexual contact has occurred. Cases are typically negative for sperm and positive for AP when the assailant had a vasectomy or is a chronic alcoholic.[37] Unfortunately, few studies have been conducted regarding the results of sexual assault examinations and the likelihood of obtaining specimens positive for sperm or AP. Today, the presence of AP is used to determine whether sufficient biological evidence to determine the DNA of the assailant is likely to exist.

In one study in which the results of 1007 rape survivors were examined, sperm was found in only 1% (n=3) of the 369 cases involving oral rape. All of the positive oral specimens were collected within 3 hours of the rape. Of the 210 cases with anal involvement, only 2% (n=4) were positive for sperm. These examinations were completed within 5 hours of the rape. In the 111 skin specimens collected, 11% (n=12) were positive. All but two of the positive specimens were collected within 5 hours of the rape. Of the 919 vaginal specimens, 34% (n=317) were positive. Of these, 263 women were examined within 5 hours and 317 women were examined within 12 hours of the rape. Only 7 of these positive specimens were collected more than 20 hours after the rape.[34]

The information collected in this study regarding the questions of when and from what orifices biological evidence can be collected helped obtain a guilty plea in a Hennepin County, Minnesota case. Five hours after being anally raped by her boyfriend, a victim came to Hennepin County Medical Center. The examining SANE found an anal tear. Laboratory results also indicated that sperm was recovered from the anus. Both the victim and her boyfriend stated that they had engaged in consenting anal intercourse 48 hours before the rape. The defendant was claiming that the tear and sperm were from this earlier sexual contact and denied any sexual contact after that time. When the prosecutor called to discuss the case shortly before going to trial, he wanted to know whether the injury could have been present 48 hours later. Though unlikely, this was possible. However, the SANE also informed the prosecutor that evidence showed that this sperm was recovered 5 hours after a rape from the anal area. The prosecutor then called the defense attorney, and within hours the assailant pled guilty.

EVIDENCE TO SHOW FORCE, COERCION, OR LACK OF CONSENT

In non-stranger sexual assaults, "consent" is likely the primary defense. In such cases, proof of force, coercion, or lack of consent becomes the most important evidence to disprove this allegation. Such evidence includes the victim's statements, especially quotes of what she told the SANE since these quotes may indicate whether she was afraid, whether she feared for her safety, or indicate the reason she did not fight back if, indeed, she did not do so. Physical injuries, both genital and non-genital, will likely become the most important evidence used to disprove this defense. When DFSA is suspected, other important evidence includes urine and blood evidence showing whether she was too intoxicated to consent or given a drug to facilitate the sexual assault.

Drug-Facilitated Sexual Assault

While alcohol has long been used to facilitate sexual assaults, today assailants use newer, memory-erasing drugs such as flunitrazepam (Rohypnol), other benzodiadepines, ketamine, gamma hydroxybutyrate (GHB), gamma butyrolactone (GBL), and many others to facilitate sexual assaults. Symptoms of DFSA include a victim's recollection of having only a couple of alcoholic beverages but quickly becoming extremely intoxicated. The survivor may remember very little of the incident other than flashes (sometimes referred to as *cameo appearances*) until she awakens. Upon waking, she may find herself undressed or partially dressed with vaginal or anal soreness, making her believe she has been raped.[5] Even though the survivor may have little memory and perhaps no certainty of a sexual assault, whenever the survivor's story remains consistent with a DFSA or suspicious of one, the forensic examiner should collect blood and urine specimen for DFSA analysis as a part of the sexual assault evidentiary examination. If the survivor calls before coming to the hospital or clinic, she should be told not to void unless necessary; if she must void, she should collect her first voided urine in a clean container and bring this container with her to the hospital or clinic.[5,24] Most experts recommend collecting urine for 72 hours after the assault, while others recommend collection for as long as 96 hours. In addition, experts recommend the collection of blood for 24 hours after the assault, because after 24 hours these drugs are not present at identifiable levels in the blood.[5,24,38]

Physical Injuries

Though most studies indicate that significant physical injury requiring medical treatment is extremely rare during a sexual assault (ie, between 3% and 5% across the studies[5,18,34]), both genital and non-genital physical injuries are probably the best proof of force and always need to be photographed, documented on body drawings, and described in writing on the sexual assault examination report.[39] Whenever an injury is documented, the SANE should record the mechanism of injury as well. Unfortunately, the myth that rape victims are injured is still widely believed, even though fewer than one-third of victims sustain even minor, non-genital injuries that do not require treatment. In addition, fewer than 1% of rape survivors require hospitalization. When injuries do occur, these injuries are more commonly found in rapes perpetrated by someone the survivor knows intimately, such as an intimate partner, rather than in date rape or acquaintance rape situations.[5,11,34,40,41] A more recent study, which surveyed 1076 sexual assault survivors, found non-genital trauma more often (ie, 67% of the time) than in previous studies.[42] Remember, though the absence of injury does prove a lack of force or coercion, it does not prove consent.

Photographing Injuries

Though important evidence, photographs of injuries should not take the place of good charting.[43] Specific consent to photograph an injury is necessary, but may be included as a standard part of the examination consent. Two sets of pictures or digital records of the pictures should always be maintained. One set of photos should remain with the chart; the second should be given to law enforcement officers along with the other

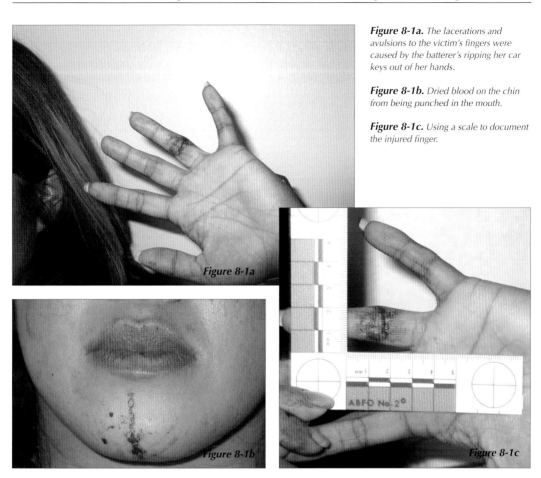

Figure 8-1a. *The lacerations and avulsions to the victim's fingers were caused by the batterer's ripping her car keys out of her hands.*

Figure 8-1b. *Dried blood on the chin from being punched in the mouth.*

Figure 8-1c. *Using a scale to document the injured finger.*

Figure 8-1d. *Photographic documentation of size of bruise located on the left thigh using tape rulers rather than a hand held ruler.*

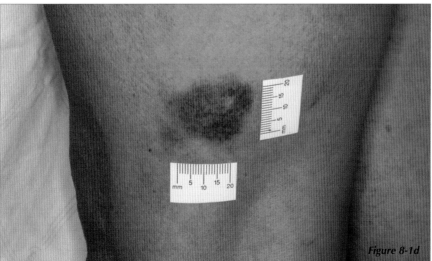

sexual assault evidence. When pictures are taken, the first picture should always be of the survivor's face as additional evidence to link the victim with the injuries **(Figure 8-1c)**. Others should follow in a systematic order (eg, head to toe or front to back) **(Figures 8-1a, 8-1b, and 8-1d to 8-2d)**. It is also important to first take a picture from further away (e.g. so as to document that the injury is on the right arm) and then to take a close-up of the injury. The close-up photographs should be taken first without a scale to show that nothing is being hidden and then with a scale to document size. While a coin (eg, a quarter) is sufficient to show scale, a gray photographic scale is recommended and also assists with color determination.

Use of Digital Photographs for Evidence Documentation

Initially, many prosecutors hesitated to accept digital photography since digital photographs could be altered; however, digital photography has quickly become the norm today. In fact, a number of advantages to digital photographs include the following:

— Photographs do not need to be sent out for processing since inexpensive, easy-to-use printers are readily available to make prints.

— Prints made from digital cameras become available to police officers during the initial investigation.

— Even inexpensive digital cameras produce superior quality pictures.

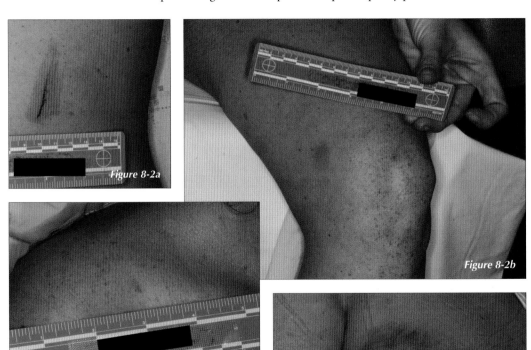

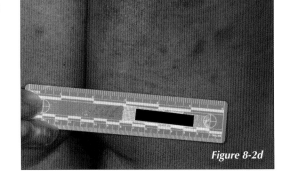

Figure 8-2a. *A fresh abrasion to the back, photographed with a scale for documentation.*

Figure 8-2b. *The fresh fingertip-sized bruises to the inner left thigh area were caused by the victim having her legs forced apart.*

Figure 8-2c. *When asked how this injury was sustained, the victim stated, "He kept poking me there. It hurts."*

Figure 8-2d. *A large bruise to the left buttock, photographed with a scale for documentation.*

When the SANE who completed the examination testifies in court, the prosecutor may ask whether the pictures being shown are an accurate representation of the injuries seen by the SANE during the examination of the victim. Today the SANE's testimony is typically all that is necessary to answer the question regarding the accuracy of digital photographs as evidence.

Figure 8-3a to 8-3c.
Photographic documentation of injuries.

Importance of Photographic Documentation of Injuries

Some examiners feel uneasy about photographing the breasts and genitals of a survivor; however, improperly documenting injuries with photographs may actually result in a liability lawsuit for the failure to accurately document injuries.[43] Examiners can maintain a survivor's dignity and still obtain proper evidence by taking close-up photographs of injuries and by properly draping exposed areas of the victim's body.

Injuries and Treatment Differences in Male and Female Rape Survivors

In a study of 351 rape survivors, physical injury occurred more frequently in male rape survivors (ie, 40%) than in female survivors (ie, 26%).[44] In this study, 25% of men and 38% of women sought medical care for their physical injuries after the rape, but only 61% of these survivors told the treating physician that they had been raped. Because male rape is extremely underreported, it is likely that the injury could be responsible for bringing the male victim to the hospital. Many more males are likely raped but do not report because they do not have injuries needing medical attention. Interestingly, women expressed a strong preference for medical treatment and counseling by a female care provider, but male survivors were less likely to express a gender preference.[44]

Documenting Bruises

Today, experts caution the SANE against trying to date the age of a bruise by its color. For people with light skin, recent bruising is red or dark blue in color and older bruising may be yellow-brown in color, but people vary greatly in their rates of bruising and healing. Additionally, medications may affect a person's bleeding and healing response as well.

Experts suggest that the size, color, and shape of bruises should be documented (eg, "1 inch x ½ inch, deep-blue–purple, oval area of bruising" without further interpretation)[5] **(Figures 8-3a to 8-9a)**. Examiners typically use metric measures in

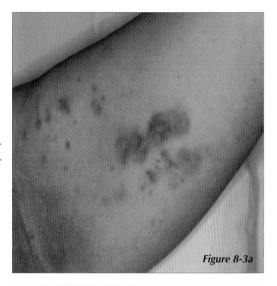

Figure 8-3a

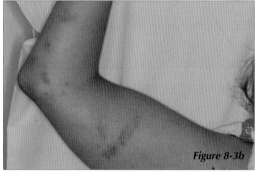

Figure 8-3b

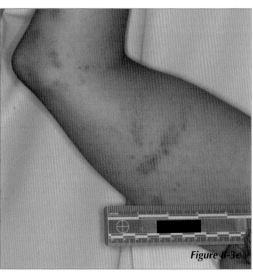

Figure 8-3c

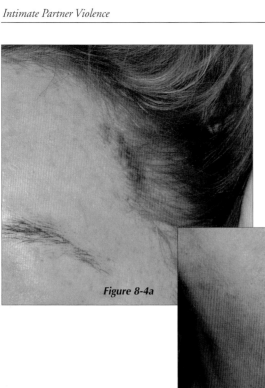

Figure 8-4a

Figure 8-4a. *A contusion to the left upper scalp area. The victim stated that she had walked into a door when questioned about this injury.*

Figure 8-4b. *Linear scratch marks and abrasions on the left neck area caused by being strangled during an argument.*

Figure 8-5a. *Scrape abrasion to the toe from being stomped on.*

Figure 8-6a. *Bruise over left eyebrow.*

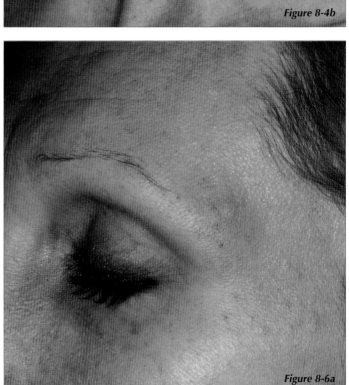

Figure 8-4b

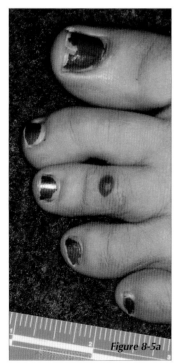

Figure 8-5a

Figure 8-6a

Figure 8-7a. *Bruises and scratches caused by being dragged across a driveway.*

Figure 8-8a. *Bruise on the arm caused by being "… grabbed and thrown around the room multiple times.*

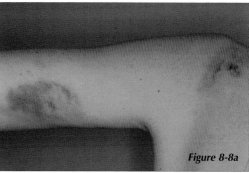

Figure 8-8a

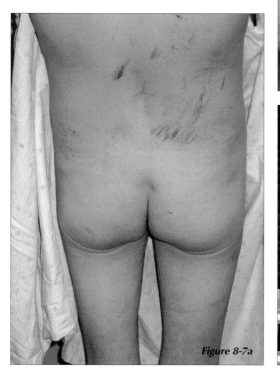

Figure 8-7a

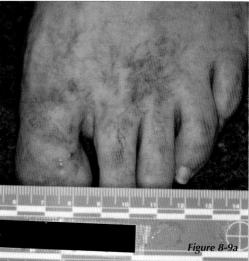

Figure 8-9a

Figure 8-9a. *Photographic documentation of an injury that was caused by a batterer's stomping on the victim's foot with boots on.*

the hospital, but in the courtroom, examiners will be asked to convert all measurements to SI units. As a result, many SANE programs chart in inches and use terminology that is more easily understood in the courtroom (eg, "bruising" rather than "ecchymosis" and "redness" rather than "erythema").

Examiners should remember that identifying bruising in dark-skinned people can be very difficult if an alternative light source is unavailable. Unfortunately, because these light sources are very expensive, most medical facilities do not have them available. The victim should always be counseled that bruises tend to become more visible after a couple of days. If this happens, she should be sure to notify a law enforcement officer so that the bruises can be photographed and the pictures entered into evidence.

Documenting Genital Trauma

Genital trauma to the involved orifice helps determine whether recent sexual contact occurred and whether force was used. Such evidence may help substantiate whether the sexual contact was consistent or inconsistent with consenting sexual contact as well as the history of the assault reported by the survivor. Genital trauma is identified by gross visualization with the naked eye, examination with a colposcope or anoscope, and staining of the tissue with a substance such as toluidine blue dye. Most SANE programs report the use of a colposcope (ie, 64%).[14] Dyes are not widely used. In fact, the national database indicates that only 17% of SANE programs report using dye and, of these programs, only 5% of additional injuries were identified by these dyes.[14]

When discussing genital trauma as evidence of force, examiners must remember that genital trauma *does not* prove rape just as whether a victim reached orgasm as a result of the sexual contact proves that the encounter was not rape. (Actually, when asked, many rape victims report having experienced an orgasm during the unwanted sexual contact of rape despite the fact that these victims were clearly raped.[45]) According to research, genital injury does occur in consenting sexual contact; however, because it also shows that more extensive injury occurs in cases of sexual assault, it is reasonable to conclude that more extensive genital trauma and injury is consistent with forced penetration and inconsistent with consenting sexual contact. When genital injuries are identified the defense attorney will likely attribute such injuries to "vigorous, consenting intercourse." The issue then becomes how many and what type of injuries can be anticipated in "vigorous consenting intercourse" when compared to "forced penetration."

Difficulty in Comparing Studies of Genital Trauma

Researchers continue to search for information showing when injuries are the result of consenting sex and when they are the result of forced penetration through studies of genital injuries and the pattern of these injuries. Researchers have difficulty evaluating the available data about genital injury since the methodology varies greatly from study to study. For example, some studies include gross visualization identification of the injury, some use colposcopy and/or anoscope visualization, and others include the use of dyes. An even more significant problem researchers find when comparing findings from various studies is that the evaluation time periods differ. For example, studies examining women who have participated in consenting sexual contact have often conducted these examinations within 24 hours of the sexual contact. Researchers may then compare these results to those of sexual assault examinations that may have occurred as long as 96 hours after the assault. However, strong data exists indicating that genital tissue heals very rapidly, so studies with differing examination times clearly do not yield comparable results.[46] Study comparison becomes even more difficult when evaluating studies that include children and adolescents, because many of them have never been sexually active and may be more easily injured when compared to sexually active adults.[47]

The following study exemplifies how these challenges present themselves in research. In one highly cited study, victims who initially reported being raped and later recanted were included in the consenting sexual contact group.[48] In this study, sexual assault victims reported a mean of 3.1 injuries in 68% of the victims examined up to 72 hours after the assault occurred. In comparison, the women in the consenting sexual contact group were examined within 24 hours of the sexual contact and showed 1 injury in 11% of the women. The decisions to include the group that recanted in the consenting contact group, and the different time frames for the two groups, clearly raises concern about how to evaluate the findings.

In another study, Rossman used a colposcope to evaluate the women and identified injury in 78% of women reporting a sexual assault and in 67% of women after consenting sexual contact.[49] Anderson and colleagues reported that 32% of rape victims were injured and that 30% of women evaluated after consenting sexual contact experienced injury.[50] By far, most injuries in the consent group were tears, while the injuries of rape victims included tears, bruises, and abrasions.[50] Clearly injury can and does occur in cases of consenting sexual contact as well as cases of sexual assault, and this is an area in need of additional research to better clarify matters.

Use of a Colposcope and an Anoscope in Examination of Injuries

When examining rectal trauma, studies have shown that both the colposcope and anoscope have proven to improve the identification of injury. In a study of 67 male rape survivors, all of whom were examined by experienced forensic examiners, 53% had genital trauma identified with the naked eye alone. This number increased only slightly (ie, 8%) when the colposcope was used; however, this number increased a significant 32% when an anoscope was used. The combination of gross visualization with the naked eye, use of the colposcope, and use of the anoscope resulted in total positive findings in 72% of the cases.[51] Larkin and Paolinetti reported a 32% increase in anal injury identification with the use of an anoscope.[36]

When used in the legal arena, the use of a colposcope is well documented as an accepted practice in the forensic examination of adults and children[52]; colposcope use for this purpose is within the scope of the nursing practice.[53] In fact, the literature suggests that colposcopic genital examination helps visualize and document genital abrasions, bruises, and tears, because these injuries are sometimes so minute that the naked eye cannot see them.[24,52] When used in the forensic examination of a sexual assault survivor to photograph the physical trauma, a colposcope only magnifies minute trauma in the genital area that is not readily visible with gross visualization and not to identify. The examiner should always document the magnification and examination positions when a colposcope is used.

Most research about sexual assault finds that the likelihood of identifying genital trauma without the use of a colposcope to magnify the trauma is similar to the likelihood of finding non-genital trauma to the body (eg arms, legs, or torso). That is, without a colposcope, examiners identify severe genital injury requiring treatment only 3%-5% of the time, and 10% to 30% of the time they identify minor genital injury such as bruises or redness, not requiring treatment.[5] In contrast, Riggs and colleagues[42] found genital trauma in 52% of the cases they reviewed. In yet another study, Briggs and colleagues identified injury in 45% of the 132 cases that they examined without colposcope magnification or use of a dye.[47] An important distinction made in their study, however, was that they separated the victims into two groups—those with previous sexual experience and those without previous sexual experience. Victims with previous sexual experience were injured 25.8% of the time, but victims who had not been sexually active before the assault were injured in 65.2% of the cases. With colposcopic examination, genital trauma has been identified in as many as 87% (n=114) of sexual assault cases.[54] Just as with non-genital trauma, the absence of genital trauma *does not* indicate consent.

Rape survivors often fear vaginal trauma and are concerned that their genitalia has been permanently damaged. Since injuries are rarely so extensive, examiners can reassure a traumatized survivor by explaining the extent of the trauma or lack of trauma after completing the forensic examination.[5] When a video colposcope is available, examiners turn the screen so that the survivor can also view the genital area during the examination. This may help reassure the victim's fears.

EVIDENCE TO CORROBORATE OR REFUTE THE SURVIVOR'S HISTORY OF THE ASSAULT

Forensic examiners must remain aware of the likely pattern of injuries from violence so that they know the appropriate questions to ask a victim, where to look for injuries based upon the history provided by the victim, and what injuries are consistent or inconsistent with the history provided by the victim regarding the assault.

Abusive injuries tend to be more centrally located and accidental injuries tend more toward the extremities. With IPV involvement, injuries are most often inflicted where the survivor can easily hide them. The most common injuries of IPV are broken ear drums from slapping; neck bruising from choking; bruising to the upper arm from punching; and injuries to the outer, mid-ulnar areas from arm "defensive posturing." Other common injuries include whip- or cord-like injuries to the back; punch or bite injuries to the breasts and nipples; punch injuries to the abdomen (especially in pregnant women); punch and kick injuries to the lateral thighs; and facial bruising, abrasions, and lacerations.[55]

Relating the location of the identified genital trauma to the victim's position during the sexual assault can be helpful in prosecution, by corroborating the victim's history of the assault. For example, since the posterior fourchette is the point of greatest stress when forceful stretching occurs and is the point of first contact of the penis with the vagina when the victim is raped in the "missionary position" (ie, the victim on her back and the assailant on top of her), this resulting injury is characterized as an "acute mounting injury." Several investigators report the posterior fourchette as the most common location for genital injuries, followed by the labia minora and labia majora.[46,47,48,54]

MALE EVIDENCE COLLECTION

Examiners must remember that men are also raped. As with female victims, male victims are sexually assaulted by strangers, non-strangers, and intimate partners; these victims can be assaulted by men or women (**Figures 8-10a to 8-10e**).

The same principles apply during the collection of evidence in the male victim of sexual assault as with female victims. As with female victims, any trace evidence from the crime scene and biological specimen from the assailant should be collected from the victim's body and clothing. The primary difference is that the penis shaft and scrotum should be swabbed for saliva or vaginal fluids, at which time the examiner must carefully avoid the urethra so as to

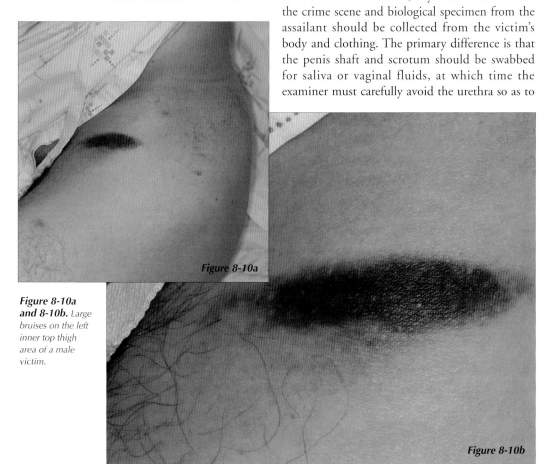

Figure 8-10a

Figure 8-10a and 8-10b. Large bruises on the left inner top thigh area of a male victim.

Figure 8-10b

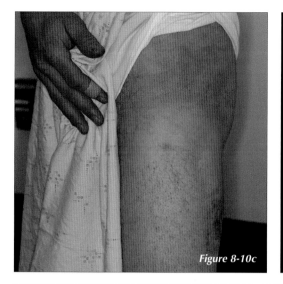

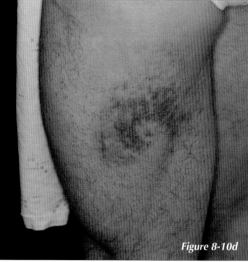

Figure 8-10c

Figure 8-10d

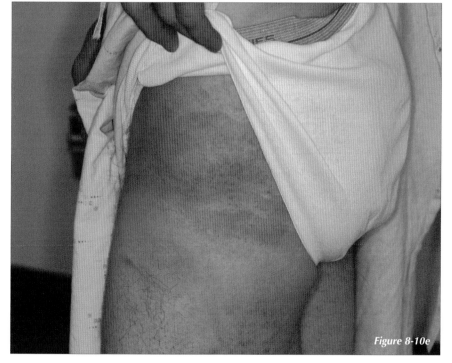

Figure 8-10e

Figure 8-10c.
Reddened area
on the outer
left thigh.

Figure 8-10d.
An older bruise on
the lower left
outer thigh.

Figure 8-10e.
A close-up
photograph of the
contusion on the
outer thigh.

avoid collecting biological fluid from the victim. When a condom was used by the assailant, scrotal swabs may still be positive for DNA of the assailant even if the swabs of the penis are negative. If the victim reports the use of a condom during the assault, the SANE should let law enforcement officers know to look for a condom at the crime scene.

MAINTAINING THE CHAIN OF EVIDENCE

Maintaining proper chain of evidence is as important as collecting the proper evidence and is the one area most often violated by non-forensically trained medical personnel. Evidence may be inadmissible in court without the complete documentation of the chain of evidence. Proper documentation includes the signature of every person who had custody of the evidence (ie, everyone from the person who originally collected the evidence to the person receiving the evidence in the courtroom).

If during the examination the SANE must leave the room for any reason, the examiner must take the evidence with him or her so that the chain of custody remains unbroken. Asking the advocate or anyone else to "watch" the evidence would be considered inappropriate and would break the chain of custody. The advocate should never be included in the chain of custody for the forensic medical evidence.

In an instance when the police officer cannot immediately return to the examination, the SANE can place the collected, sealed, and documented evidence in a locked storage area that has limited accessibility. When the police officer does return, then any available nurse can transfer the evidence to him or her. Of course, both the nurse releasing the evidence and the law enforcement officer accepting the evidence must sign the chain-of-custody form documenting this transfer of custody.[3]

MAINTAINING EVIDENCE INTEGRITY

Dry evidence kits (ie, kits without whole blood evidence) can be stored at room temperature indefinitely. Though evidence should be refrigerated for long-term storage to prevent deterioration of the specimens when whole blood is collected, an air-conditioned room is sufficient for short-term storage.[5] Today, even deteriorated specimens can be processed and DNA recovered using mtDNA analysis.

DOCUMENTATION

Documentation by the SANE should be concise and objective, describe what the SANE sees, and not interpret the findings. The SANE is not an investigator; as a result, the SANE does not collect detailed, investigative information about the assault or assailant. The SANE should ask a victim for information necessary to medically evaluate and treat the survivor's immediate physical and psychological needs, collect the proper

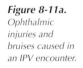

Figure 8-11a. *Ophthalmic injuries and bruises caused in an IPV encounter.*

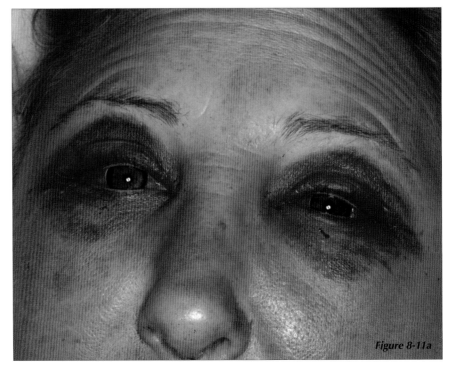

Figure 8-11a

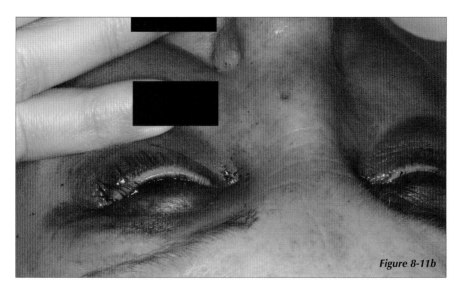

Figure 8-11b. *Ophthalmic injuries and bruises caused in an IPV encounter.*

Figure 8-11b

medical evidence, **(Figures 8-11a and 8-11b)** and collect and interpret the physical and laboratory findings. While the SANE is conducting a medical examination of the survivor for the purpose of evaluation and treatment, this examination is not a routine medical evaluation. The survivor's complete medical history should not be recorded if not pertinent to the sexual assault, and such history is rarely pertinent. Examiners must also remember that they are conducting a medical interview that centers on the survivor rather than on other assault details or investigative information (eg, not the assailant's height or weight). Any such details reported by the victim to the nurse should, of course, be recorded if these details relate to the assault. The only necessary information is, however, the information needed to guide the examination and medically evaluate and treat the survivor.[5]

The SANE must maintain focus on the medical models. In 2004, the US Supreme Court decision regarding *Crawford v Washington* reinforced this.[56] In this decision the court ruled that if the witness (ie, victim) made a statement for medical treatment rather than for later use as testimony, then the SANE could testify about such statements under the usual medical exception to the hearsay rules relating to medical treatment and diagnosis without the victim needing to be available for cross examination. However, if the witness (ie, victim) made any statements under circumstances that could be deemed "testimonial," that is, statements that she could expect would be later used at trial, then they could only be admitted if the victim testified and was available for cross examination.[57]

Basic documentation should include:

— Site and time of assault

— Nature of physical contact(s)

— Race of assailant and number of assailants

— Relationship to assailants(s)

— Weapons and restraints used

— Actual and attempted penetration of which orifice by penis, foreign objects, or fingers

— Ejaculation, if known, and where

— Use of a condom

— Activities of the survivor that may have destroyed evidence (eg, bathing, douching, bowel movement)

— Consenting sexual contact within the last 72 to 96 hours

— Use of a tampon

— Change of clothing

— Contraceptive use

— Current pregnancy status

— Allergies

— Survivor's general appearance and response during examination

— Survivor's mental status (eg, orientation to person, place, and time; ability to remember recent and past events)

— Signs of intoxication or lack there of (eg, steady or unsteady gait, clear or mumbled speech, patient's statements about drug or alcohol use)

— Physical injuries (eg, size, shape, color, location)

When documenting injuries, the SANE must objectively document what she sees; that is, she must document the size (as measured), shape, color, and location of injuries (eg, "Red and blue area of discoloration, ½ inch by ½ inch, rectangular in shape, located on left upper arm"). The examiner should never interpret (eg, "small bruise") an injury during its documentation. Whenever an injury is documented, the mechanism of injury should also be documented (eg, "Victim grabbed on left upper arm when assailant was standing in front of her with his right hand"). The location of the injury should also be documented on a body drawing, and photographs should be taken both with and without a measuring instrument.

As a result of advances in DNA recovery, crime laboratories can now identify a person's DNA from a small drop of blood on a piece of paper instead of from a tube of blood as before. These advances have encouraged most crime laboratories to use dry kits that do not include samples of whole blood for the victims' DNA identification since storage is easier with the dry kit. As previously mentioned, dry kits do not require refrigeration for long-term storage.

Because of the more frequent use of dry kits, the SANE no longer routinely draws a tube of whole blood or urine on all cases for future use as a toxicology screen. Instead, blood and urine samples are now only recommended when DFSA is suspected; the SANE usually collects these samples in a separate blood and urine kit. This change impacts all cases because blood and urine evidence are no longer routinely available to prosecutors and officers. In case the issue of drug use would emerge as the case develops, examiners must become especially diligent about documenting other evidence. As a result, SANEs must document *all* evidence that could be used at a later time to evaluate a claim that "the victim was too intoxicated (from drug or alcohol use) to remember consenting to the sex" or that "she was exchanging sex for drugs;" both of which are typical defense tactics in consent cases. The SANE does this by routinely documenting the victim's mental status while conducting the examination. In addition, the SANE should always document the victim's ability to recall recent and past events, whether her gait is steady or unsteady, and whether her speech is clear or garbled. If the victim's breath smells of alcohol, the examiner should always ask the victim whether she was drinking and, if so, how much she drank. Whenever a victim was drinking or using drugs or whenever DFSA is suspected, the SANE should collect blood and urine according to local policy.

Remember that, in addition to the SANE assault examination report, the entire chart completed at the time of this examination becomes part of the legal record and may be submitted as evidence if the case goes to trial. This includes all emergency department records made at the time of the examination. The examiner must accurately, completely, and legibly record all statements, procedures, and actions. In addition, the SANE should also accurately and completely document the survivor's emotional state and quote important statements made by the survivor (eg, threats made by the assailant).[5,55] Whenever appropriate, the examiner should use qualifying statements such as "patient states" and "patient reports." If the examination findings match the history provided by the survivor, then the examiner should also document that "there is congruence between the survivor's report and her injuries" or "the injuries are consistent with the history of the assault that the victim reports." Since consent is a likely defense in intimate partner sexual assault, it becomes especially important to clearly document and quote the victim whenever possible if she says anything that may explain the reason she felt threatened or coerced and, if necessary, explain the reason she did not try to resist, get away, or yell for help during the assault.

The term "alleged sexual assault" should *never* be used when documenting a sexual assault. This phrase carries negative connotations and may be misinterpreted by judges and juries as an indication that the survivor exaggerated or lied about the assault.[55]

NON-FORENSIC EXAMINATION COMPONENTS

SEXUALLY TRANSMITTED INFECTIONS

Often, sexual assault survivors fear the contraction of STIs. Examiners must always address this concern during the initial examination; however, when a woman is sexually assaulted by an intimate partner, she is usually not as concerned about contracting an STI, especially human immunodeficiency virus (HIV), because she usually knows the assailant's HIV status. Regardless, the examiner should always tell the woman about her options and allow her to make an informed decision about prophylaxis. Examiners should remember that if a woman chooses not to take medications to prevent an STI, this does not mean that she was not raped.

Likelihood of Victims Returning for Follow-Up Care

Though an early study found that 36% of rape survivors who go to the emergency department state that their primary reason for coming is concern about having contracted an STI,[58] the actual risk is rather low. Testing for STIs is expensive and time-consuming for the survivor, who must return 2 or 3 times and, unfortunately, most survivors do not return. In fact, this study also found that only 25% of the survivors seen in the emergency department returned for the initial STI follow-up visit.[58] In another study, only 15% of survivors returned. The researcher of this second study contacted 47% of those victims who had not returned for follow-up and learned that an additional 11% of these went elsewhere for medical follow-up; however, only 14% told the physician seen for their follow-up about the rape.[59]

Prophylactic Care Versus Testing

In the past, medical professionals tested for STIs in the emergency department and then again during the follow-up examination. The rationale was that if a survivor initially tested negative for STIs and positive upon follow-up, then the assailant could be tested as well, if apprehended. If he was positive for the same STI, then this could then link him to the crime. As a result of the many variables that could account for a positive STI test, this practice has not proven useful forensic evidence and is no longer recommended practice for adult or adolescent examinations. In addition, while the Rape Shield Laws in all states were designed to limit the ability of defense attorneys to use information about previously acquired STIs to discredit a rape victim, these findings can often still be used against victims in court. This is another reason for the clinician to defer testing and treat for STIs with prophylactics. Initial testing is, however, recommended for ongoing child sexual abuse.[24,5,60]

Even though the risk of contracting an STI as a result of rape remains low, prophylactic treatment for STIs is generally recommended as a part of the initial care for adolescents and adults since most victims do not return for follow-up testing or treatment and such preventive treatment is safe and effective.[5,24,25] Although the recommended standard, prophylactic treatment is not yet the norm in medical facilities when treating rape victims. One study showed that 62% of sexual assault victims received STI prophylaxis,[61] which is nearly double the 34% prophylaxis rate found in a national study.[62] Studies show that this situation improves under care provided to sexual assault victims by SANE programs. In a survey of 61 SANE programs, 90% offered STI prophylactic care.[63]

Prophylactic Care Recommendations

Recommended prophylaxis includes coverage for chlamydia, gonorrhea, syphilis, trichomoniasis, and hepatitis B (for individuals who have not already been vaccinated for hepatitis B, the first dose of the hepatitis B vaccine should be given, without hepaatitis B immune globulin [HBIG]). Chlamydia, syphilis, and gonococcal infections in women are of particular concern, because these STIs carry the possibility of ascending infections that lead to pelvic inflammatory disease (PID).[60] The benefits and side effects of these medications should, of course, be discussed with the survivor so that she can make an educated decision.

Post-exposure prophylaxis for HIV remains controversial; as a result, a widely accepted recommendation does not exist.[60] Examiners need to discuss the risk and options regarding HIV with all sexual assault survivors so that they can make educated decisions regarding care. Except in high-risk cases, routine HIV prophylaxis is not recommended.[5,25,60] The following factors should be considered when determining whether a sexual assault should be considered high-risk:

— Anal penetration occurred

— Ejaculation occurred on mucous membranes

— Multiple assailants involved

— Mucosal lesions present

— Assailant is a suspected or known intravenous (IV) drug user

— Assailant is suspected or known to be HIV positive

Human Immunodeficiency Virus

Since the early 1980s, rape survivors have shown concern about contracting HIV even though the actual risk appears low. In fact, the Centers for Disease Control and Prevention (CDC) estimates the risk of a rape survivor contracting HIV at 1 in 500 nationally.[64] One study tested 412 rape survivors in the Midwest for HIV while in the emergency department as well as 3 and 6 months after their rapes. These assaults had involved vaginal or anal penetration. The study found that not one of these women became positive for HIV. In addition, the study demonstrated that even if the survivor did not initially ask about HIV while in the emergency department, within 2 weeks after the assault, HIV had become a concern of theirs or of their sexual partners. Although the researchers did not recommend routine HIV testing, they did recommend that, even if survivors do not raise the issue of HIV in the emergency department, SANEs should provide survivors with information about their risk, testing, and safe-sex options. This will allow survivors to make decisions based upon facts, rather than fear.

If a survivor is considering antiretroviral post-exposure prophylaxis, then an HIV professional should be consulted.[60] Also, the CDC recommends that if antiretroviral post-exposure prophylaxis is offered, the SANE should discuss the following with the survivor[60]:

— The unknown efficacy of the drugs

— The known toxicities of the drugs

— The necessary close follow-up required

— The importance of strict compliance with the complete recommended course of therapy

— The need to immediately initiate treatment for maximal likelihood of effectiveness (ie, as soon as possible and within 72 hours of exposure)

How to best deal with the issue of HIV remains complicated and controversial. Because rates of infection vary from state to state, the actual risk of infection varies, too. The antiviral agents used after possible exposure are toxic and have side effects that will likely make the survivor very nauseated. In addition, these prophylactic agents' efficacy is still uncertain and they are not routinely recommended.[24,65]

PREGNANCY

Although the risk of pregnancy from a rape remains the same as the risk of pregnancy from a one-time sexual encounter (ie, 2% to 4%), pregnancy is a concern of most sexual assault survivors and must be addressed during the initial examination even if the treating medical personnel or medical facility does not support the termination of an existing pregnancy. The National Conference of Catholic Bishops has even agreed "A female who has been raped should be able to defend herself against a potential conception from the sexual assault. If, after appropriate testing, there is no evidence that conception has occurred already, she may be treated with medication that would prevent ovulation or fertilization."[66] Despite the controversy surrounding this issue even in cases of sexual assault, Ronald Hamel, Senior Director of Ethics within the Catholic Health Association, published an opinion supporting the prevention of pregnancy through emergency contraception (EC).[67]

According to a national study, only 20% of rape survivors nationally receive EC.[62] When SANE programs are evaluated separately, this statistic improves noticeably. For example, a Canadian study found that 45% of rape victims seen by a SANE program received EC, though the percentage of victims offered EC was not included.[61] Ciancone and colleagues found that 97% of sexual assault victims seen in the 61 SANE programs surveyed were offered both pregnancy testing and EC, but researchers did not report the number of women who chose not to accept the EC.[63]

Because the US Congress has not successfully passed a bill requiring sexual assault survivors be offered EC within the United States, many states have tried to require victims of sexual assault to be informed about their option of EC and be provided with EC if they decide that this is their best option. Currently, several states have passed legislation requiring that sexual assault victims be informed about EC or given the medications when they request. Most states do not legislate whether victims receive EC after their sexual assault. In addition, such a recommendation remains noticeably absent in the *National Protocol for Sexual Assault Medical Forensic Examinations*.[25] Despite this, nearly all SANE programs recognize that the best medical practice is to inform the rape victim about the option of EC. These programs contend that if a victim is at risk for becoming pregnant, has been seen within 5 days of the rape, and had a negative pregnancy test while in the emergency department, then she should have the right to decide whether she wants to take EC to lower her risk of pregnancy.

Oral contraceptives (eg, *Ovral, Lovral*) have been used for EC for many years.[24] In the past, the regimen that used a combined oral contraceptive, called the Yuzpe regimen, was the most common EC. Use of such contraceptives reduces the risk of pregnancy between 60% and 90%. More recently, clinicians have begun using the progestin-only contraceptive, levonorgestrel 0.75 mg (ie, Plan B). Plan B reduces the risk of pregnancy slightly more than the Yuzpe regimen. Unlike other forms of EC, Plan B can be given in one dose in the emergency department. In fact, research indicates that Plan B is slightly more effective still when given this way, rather than having the victim take a second dose 12 hours later. One study showed that when taken within 72 hours of unprotected intercourse, 85% of pregnancies were prevented with Plan B in comparison to 57% prevented with the Yuzpe regimen.[68,69]

Plan B is usually offered for up to 5 days after a sexual assault; however, the effectiveness of both methods decreases as the time between the assault and the administration of the first dose increases. When given within the first 24 hours, Plan B reduced the risk of pregnancy by 95%, but only by 61% when given between 48 and 72 hours after unprotected intercourse. The significant difference between the two methods is in the only side effect (ie, nausea and vomiting); 50% of women experience nausea and vomiting after using the Yuzpe method, while only 23.1% experience these side effects with the use of Plan B.[69,70] The care provider must explain to the victim that Plan B will *not* interfere with an established pregnancy or cause an abortion. Unfortunately, even medical professionals sometimes misunderstand this medication's mechanism of action.

The importance of offering complete care to sexual assault survivors, which includes care to prevent pregnancy when the survivor wants this care, was further strengthened by the fine against a New York City hospital. In addition to other errors, this hospital did not ensure that the victim received the full birth-control regimen in order to prevent pregnancy.[71]

CRISIS INTERVENTION AND SUPPORT
Some basic components of the evidentiary examination for all survivors is crisis intervention and support, mental health assessment, and referral for follow-up counseling. Although primarily the role of the rape crisis center advocate, the SANE is also responsible for providing crisis intervention and support and ensuring the availability of follow-up counseling services.[2,25,72] Providing information and support has always been an important role for medical professionals and remains part of the SANE's clinical role. This role does not imply that a SANE is biased or an advocate and should not challenge the SANE's ability to testify in court about what the victim said during the medical interview.

In Malloy's study, 85% of 70 rape victims reported that the SANE's willingness to listen to them helped them the most during the examination.[73] In a survey of sexual assault survivors seen by trained forensic examiners in a specialized program, Erickson and colleagues found the following aspects of the care significant for the survivor[74]:

— Being respected and cared about as a whole person and having concrete needs met

— Having the nurse present throughout the process

— Feeling a sense of safety and being physically touched by the SANE

— Being given options to feel in control of the situation

— Being reassured that she had done the best she could

— Knowing the SANE was an expert in providing care to rape victims

— Receiving clear information about the care and treatment options available

When domestic violence is suspected or if substantial drug or alcohol abuse appears to be an issue, medical facilities should have protocol in place for screening and referral. Many medical facilities have domestic violence advocates or rape crisis center advocates available who can be called to the hospital for a sexual assault victim. If available, health care providers should use these services. In addition, health care providers should remain aware of shelter availability for domestic violence survivors who may need a safe place to go after the evidentiary examination.

Continued fear and anxiety resulting from the rape can significantly affect the survivor's life (eg, work, school, and relationships) far into the future.[5] The psychological impact and treatment needs of survivors have been addressed extensively in the psychological literature; review of which is beyond the scope of this chapter. Self-help books, such as *Recovering from Rape*,[45] are available for rape survivors who do not return for counseling. Since most victims do not return for follow-up support and counseling, many SART programs provide this book to victims in the emergency department.

CONCLUSION

The SANE has 2 related and overarching goals during the initial examination of a sexual assault victim during the initial 72 or 96 hours after the rape: 1) medical evaluation and treatment and 2) evidence collection. The medical examination includes an initial interview to guide the examination; evaluation for the risk of STD (including HIV and pregnancy) and offering preventive care; the evaluation and treatment of physical injuries; and crisis intervention and support. Based upon the initial interview, the SANE also collects all potential evidence and should think "outside the box" to ensure that valuable evidence is not missed. Other critical roles for the SANE include properly documenting and identifying the collected evidence, maintaining the chain-of-custody, and ensuring the integrity of the collected evidence.

The SANE should always carefully assess each case individually and keep in mind how the collected evidence may be used. In sexual assault cases involving IPV, with the exception of DFSA cases, evidence used to identify the assailant is not likely to be helpful. Likewise, proof of recent sexual contact is less likely to be useful since assailants commonly use the "consent" defense whenever sperm or semen is identified. The most important evidence in IPV cases shows the sexual contact resulted from force, coercion, or lack of consent. Evidence to corroborate the victim's history of the assault is also likely to be important in these cases since they often involve the word of one person against another. Any evidence to support the victim's credibility will be significant in this type of case since the defense will likely attempt to make the victim look like a less credible witness.

Although the SANE always collects all possible evidence available, thinking "outside the box" helps identify potential evidence not specifically requested. The SANE must carefully document all such potential evidence that may relate to the case regardless of the implications. After all, the SANE must always remain objective.

REFERENCES

1. Datner EM, Asher JB, Rubin BD. Domestic violence and partner rape. In: Giardino AP, Datner EM, Asher JB. *Sexual Assault Victimization Across the Life Span: A Clinical Guide.* St. Louis, Mo: GW Medical Publishing; 2003:347-362.

2. Speck P, Aiken M. 20 years of community nursing service: Memphis Sexual Assault Resource Center. *Tenn Nurs.* 1995;58:15-18.

3. Ledray LE. Sexual assault nurse clinician: an emerging area of nursing expertise. *AWHONNS Clin Issues Perinat Womens Health Nurs.* 1993;4:180-190.

4. Antognoli-Toland P. Comprehensive program for examination of sexual assault victims by nurses: a hospital-based project in Texas. *J Emerg Nurs.* 1985;11:132-135.

5. Ledray LE, for the Sexual Assault Resource Service. *Sexual Assault Nurse Examiner (SANE) Development & Operation Guide.* Washington, DC: US Department of Justice, Office for Victims of Crime; 1999. NCJ 170609.

6. Campbell R, Townsend SM, Long SM, et al. Washington, DC: US Bureau of Justice; 2002. Criminal Victimization Series. NCJ 194710. Organizational characteristics of Sexual Assault Nurse Examiner programs: results from the national survey project. *J Forensic Nurs.* 2005;1:57-64, 88.

7. Resnick HS, Holmes MM, Kilpatrick DG, et al. Predictors of post rape medical care in a national sample of women. *Am J Prev Med.* 2000;19:214-219.

8. Bachar K, Kass MP. From prevalence to prevention: closing the gap between what we know about rape and what we do. In: Renzetti CM, Edleson JL, Bergen RK. *Sourcebook on Violence Against Women.* 2001;117-142.

9. Rennison C. *Criminal Victimization 2001: Changes 2000-01 With Trends 1993-2001.* US Bureau of Justice Statistics. Washington, DC: US Bureau of Justice; 2002. Publication NCJ 194710.

10. Hessmiller J, Ledray L. Violence. In: Condon MC. *Women Health: Body, Mind, Spirit: An Integrated Approach to Wellness and Illness.* Upper Saddle River, NJ: Prentice Hall; 2004:516-536.

11. Moynihan B. Domestic violence. *Forensic Nursing.* St. Louis, Mo: Elsevier; 2006:260-270.

12. Campbell R. *The Effectiveness of Sexual Assault Nurse Examiner (SANE) Programs.* Harrisburg, Pa: National Online Resource Center on Violence Against Women; 2004.

13. Campbell R, Ahrens CE. Innovative community services for rape victims: an application of multiple case study methodology. *Am J Community Psychol.* 1998;26:537-571.

14. Available at: www.sane-sart.com. Accessed on December 15, 2005.

15. Available at: www.iafn.com. Accessed on December 15, 2005.

16. Ledray LE, Simmelink K. Efficacy of SANE evidence collection: a Minnesota study. *J Emerg Nurs*. 1997;23:75-77.

17. Crandall CS, Helitzer D. Impact Evaluation of a Sexual Assault Nurse Examiner (SANE) Program. Washington, DC: US Dept of Justice; 2003. NCJ 203276.

18. Little, K. (2001) *Sexual assault nurse examiner programs; Improving the community response to sexual assault victims*. Office for Victims of Crime Bulletin, 4, 1-19.

19. Campbell, R., Long, S., Townsend, S., Kinnison, K., Pulley, E., Adames, S. B. & Wasco, S. (2007) "Sexual Assault Nurse Examiners' Experience Providing Expert Witness Court Testimony." *Journal of Forensic Nursing*, (3)1, 7-14.

20. Logan, T.K., Cole, J. & Capillo, A. (2007) "Sexual Assault Nurse Examiner Program Characteristics, Barriers, and Lessons Learned." *Journal of Forensic Nursing*, (3)1, 24-34.

21. Lt Ted Smith, WV State Police: November 15, 2005, Parkersburg, WV SANE Training [oral communication].

22. Lopez-Bonasso D, Smith T. Sexual Assault Kit Tracking Application (SAKiTA): technology at work in West Virginia. *J Forensic Nurs*. 2006;2:92-95.

23. Arndt S. Nurses help Santa Cruz sexual assault survivors. *Calif Nurse*. 1988;84:4-5.

24. American College of Emergency Physicians. *Evaluation and Management of the Sexually Assaulted or Sexually Abused Patient*. Dallas, Tex: American College of Emergency Physicians; 1999.

25. US Department of Justice Office on Violence Against Women. *A National Protocol for Sexual Assault Medical Forensic Examinations: Adults/Adolescents*. Washington, DC: US Department of Justice Office on Violence Against Women; September, 2004. NCJ 206554.

26. McClain KC. The military response to sexual assault: the new Department of Defense Sexual Assault Prevention and Response Policies. Paper presented at: Third National SART Training Conference; June 2, 2005; San Francisco, Calif.

27. Ledray L. 2005. Investigative & Forensic Contributions of the Sexual Assault Nurse Examiner (SANE). *"Rape Investigation Handbook" Editors: Det. John O. Savino, NYPD Manhattan Special Victim's Squad (MSVS), Brent E. Turvey, MS, Knowledge Solutions LLC*. 119-146.

28. Lewis R. DNA fingerprints: witness for the prosecution. *Discover*. June 1988:44-52.

29. Ledray LE, Netzel L. DNA evidence collection. *J Emerg Nurs*. 1997;23:156-158.

30. Miller P. Sexual violence and the gay and lesbian communities. In: *Minnesota Coalition Against Sexual Assault Training Manual*. Minneapolis, Minn: Minnesota Coalition Against Sexual Assault; 1997.

31. Loftus P, Niezgoda S, Behun J. DNA and CODIS project. In: Lynch V. *Forensic Nursing*. St. Louis, Mo: Elsevier; 2006.

32. Office of Victims of Crimes/DOJ (2008) DNA collection and Use in Sexual Assault Cases: The Role of the First Responder.

33. *The Crime Survivor Report: Legal Reviews*, Kingston, NJ: Civic Research Institute; 2001;5:55-63.

34. Tucker S, Claire E, Ledray LE, Werner JS, Claire E. Sexual assault evidence collection. *Wisc Med J.* 1990;89:407-411.

35. Groth AN, Burgess AW. Sexual dysfunction during rape. *N Engl J Med.* 1977; 297:764-766.

36. Larkin H, Paolinetti L. Pattern of anal/rectal injury in sexual assault victims who complain of rectal penetration. Paper presented at: International Association of Forensic Nurses Annual Scientific Assembly; October 1-5, 1998; Pittsburgh, Pa.

37. Enos WF, Beyer JC. Prostatic acid phosphatase, aspermia, and alcoholism in rape cases. *J Forens Sci.* 1980;25:353-356.

38. LeBeau, M & Ashrav Mozayani, 2001. *Drug facilitated Sexual Assault: A forensic Handbook.* Academic press of London.

39. Ledray L, 2006. *Forensic Nursing: Sexual Assault.* Chapter 26 pp279-291. Virginia Lynch (editor) Elsevier Mosby.

40. Bownes IT, O'Gorman EC, Sayers A. Rape—a comparison of stranger and acquaintance assaults. *Med Sci Law.* 1991;31:102-109.

41. Marchbanks PA, Lui KJ, Mercy JA. Risk of injury from resisting rape. *Am J Epidemiol.* 1990;132:540-549.

42. Riggs DS, Kilpatrick DG, Resnick HS. Long-term psychological distress associated with marital rape and aggravated assault: a comparison to other crime victims. *J Fam Violence.* 1992;7: 283-286.

43. Pasqualone GA. Forensic RNs as photographers: documentation in the ED. *J Psychosoc Nurs Ment Health Surv.* 1996:34:47-51.

44. Petrak JA, Skinner CJ, Claydon EJ. The prevalence of sexual assault in a genitourinary medicine clinic: service implications. *Genitourin Med.* 1995;71:98-102.

45. Ledray L. *Recovering from Rape.* New York, NY: Holt & Company; 1994.

46. Adams JA, Girardin B, Faugno D. Adolescent sexual assault: documentation of acute injuries using photocolposcopy. *J Pediatr Adolesc Gynecol.* 2001;14:175-180.

47. Briggs M, Stermac LE, Divinsky M. Genital injuries following sexual assault of women with and without prior sexual intercourse experience. *CMAJ.* 1998;159:33-37.

48. Slaughter L, Brown CR, Crowley S, Peck R. Patterns of genital injury in female sexual assault victims. *Am J Obstet Gynecol.* 1997;176:609-616.

49. Rossman, D, (2002) paper presented Friday Oct 11, 2002 at IAFN 10th Annual Scientific Assembly: "A Decade of Change", Minneapolis, MN, October 9-13, 2002. "Pattern of Injury is Sexual assault cases"

50. Anderson SA, McClain N, Riviello RJ. Genital findings of women after consensual and nonconsensual intercourse. Journal of Forensic Nursing 2(2):59, 2006.

51. Ernst AA, Green E, Ferguson MT, Weiss SJ, Green WM. The utility of anoscopy and colposcopy in the evaluation of male sexual assault victims. Ann Emerg Med. 2000;36:432-437.

52. IAFN Statement. Utility of the colposcope in the sexual assault examination. Fourth Annual Scientific Assembly of Forensic Nurses; November 1-4, 1996; Kansas City, Mo.

53. Ledray L. Is the SANE role within the scope of nursing practice? On "pelvics," "colposcopy," and "dispensing of medications." *J Emerg Nurs*. 2000;26:79-81.

54. Slaughter L, Brown CR. Colposcopy to establish physical findings in rape victims. *Am J Obstet Gynecol*. 1992;166(pt 1):83-86.

55. Sheridan DJ. The role of the battered woman specialist. *J Psychosoc Nurs Ment Health Surv*. 1993;31:31-37.

56. Crawford v Washington. (2004) March 8. 158 L Ed 2nd 177; 124 S Ct 1354.

57. Phillips A. Weathering the storm after *Crawford v. Washington*. Update [serial online]. 2004;17(pt 2). Available at: http://www.ndaa-apri.org/publications/newsletters/update_volume_17_number_6_2004.html. Accessed January 12, 2007.

58. Ledray, 1991. Sexual Assault and Sexually transmitted Disease: The Issues and Concerns. In Ann Wolbert Burgess (ED), *Rape and Sexual Assault III: a Research handbook*. New York & London: Garland Publishing, Inc 1991.

59. Tintinalli JE, Hoelzer M. Clinical findings and legal resolution in sexual assault. *Ann Emerg Med*. 1985;14:447-453.

60. Sexually transmitted diseases treatment guidelines 2002. Centers for Disease Control and Prevention. *MMWR Recomm Rep*. 2002;51:1-78.

61. Stermac, Dunlap, Bainbridge, 2005. Stermac, L., Sheridan, P. Davidson, A. & Dunn, S. (1996) Sexual assault of adult males." *Journal of Interpersonal Violence*. Vol 11, (1) (pp 52-64).

62. Amey AL, Bishai D. Measuring the quality of medical care for women who experience sexual assault with data from the National Hospital Ambulatory Medical Care Survey. *Ann Emerg Med*. 2002;39:631-638.

63. Ciancone, Wilson, Collette, Gerson, 2000. Ciancone, AC., Wilson, C. & Gerson, LW. (2000) Sexual assault nurse examiner programs in the United States. *Annals of Emergency Medicine*. 35(4): 353-7

64. Centers for Disease Control and Prevention. NHCHSTP-Division of HIV/AIDS/Prevention. www.ede.gov/hiv/topics/prev_prog 2008.

65. Hampton HL. Care of the woman who has been raped [published correction appears in *N Engl J Med*. 1997;337:56]. *N Engl J Med*. 1995;332:234-237.

66. National Conference of Catholic Bishops. Ethical & Religious Directives for Catholic Health Care Services [pamphlet]. Washington, DC: National Conference of Catholic Bishops; 1995:14-17.

67. Hamel RP, Panicola MR. Emergency contraception and sexual assault. Assessing the moral approaches in Catholic teaching. *Health Prog*. 2002;83:12-9, 51.

68. Hertzen, H., Piaggio, G., Ding, J., Chen, J., Song, S. & Bartfal, G. (2002) "Low dose mifepristone and two regimens of levonorgestrel for emergency contraception: a WHO multicentre randomized trial." The Lancet. 360:1803-1810.

69. Task Force on Post-Ovulatory Methods of Fertility Regulation. Vol:1(5) 2000 http://www1.elsevier.com/cdweb/journals/00107824/viewer.

70. Available at: www.go2planb.com/ForConsumer/Index. Accessed on February 24, 2004.

71. Chivers CJ. In sex crimes, evidence depends on game of chance in hospitals. *The New York Times*. August 6, 2000:1-6.

72. Ledray LE, Faugno D, Speck P. SANE: advocate, forensic technician, nurse? *J Emerg Nurs*. 2001;27:91-93.

73. Malloy M. *Relationship of Nurse Identified Therapeutic Techniques to Client Satisfaction Reports in a Crisis Program* [master's thesis]. Minneapolis, Minn: University of Minnesota; 1991.

74. Ericksen J, Dudley C, McIntosh G, Ritch L, Shumay S, Simpson M. Clients' experiences with a specialized sexual assault service. *J Emerg Nurs*. 2002;28:86-90.

Chapter 9

SOCIAL WORK INTERVENTION IN INTIMATE PARTNER VIOLENCE

Jennifer B. Varela, LCSW
Eileen Giardino, RN, MSN, PhD, MSN, FNP-BC
Angelo Giardino, MD, PhD, MPH, FAAP

Social workers encounter many situations that involve domestic violence, whether it be with a client who has experienced or is currently experiencing violence or within a system that tends to support the oppression of women. As a result, all social workers should have training in basic intimate partner violence (IPV) issues and remain aware of the major theories related to it.

The intervention of social workers within IPV situations varies according to the site in which that social worker practices. According to the code of ethics for the National Association of Social Workers (NASW), social workers must maintain certain skills and a common mindset when working with people who have IPV issues.[1] All social workers are trained to respect their clients, use a person-in-environment approach (ie, consider the individual client within the context of his/her culture, environment, and society), and work with clients "where they are" (ie, begin with the client's perspective and work from there). To remain effective, social workers must first understand the nature of IPV, as well as the complex and confusing ways it impacts individuals, families, and society.

Often, a family experiencing IPV also suffers from the compounding problems of mental illness, substance abuse, discrimination, unrealistic cultural or community expectations, and poverty. While helping to meet a client's basic needs (eg, safety, shelter, food, health care), social workers should use empowering and supportive techniques that are diametrical to the shaming and controlling techniques used by batterers. Batterers use shame, power, violence, and control to force their partners to do what they want. The road to true safety, freedom, and peace does not involve the use of shame and threats. Social workers must be careful not to cross the line between using batterer-style control techniques and remaining firm, following the law, setting limits, and reality testing. This chapter explores the interventions used by social workers when faced with an individual IPV situation. Social workers also can work in political and broader social arenas to eradicate IPV. In working with individuals who have experienced IPV, social workers should use the values of competence, service, social justice, dignity, and self-worth, as well as the importance of human relationships and integrity, as defined by the NASW's code of ethics.[1]

Competence

Case Example

Mary† had done what society expected of her by leaving her violent, crack-abusing husband to protect her child. She applied for a protective order, filed for divorce, and began talking with a supportive and caring social worker. Her husband saw the change in her and knew that Mary was committed to extracting him from her life.

Mary felt better about her life as she and her 10-year-old son headed out the door one morning for work and school. That morning, her husband waited for her and shot her in the driveway of the family's home. As she died, surely Mary's last thoughts were about her son. After all, she had taken the dangerous step of separating from her husband primarily for the sake of her son so that he would not be exposed to any more violence. When emergency help arrived, they found Mary's son hugging her body. Mary's estranged husband did not resist arrest. He had accomplished what he set out to do—control Mary.

Understanding Intimate Partner Violence

One of the most important things to understand about IPV is that all victims of family violence are ultimately alone. Perhaps feminist writer and activist Andrea Dworkin best expressed this statement when she wrote, "The governing reality of women of all races is that there is no escape from male violence, because it is inside and outside, intimate and predatory. While race hate has been expressed through forced segregation, women hate is expressed through forced closeness… For this reason, no matter how many women are battered… each one is alone."[2] Support, referrals, and counseling can help battered women tremendously, but they do not change the fact that when she comes home at night and puts her key in the door, she is alone and must rely upon herself to remain safe.

Lenore Walker's theory of the cycle of violence is critical to understanding the dynamics in an IPV relationship and should be read and understood by social workers.[3] In her work, Walker describes the phases in a battering cycle as "the tension building phase; the explosion or acute battering incident; and the calm, loving respite."[3] A relationship that includes intimate partner violence is complex, in that both people in the abusive relationship exhibit low self-esteem, poor impulse control, unrealistic ideas, unhealthy role models, immature coping techniques, and unregulated or poorly regulated expressions of emotion. This relationship is often further complicated by mental illness and substance abuse and reinforced by societal norms, religion, and economic necessity. Walker posits that one of the most opportune times to intervene in IPV is shortly after a violent, explosive incident. Once the couple enters the "calm" stage, intervention becomes more difficult because both the batterer and victim enter a denial period and become more closely bonded together.[3]

Mary Ann Dutton proposes the need to understand the "social, political, cultural, and economic context"[4] in which a battered woman finds herself. Considering these paradigms will lead to understanding a survivor's sources of strength, support, or barriers. Dutton contends that a professional may encounter an abused woman who is currently in an IPV relationship, but who also has been victimized in the past. This victim's current, abusive relationship may have begun with a man whom she initially thought of as strong and protective, but later learned was controlling. Dutton states that other factors (eg, institutional response, personal and tangible recourses, social support), additional stressors, and even positive aspects of the relationship all play crucial roles in a battered woman's response to the abuse.

---

† *Unless noted, all cases described in this chapter are true, though the identifying information has been changed for privacy.*

Sarah Buel, a law professor and IPV survivor, trains attorneys and judges regarding intimate partner and sexual violence. She states that a battered woman's job is to stay alive, and that the victimized woman will do what she needs to do to avoid being murdered.[5] Battered women want their abusers to stop hurting them. They want them to be the men they initially met, or the men that the women think they can become.

In his book, *Vital Lies, Simple Truths*, psychologist Daniel Goleman writes about the necessity to ignore "the terrible truth."[6] He references R. D. Laing, who describes the ways families that experience even the worst types of abuse play "the game of happy family."[7] Not only is the battered woman in denial about the abuse, but the whole family as well as the family's friends and extended family members also accept the "happy family" version rather than the true, pathological version of the family.

Goleman writes that these families "go on amid a collusive fog. Such families often go through a cycle of denial and guilt."[6] Families can function like this for years until a crisis occurs that cannot be managed and destroys the façade. Such a crisis could occur when an abuser turns his violence on a child when he had previously only physically abused the mother, when an arrest occurs, when a child physically intervenes in an assault, or when the abuse becomes too public to ignore. For one formerly battered woman, this crisis occurred when she overheard her 10-year-old daughter tell friends that she was never getting married or having kids, because she did not want her husband to tell her what to do and how to act all the time. The woman then knew that she must leave the relationship for her daughter's sake so that her daughter would not think that all marriages are abusive. For another woman, the crisis occurred when her 4-year-old son called her a "stupid f**king bitch," just like his father. Some people wait until they feel they have tried "everything" (eg, going to counseling, calling the police, trying to be "good enough" to avoid violent situations) and then leave. Some battered women are lucky when their abuser leaves them for another woman, but then often find that the batterer still wants to maintain control over them, as well as be with the other woman. No matter the reason for ending the abusive relationship, all women want to leave safely, but realize that, by doing so, they are absolutely challenging the batterer's control, which places these women in danger.

Risk Factors

Social workers must remain aware of the major risk factors when determining lethality of a situation. The most dangerous time for a woman who has been in an IPV relationship is during the separation process. Sometimes remaining in the abusive relationship is safer for the woman than leaving. When the victim leaves, this shows that the batterer has lost control, and he will not tolerate her departure. One must only notice stories in the local media to confirm this fact. Very often when an IPV murder is reported, there is a comment that the woman just separated from her partner.

The National Institute of Justice (NIJ), which is the research agency of the US Department of Justice (DOJ), is an excellent source of information regarding IPV. In 2003, the NIJ published research detailing the risk factors for intimate partner homicide.[8] This research shows that high-risk lethality indicators include a history of use or threats with a weapon, access to a gun, threats to kill the woman or her children, violence during pregnancy, strangulation, stalking, forced sex, substance abuse, extreme control, and jealousy. **Table 9-2** provides a checklist used to determine the danger level of the situation. **Figures 9-1 through 9-22** are drawings by a number of anonymous children and adults who had witnessed violence. They were drawn as part of a domestic violence awareness project presented by the Harris County District Attorney's Office.

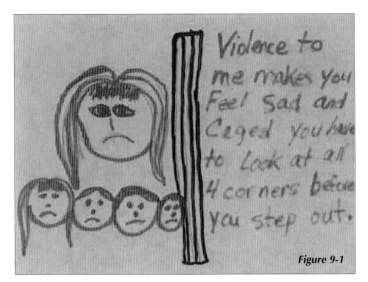

Figure 9-1

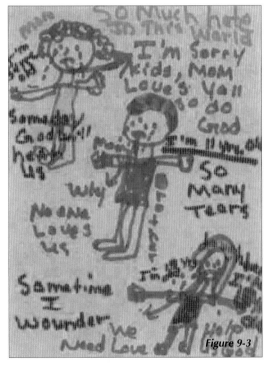

Figure 9-3

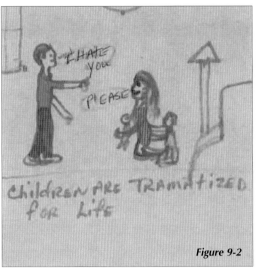

Figure 9-2

Figure 9-1. *This drawing conveys a family's feeling of being caged by violence.*

Figure 9-2. *"Children Are Tramatized for Life"*

Figure 9-3. *This drawing communicates the thoughts and questions violence causes in both children and adults.*

Figure 9-4. *A comparison of life before and after violence.*

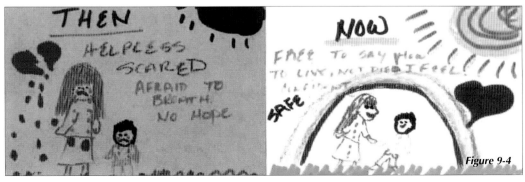

Figure 9-4

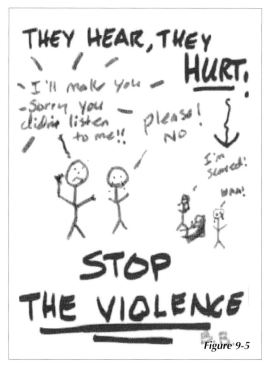

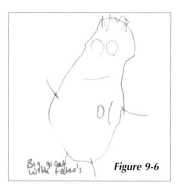

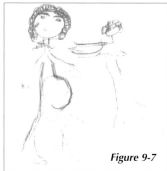

Figure 9-5

Figure 9-6

Figure 9-7

Figure 9-5. *"They hear, they Hurt. Stop the Violence"*

Figure 9-6. *"Big Giant with Tattoos"*

Figure 9-7. *This drawing depicts a scene in which a pregnant woman is being strangled.*

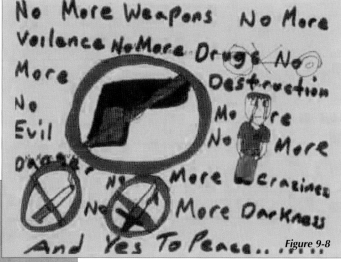

Figure 9-8

Figure 9-8. *"No more weapons, no more voilence, no more drugs, no more destruction, no more evil, no more danger, no more crazines, no more darkness, and yes to Peace"*

Figure 9-9. *"Where is he? That's me! Always looking over my shoulder! I never feel safe! He has changed my whole daily routine! He has changed my Life!"*

Figure 9-9

ASSESSMENT

Social workers are experts at knowing where and how to obtain help for their clients. To determine the needs of a battered woman, the social worker first meets with the client to assess her status (ie, lethality and/or danger risk assessment, strengths, pressure points, concerns, physical, mental, cognitive), resources (ie, a safe place to stay, family support, employment status, access to money), and needs (ie, safety, family court help, employment, counseling). Then the social worker helps the client create a treatment or action plan, implement that plan, and continue monitoring the situation and adjusting the plan as needed. See **Table 9-1** for more information on assessment techniques.

The woman may not be willing to tell the social worker everything that has happened to her because she feels shame, confusion, or even manipulation. If the social worker starts "where the client is," then the social worker will learn of the client's main concerns (eg, safety, children, meeting basic needs). The social worker must also determine the client's available resources, her needs, and the available community resources.

The social worker must be prepared to ask the client questions in a way that will elicit the information necessary to help the abused woman because her feelings of shame or lack of information about what abuse actually is may make disclosure difficult. For example, one woman went to the police after her boyfriend broke her ribs and jaw by savagely beating her. In addition, he forced her to have sex with him during the beating. The abused woman did not realize that this was considered sexual assault; she thought that, because she had had consensual sex with him in the past, he could not be charged with raping her. She thought she was only reporting the physical abuse, but was surprised when her ex-boyfriend was charged with aggravated assault with serious bodily injury and aggravated sexual assault.

Intimate partner violence survivors within gay, lesbian, bisexual, or transgendered (GLBT) relationships face additional barriers (eg, fear of homophobia, actual homophobia, being "outed" at work or with their families). Such victims may fear being taken seriously[9] or simply being told to fight back against their batterer. Social workers should be aware of these additional barriers faced by GLBT clients. It is important to be able to link these clients with agencies that are equipped to meet their needs, including advocacy.

PLAN DEVELOPMENT

Because clients are often in crisis mode, social workers can help them organize and prioritize their needs. Social workers should recognize and utilize the battered woman's strengths, as well as identify and address her concerns. When planning anything with someone who has experienced IPV, safety planning is the first priority. Usually safety planning is integral in planning basic needs (eg, shelter, food, clothing, children's needs [eg, schooling]) as well. Careful thought should be given to ways in which the abuser's contact with the survivor is limited.

McFarlane and colleagues' research shows that when offered information about safety behaviors, abused women quickly adopted the new behaviors.[10] Other important priorities include making police reports, filing criminal charges, and filing orders of protection or other legal documents that will help the survivor and her children remain safe. Planning should also include treatment for mental health and supportive counseling for anyone in the family impacted by the violence. If a social worker encounters a batterer who wishes to receive treatment for his violent behavior, he should be referred to a batterer's intervention program and encouraged to leave the home until he is able to choose not to use violence and control.

Table 9-1. Social Work Interaction Scenarios

Scenario	Controlling, Shaming, or Disempowering Responses	Empowering Responses
Social worker must involve CPS. Knows that involving CPS will cause mother to feel very threatened, which will damage the social worker–client relationship.	*If you go back to him, I'm calling child protective services, and we'll see what they have to say.* *Fine. I'll just call child protective services.*	*I know you love your kids and worry about them. I'm worried about them too, so I need to call [or I called] child protective services. I know that is probably scary to you, but maybe we can talk about your fears and concerns.*
Batterer is dangerous and victim wants to return to the relationship. Client makes decisions that are unsafe.	*He's going to kill you.* *He's going to kill your children.* *Don't you care about yourself or your children?* *You need to… (ie, making demands of the client)*	*I'm very worried for your safety and the safety of your children. He seems like he could really hurt you, and none of you deserve that.* *How will you live in safety and peace if you make the decision to (fill in the blank).*
Client wants social worker to make choices and decisions for her. Client is unreasonably demanding.	Social worker does most of the work; client puts forth little effort. Client does not like the options available; social worker makes impractical changes to accommodate client.	Social worker verifies that she is being reasonable and tells client: *Well, these are the options I can think of and have available. Would you like to consider any of them?* *I wish I could accommodate all of your needs, but this is what I can do. Would you like to try it?* *Can you think of something else to try?* Refer client to other agencies and suggest that client check out other sources for different options.
Client will not follow agreed upon safety plan that she and her social worker created.	*If you don't do it this way, then I can't work with you.* *I don't understand why you don't do what is good for you.*	Recognize that the plan really may not be the best, and the victim is doing what she needs to do to remain safe. Accept that people will simply do what they want to do or feel they need to do. When done with compassion, confrontation is good.
Mental illness or substance abuse is present.	Social worker allows batterer or victim to shift responsibility for the violence to other problems.	Clients should be taught that violence is a choice. Mental illness or substance abuse may amplify the violence but generally does not cause the violence. Social worker can help client obtain treatment.

Figure 9-10. *"Dear Mommy, when your not here, he unloads on me. Please don't let him come back."*

Figure 9-11. *A message of hope to victims of violence.*

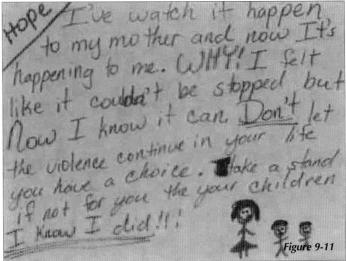

Figure 9-11

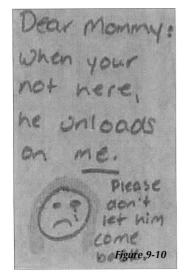

Figure 9-10

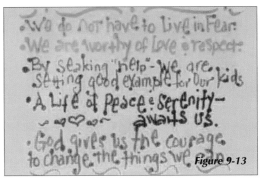

Figure 9-13

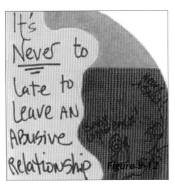

Figure 9-12

Figure 9-12. *"It's Never to late to leave an abusive relationship. Baby Come Back! Never Again!"*

Figure 9-13. *"We do not have to Live in Fear. We are worthy of love and respect. By seaking 'help' - we are setting good example for our kids. A Life of peace and serenity awaits us. God gives us the courage to change the things we can."*

PLAN IMPLEMENTATION AND MONITORING

After the social worker and client agree upon a safety plan, they begin to work the plan and make adjustments as needed. Social workers realize that their clients will ultimately make their own choices but also understand that maintaining open lines of communication with their clients remains most important. As time goes by, more problems may arise or, as the client trusts the social worker more, issues may be discussed more freely. For example, a battered woman may not have disclosed her substance abuse problem to the social worker at first, because she felt embarrassed or was not ready to address her addiction. Over time and with open lines of communication, the client may come to a point where she is ready to address this issue and mention the problem to her social worker. **Table 9-1** gives examples of common social work interaction scenarios.

Table 9-2 provides descriptions of some common issues that arise when working with clients who have experienced IPV. In addition, it addresses some ways that social workers can effectively obtain the information they seek.

Depending upon the setting in which a social worker works, the intervention into IPV cases varies. **Table 9-3** lists intervention strategies based upon the setting in which the social worker practices.

SERVICE

Case Example

Jackie lived in an abusive marriage for 6 years when she met the district attorney social worker. Jackie had a high school education, not much work experience, and a 4-year-old son named David, whom she adored. Her husband was charged with assault, and she was asking for the charges to be dropped.

The social worker knew that Jackie's attorney was not actually helping her. Her husband had money and had hired an attorney to "represent" her in order to keep her from disclosing family matters to the district attorney's office that could help prosecute him and hold him accountable for his actions. Upon the advice of her attorney, Jackie spoke very little.

Jackie's silence did not matter, because the social worker started with Jackie where she was. The social worker verbalized her realization that Jackie was not prepared to talk, and asked her simply to listen. The social worker told Jackie that it was wrong for her to be hurt, that she did not deserve such treatment, and that she and her son deserved to live in a place where they would not experience constant fear. The social worker helped Jackie develop a safety plan and told Jackie that she and other organizations, such as the local women's center, were available whenever Jackie needed help. Because Jackie could not confirm the abuse under the advice of her attorney, she simply embraced the social worker. With that embrace the social worker and Jackie shared an unspoken, but powerful moment of alliance, hope, and promise. During the next 3 years, Jackie and the social worker met many times, and sometimes they met secretly.

Like most social workers, her caseload was so heavy that she could not give her cell number to all of her clients, because she would have been inundated with telephone calls. Instead, she usually gave her clients the telephone numbers for 24-hour help lines and made plans with her clients for emergency situations. In some cases, she gave her cell phone number to clients who needed extra support. Jackie was one such client. Her social worker talked with Jackie whenever she could, and was open with her whenever she needed to involve child protective services (CPS).

Jackie left her abusive husband but returned a couple of times during that 3-year period. Jackie eventually left for good, obtained a protective order against her husband, and fought her ex-husband for custody. Jackie and her son entered counseling. Fortunately, they have a supportive extended family, and a judge who understood IPV heard her case.

Figure 9-14. *"Domestic violence hurts the way our children choose their HEROS. Stop it today. You should be his hero."*

Figure 9-15. *"It's okay to say no!"*

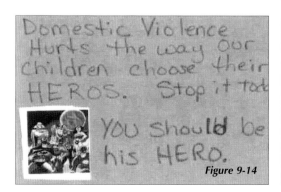

Figure 9-14

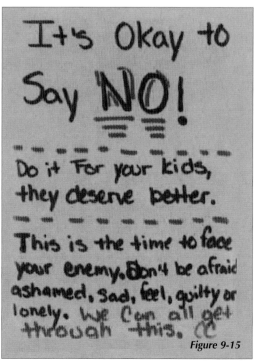

Figure 9-15

191

Table 9-2. Assessment Techniques		
ISSUE	UNCLEAR OR INADEQUATE QUESTIONS AND TECHNIQUES	BETTER OR MORE SPECIFIC QUESTIONS AND TECHNIQUE
Client's Needs	Social worker never asks client what she needs, rather assumes what she wants or needs. Social worker determines what the client needs or wants based upon what the social worker or the agency "usually does" in similar situations.	*How do you feel that we can help you?* *How can I help you?* *What is it that you would like to see happen?* *What most concerns you?* *What are you most afraid of?* *How do you see yourself and your children 6 months or 1 year from now?*
Extent of Physical Violence	*Have you or your children been physically assaulted?* Clients sometimes think this question only refers to being punched, so they do not think about hair pulling, shoving, kicking, or other types of physical assaults.	*Have you or children been hurt?* *When was the first time, last time, and worst time he hurt you.*[5] Ask specific questions about different types of assaults (eg, *Have you been punched? kicked? had your hair pulled?*). Ask questions about more severe types of abuse (eg, *Has he strangled you? Has he become increasingly more violent? Used a weapon? Assaulted you when you were pregnant? Threatened to kill you or your children? Has he become more violent since you left?*).
Sexual Assault	*Have you been raped?* *Have you been sexually assaulted?* These seem like straightforward questions, but they are not. The victim may not even identify "forced sex" because she may feel that she cannot say no to her partner, or she may feel too embarrassed because of the nature of the question.	*Have you had sex when you did not want to?* *Can you tell me about that experience?* *If he wanted to have sex, and you did not want to, what happened?* *Have you ever been beaten right before having sex with your partner?*
Threats of Violence	*Did he threaten to kill you or your children?* This question is good to ask, but needs follow-up questions such as when, under what circumstances?	*What has he told you he would do if you ever left him?* *What has he said about the children?*

(continued)

Table 9-2. *(continued)*

ISSUE	UNCLEAR OR INADEQUATE QUESTIONS AND TECHNIQUES	BETTER OR MORE SPECIFIC QUESTIONS AND TECHNIQUE
Weapons	*Has he ever used or threatened to use a weapon on you or your children?* Many people only think of a gun and forget about other types of weapons (eg, knives).	Be specific. *Has he shown a gun or a knife to you or your children? What did he say when he did that?* *Where was the gun or knife?* *Has he ever hit you or threatened to hit you with any other object, like a piece of wood or a belt?* *Does he own or have access to a gun?*
Substance Abuse	*Do you have a substance abuse problem?* *Are you an alcoholic and/or a drug abuser?* It is hard to say "yes" to these questions even if a person has a problem.	Explain more about the reason this information is needed in order to assist the client. Ask about the victim's or abuser's substance use or abuse. Tell clients it is common for people who have been hurt to "self-medicate," and ask them whether they ever did this. *Have you ever drank, smoked marijuana, or used a drug just to feel better about your situation? If so, details?*
Mental Health	*Do you have mental health problems?* It is hard to say yes to this question.	Explain that it is normal for people who have been hurt to suffer emotionally and mentally, and there is no shame in this suffering. Ask about the mental health of the victim, abuser, and children. *How have you and your children been sleeping, acting, and coping?* *What helps you the most in this situation?* *Have you ever taken or felt like you needed to take any medicine for depression? If so, what kind of medication was taken?* *If you have been to a physician for this type of medicine, did the doctor tell you a name for what was going on with you, for example, did you hear the word "depression"?* *Do you feel like your emotions are out of control, for example, do you start crying without a reason?*

(continued)

Table 9-2. *(continued)*

ISSUE	UNCLEAR OR INADEQUATE QUESTIONS AND TECHNIQUES	BETTER OR MORE SPECIFIC QUESTIONS AND TECHNIQUE
Suicidal Risk	Client gives signs of suicidal thoughts (eg, *Sometimes I just can't go on.*), but social worker does not respond to these signs.	Find out about the risk of suicide for both the abuser and victim. Understand people often commit suicide because they believe suicide is the only way out of an unmanageable situation. Sometimes battered women and abusers reach this point and start to see suicide as an option. If clients are depressed or make statements that they can't go on, perform a suicide risk assessment.
Safe Home, Workplace, or School	*Do you have a safe place to stay?* The social worker and client can have different definitions about what "safe" means.	Be more specific (eg, *Do you have a place to stay that he does not know about?*). If the client is staying someplace that is not confidential, ask her about her plans if her batterer comes to that place. Ask about workplace and school safety.
Strengths	Her strengths may not be addressed by the social worker. Sometimes mental health professionals get stuck in a pathological model and completely leave out the victim's strengths.	The client's strengths may be determined during the assessment process (eg, good coping skills, access to money, supportive family, supportive church). Point out these strengths to the client, and encourage her to use these strengths and build on them.
Pressure Points	Her pressure points may be assumed or touched upon by the social worker, but not specifically addressed	Work with the client to find out what concerns her most. Ask her, *What scares you the most? What is the worst thing that might happen?* Possible answers include: — Her abuser is her sponsor for immigration — She will not have access to money — She is afraid to lose her children — She is afraid of "taking the father away" from her children — She feels sorry for her abuser — She has previous mental health concerns — She has a substance addiction — Her religion prevents her from divorcing — The relationship is a same-sex relationship and the client is afraid of being "outed." — She and her children will be homeless

For more than 2 years after leaving her abusive relationship, Jackie had kept herself and David safe. Jackie and her social worker understood that Jackie could not simply walk out the door and leave a batterer such as her husband. Jackie knew that she would have to have the strength and money not only to leave, but also to fight. Her abusive husband had always told Jackie that he would go after custody of their son, and, true to his word, when he realized Jackie would not return, he did. Prepared for the fight, Jackie rallied and won. Throughout her ordeal, Jackie had the support of many people including her family members, counselors, and law enforcement officers.

Service means being available to work with the client in a manner that assists and supports that client while putting personal interests aside. Social workers must remain careful to not cross the line between service and blind servitude. For example, if the social worker takes control and makes important decisions for the client, even if the client wants, requests, or demands such action, he or she isn't really helping the client. By using an empowerment and strengths model, that is a model that empowers former victims to learn to do things for themselves and recognize their inherent strengths, social workers can teach their clients to become advocates for themselves, as well as make decisions and plans that will allow them to exercise control and responsibility in their own lives and the lives of their children.

The value of service in social work also extends to pro bono work. Many social workers become tense at the thought of providing free work in addition to their usually stressful paid work; however, pro bono work can be simple. The following lists some examples that do not require a large time commitment:

— Providing opportunities for public education about family violence

— Keeping abreast and voting for elected officials who support pro women and children policies

— Placing brochures about IPV where survivors might see them (eg, in a public bathroom, at a place of worship)

— Volunteering time to make a presentation about IPV and domestic violence to a local NASW chapter or to another group

The possibilities for pro bono opportunities are numerous for social workers who can donate more of their time. One example would be providing volunteer counseling services at a local women's shelter.

SOCIAL JUSTICE

Case Example

An experienced social worker was in court with her 45-year-old Hispanic client, Marisol. Marisol was seeking a protective order against her ex-husband on behalf of herself and her 2 young children. Marisol's ex-husband, a white state trooper, had been violent with her in the past. He had forced his way into her home one evening and refused to leave or to allow her to leave the home. Marisol described her feelings as a mixture of fear and outrage. She and her husband had already divorced, and she knew that he had no right to be in her home. Marisol thought that her problems with her ex-husband would be over once their divorce was finalized; however, she learned that the divorce only made him desperate for a last grasp of control over her.

During the incident, Marisol yelled at her ex-husband and expressed her justifiable anger. Standing up for

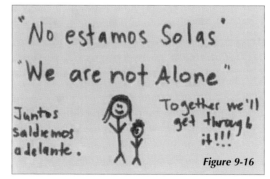

Figure 9-16.
"No estamos solas. We are not Alone"
"Juntos saldemos adelante. Together we'll get through it!!!"

Figure 9-16

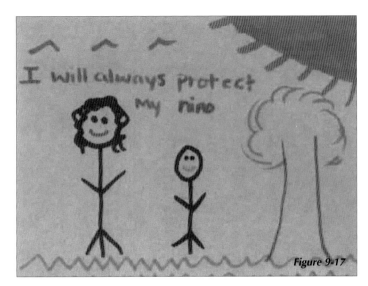

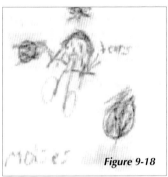

Figure 9-17. *"I will always protect my nino."*

Figure 9-18. *"tears and noises"*

Figure 9-17

Figure 9-18

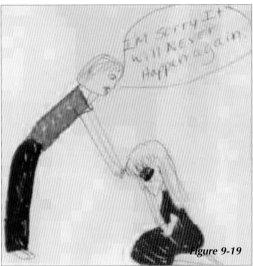

Figure 9-19

Figure 9-19.
This picture portrays a scene in which a man stands over a woman shown with a black eye, the man promises to never use violence again by saying, "I'm sorry. It will never happen again."

herself came back to haunt her, however. The children's ad litem attorney, a man who had little or no understanding about IPV, criticized Marisol for scaring her children by yelling at her ex-husband. The judge agreed with the ad litem attorney; in open court and in front of her batterer, the judge told her, "Lady, you're a hothead."

Marisol and her social worker talked after the hearing. Both had interpreted the unspoken word at the end of the judge's statement—"Mexican – Lady, you're a hotheaded Mexican." Although Marisol felt humiliated in court, it was far worse that the ad litem attorney had recommended unsupervised visitation for her abusive ex-husband, and that the judge had agreed. Such a recommendation further clarified the attorney's lack of understanding regarding IPV, especially since he had only met with her children briefly (about one hour).

Although the events that occurred in that courtroom were unacceptable, Marisol resolved to focus on her future. Her life eventually improved. By remaining beside Marisol even after the hearing, the social worker was able to help Marisol view the justice system more clearly, which helped diffuse some of her feelings of shame. Marisol also found a counselor who understood IPV. With this counselor's help, she and her children began to heal emotionally.

SOCIAL WORKERS WITHIN FAMILY COURTS

Social workers work within various parts of the court and justice systems to advocate on behalf of clients and to educate judges, attorneys, jury members, and other court staff members regarding IPV issues. They also work to promote laws that provide protection and empowerment to IPV victims. Cecelia Burke, the Director of the Travis County Domestic Relations Office in Austin, Texas, says their office has realized the value of involving social workers in the family court system (Oral communication, October 2005).

While many family court systems use attorney guardian ad litems (ie, attorneys hired to represent the best interest of the child in family cases), in Travis County the courts use social worker ad litems. Even in the best of situations, attorney guardian ad litems are trained regarding IPV issues, but they do not have the type of training that really allows them to investigate all the complicated issues that arise in family court, much less the specialized issues that arise with families in which IPV has been a factor. In contrast, these social workers must have a master's degree and several years of experience with family issues, including IPV. Social workers have experience and specialized training in child development, mental health, and substance abuse. In addition, they know how best to communicate with the child whom they represent and can work with the parents to resolve the cases with less conflict than attorney ad litems. Moreover, the social work guardian ad litems can conduct psychosocial evaluations and make recommendations when further psychological evaluations are necessary. In such situations, these social workers can even select the therapists and monitor that therapy. This is especially important because, in the author's experience, mental health professionals often have surprisingly little or no training regarding IPV. Social workers have been trained to understand and interpret psychological reports and make insightful recommendations and comments.

In 2003, the Travis County Domestic Relations Office conducted a 3-month pilot study in which their social worker guardian ad litems interviewed 39 children older than 6 years who had a parent who applied for a protective order.[11] They learned the following from their interviews:

— 80% of the cases involved substance abuse.

— 74% of the children reported failing grades or trouble concentrating.

— 61% of the children reported intervening during a violent incident.

— 56% of the children reported trouble sleeping.

— 13% of the children were in counseling, though 18% had serious issues that
    required referrals to counseling.

— 12% of the cases involved CPS.

These findings underscore the importance of having social workers available to work with family violence victims at the points in which such victims enter the court system.

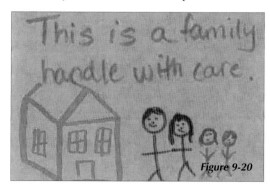

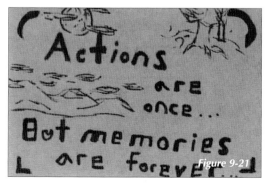

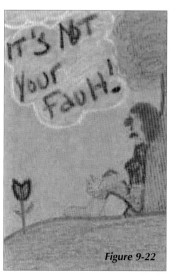

Figure 9-20. *This drawing illustrates the ideal family, free from danger and violence.*

Figure 9-21. *"Actions are once… but memories are forever."*

Figure 9-22. *"It's Not your Fault!"*

Even though CPS is the agency that typically intervenes with families experiencing IPV in many places, protective services clearly cannot shoulder this burden. If more locations appointed social work guardian ad litems in the family courts, these social workers could identify, assess, evaluate, implement, and monitor potentially damaging or explosive situations.

SOCIAL WORKERS WITHIN CRIMINAL JUSTICE AGENCIES

Many family violence victims are reluctant to seek services. As a result, social workers need to work in non-traditional settings where they will encounter family violence survivors (eg, prosecution offices, police agencies, parole departments, probation departments).

One such program exists through the Family Criminal Law Division of the Harris County District Attorney's Office in Houston, Texas. Using a multidisciplinary approach, prosecutors, police officers, social workers, and caseworkers work together to determine policies and procedures for intervening in IPV situations. The chief prosecutor, Jane Waters, leads the team. She frequently says that everyone who comes to the division wants the same thing—safety. The Director of Family Violence Services is a clinical social worker and designed the programs using a social work perspective. Applicants for protective orders and complainants in family violence criminal cases are asked to meet with a social worker before proceeding to work with the legal staff.

Often complainants in family criminal violence cases request that charges be dismissed and do not seek services when they are in the "respite" phase of the cycle of violence. When meeting with the client, the social worker gathers a brief social history, discusses the pending criminal case, addresses the possibility of filing a protective order, discusses risk issues, and outlines the client's options. The social worker uses an empowerment model, points out the client's strengths, and talks about how the client deserves peace and safety. In addition, the social worker works with the client to design a safety plan and works with outside agencies for continued support for the client. After meeting with the client, the social worker recommends probation conditions to prosecutors, which include mental health and IPV counseling and substance abuse treatment.

THE DIGNITY AND WORTH OF THE ABUSE VICTIM

In her fictional novel, *Black and Blue*,[12] Anna Quindlen describes how her main character, Fran Benedetto, goes into hiding from her abusive husband. The caseworker in the book attempts to force Fran to move in order to avoid her husband. When Fran refuses, the caseworker tells her, "Do you want to stay alive?" Fran then thinks about how her caseworker and abusive husband have often made the same types of statements.

Social worker Brené Brown writes about how "silence, secrecy, and judgment" contribute to women's feelings of shame and isolation.[13] She writes that the anecdote to shame is empathy and how empathy leads to "freedom, power, and connection."[13]

Social workers must ask themselves about the price of working with family violence victims in order to help these victims change their circumstances. As shown in the *Black and Blue* example, when social workers use threats, coercive behavior, intimidation, or humiliation, they need to ask how they differ from the batterer. Social workers must consider whether the abused woman feels as though she were first forced to do something by her batterer and now feels forced into another situation by her social worker. This is not empowerment, and such tactics do not work. Social workers can be firm and empowering at the same time, particularly when it comes to addressing the safety of children. **Table 9-3** describes some common scenarios and types of actions and comments, which are controlling and empowering, that social workers can mistakenly make.

Table 9-3. Common Practice Settings for Social Work Intimate Partner Violence Intervention

Scenario	Intervention Opportunity	Options	Cautions and/or Concerns
General (ie, all types of settings)	— Outcry made by client. — Depending upon the setting, ask client open screening questions: — *How safe do you feel at home?* — *Has anyone hurt you?* — *When have you been hurt?* — *How have you been hurt?* — Teach positive family, parenting, and relationship skills.	— Display posters, fliers, or handouts in the appropriate languages regarding domestic violence and referral information. — Have an agency plan that addresses domestic violence, including when to contact law enforcement and child protective services.	— When talking with a client about abuse, speak with them alone. They may not disclose any information at all or disclose information incompletely in front of others (especially in front of the abuser). — Use a person-in-environment approach to understand domestic violence in an individual and societal context. — Know what to tell a client if the client does disclose. — Be ready to help formulate a safety plan. — Know the risk factors and lethality significance. — Know where to refer clients. — Use non-shaming, non-threatening, and respectful intervention techniques. — Especially if testifying in criminal or family court, know the important research and theories regarding IPV. — Know that children do not need to be physically abused in order to suffer damaging effects from violence.
Adult Protective Services	— Report made for domestic abuse. — Report made for any other reason.	— Routine screening for Intimate Partner Violence.	— Clients may deny or minimize the violence experienced. Know how to use collateral resources (eg, police officers, prosecuting attorneys, close friends, relatives) to determine whether abuse has occurred. — Client's disability (ie, cognitive or mental health issues) may prevent her from disclosing. Be aware of collateral sources (caregivers, friends, family apart from the suspected abuser).

(continued)

Table 9-3. *(continued)*

SCENARIO	INTERVENTION OPPORTUNITY	OPTIONS	CAUTIONS AND/OR CONCERNS
Child Protective Services	— Report made for child physical or sexual abuse.	— Routine screening for Intimate Partner Violence.	— See "Adult Protective Services" above. — Speak with the child's teacher or caregiver. — Domestic violence may or may not be noted at the time of the report.
Community Agency	— A family experiencing Intimate Partner Violence goes to a community agency for services. This family may not be seeking services for IPV, but may identify this as an issue once trust has been established.	— Discuss techniques for solving healthy problems. — Teach non-violent communication skills and anger resolutions tactics. — Offer parenting tips and support.	— Batterer uses control with his partner and other family members. If he feels threatened, he may not allow his partner and family members to participate in agency activities. — A community agency may be one of only a few safe places in the family's life.
Criminal Justice– District or County Attorney Offices	— Criminal charges filed for cases involving IPV. — District or county attorney may file protective orders. — Work with the prosecution team.	— Take IPV seriously, treating it like the crime that it is. — Educate prosecutors, police officers, and judges. — Advocate for the safety of the victims and accountably for the offenders.	— Social workers working in criminal justice centers must remain cautious about being co-opted by the agency's beliefs, which are sometimes at odds with social work values. — Important to working within the system, respect coworkers with different viewpoints.
Criminal Justice– Police Agencies	— Investigations for cases involving IPV.	— Educate police officers about IPV issues. — Advocate for the victims.	— See "Criminal Justice– District or County Attorney Offices" above.
Criminal Justice– Probation and/or Parole	— Perpetrators may be on parole or probation. — Victims may be on parole or probation.	— Educate co-workers who may not have social work or human services backgrounds.	— See "Criminal Justice–District or County Attorney Offices" above. — If working as a probation officer, hold batterer accountable to improve the safety of his victims.

(continued)

Table 9-3. *(continued)*

Scenario	Intervention Opportunity	Options	Cautions and/or Concerns
Criminal Justice– *(continued)*		— See other "Criminal Justice" areas above.	— Understand that batterers can use the fact that their victims are on probation or parole in order to control them.
Family Courts	— Intimate Partner Violence reported at the time the divorce or child custody case is filed. — Social worker may suspect IPV based upon interaction between the parties. — Social workers can work as guardian ad litems for children (instead of having attorney ad litems appointed). — Social workers perform home studies in order to determine custody and visitation issues.	— Depending on role, investigate allegations or advocate on behalf of victims. — Testify as an expert witness regarding IPV, common characteristics of batterers and victims, and the impact on children. — Help arrange custody and visitation agreements that increase the safety of children, and lessen the contact between the batterer and abused partner.	— Because of power and control issues involved in IPV, advocate against the use of medication or unsafe depositions in IPV cases. — Be prepared to advocate for child's safety over the rights of parental visitation. — Be aware that custody is one of the batterer's most powerful weapons.
Health Care– Hospital	— Victim seeks medical treatment when assaulted. — Victim may be at the hospital for another reason. — The victim or batterer may seek mental health services.	— Work with the management to have clear policies regarding reports made to police officers and protective services agencies. — Document medical treatment or the suspicion/confirmation of IPV in the records. — Perform routine IPV screenings when client comes to the hospital with injuries.	— If abuse is suspected, give the client information in case she should ever become a victim. — Have information displayed for safety referrals. Client may not disclose, but may contact the agency when she can. — Be prepared to work with batterers or victims to address their needs. — When working with the batterer, advise that a mental health diagnosis is not an excuse for IPV.

(continued)

Table 9-3. *(continued)*

Scenario	Intervention Opportunity	Options	Cautions and/or Concerns
Health Care– Physician's Office or Clinic	— Victim seeks medical treatment when assaulted or may be at physician's office or clinic for un-related reason.	— See "Health Care– Hospital" above. — For any type of examination, ask safety and IPV routine questions.	— See "Health Care– Hospital" above.
Homeless Shelters and Programs	— Victim seeks shelter because she is fleeing IPV.	— Screen for safety and IPV.	— Develop and maintain procedures intended to provide for the safety of families fleeing violence.
Immigration Work	— Victim may report that she has experienced IPV at the hands of her immigration sponsor. — Social worker may suspect abuse based upon interaction between the parties.	— Know about Violence Against Women Act (VAWA) or other legislation that impacts immigrant victims of family violence. — Have information available in appropriate languages that informs immigrants about their right not to be abused and what laws help protect them. — Include questions about abuse in routine screening.	— Because IPV is based upon power and control, know that controlling someone's immigration status is a powerful threat.
Political Setting (eg, Elected Official, Political Staff Member)	— Work to enact and support legislation to strengthen systems that support healthy, safe families.	— Keep track of legislation that can impact IPV as well as empower women and children.	— Be aware that legislation impacts poverty, basic needs, and housing, which all affect a victim's ability to leave and stay away from her violent partner.
Private Practice Counseling and Therapy	— Individuals, couples, or families seek services and may or may not identify their IPV issues.	— Know how to screen and identify for IPV.	— Oftentimes, both partners take responsibility for the violence, or an abuser portrays himself as the "victim" and portrays the true victim as "crazy." *(continued)*

Table 9-3. *(continued)*

SCENARIO	INTERVENTION OPPORTUNITY	OPTIONS	CAUTIONS AND/OR CONCERNS
Private Practice Counseling *(continued)*		— Have a plan in place when the issue of IPV arises, which includes talking with the parties alone. — Discuss healthy relationship values and practices.	— Have a safety plan in place for the family. — Work with the abuser to get him into a batterers' treatment group. — If diagnosing, consider history of abuse, that is, symptoms for posttraumatic stress disorder (PTSD), which may look similar to bipolar disorder. Know how to evaluate such disorders.
Religious Setting– Church Youth Group and Family Supportive Counseling	— Religious leader may be approached regarding "family problems."	— See "Private Practice and Health Care– Hospital" above. — Talk about and teach about healthy, respectful family relationships from the pulpit.	— See "Private Practice and Health Care– Hospitals" above. — Be aware that some religious doctrines can be misinterpreted in order to state that men have absolute control over women.
School	— Child may disclose the violence or abuse to a teacher or a school social worker. — Child may present with other problems (eg, sadness, aggression).	— Provide healthy, non-violent options for problem and anger resolution. — Teach children to call emergency personnel by dialing 911 if they become afraid.	— Know what to say to a child if the child discloses information about abuse or violence. — Use caution when giving general safety information. Some parents, especially batterers, will be uncomfortable with children receiving this type of information. — Have a protocol in place for reporting these situations to protective services.
Substance Abuse Treatment	— The abuser or victim may seek treatment for a substance abuse problem.	— See "Private Practice and Health Care– Hospital" above. — Address abuse and self-esteem issues as part of a recovery plan.	— See "Private Practice and Health Care– Hospital" above. — Substance abuse is no excuse for family violence.

THE IMPORTANCE OF HUMAN RELATIONSHIPS

On November 3, 2005, country singer Mindy McCready appeared on the Oprah Winfrey show. Despite her fame, money, and resources, she described a situation that is shared by thousands of battered women. That is, she described how her boyfriend threatened that he would kill her, beat her severely, and strangled her to the point of near unconsciousness. This did not occur during the first beating, just during the worst one. Though she felt devastated by this attack, she got back together with him and claimed to have become accidentally pregnant. She talked about how she felt compelled to "save" him each time he beat her. Like many women in IPV relationships, McCready struggled with depression and substance abuse. She also tried to kill herself. One of her suicide attempts occurred after her realization that her abusive boyfriend did not show remorse.

INTIMATE PARTNER VIOLENCE RELATIONSHIP

Sometimes people say that women who remain with their batterers "must like being hit," which is ridiculous. Raised to be caregivers, some women feel compelled to help the men who hurt them. They confuse this idea of "saving" their abusers with love. Though nurturing is a good thing, a virtue, and a skill, nurturing taken too far has a dark side. Some women believe they don't have a choice, that that's just the way men are.

The heading on *Seventeen* magazine's May 2005 cover read "Bad B♥ys—Is Loving One Worth It?"[14] Inside was a mere 1-page article in which a young woman discussed her "bad" boyfriend and how she feels good when he needs her and how she wants to save him. Even the title of the article conveys the mixed message that young girls receive. Clearly someone who is "bad" is not good for a young woman. But, even the title of the article, with a heart in place of the "o" in "Boys," implies that they are worth it, and fun to boot. The magazine did not offer insight or commentary from a professional, who could have provided insight into such an abusive relationship or suggestions for girls who find themselves in such situations. Instead, readers were simply encouraged to visit a Web site and make comments.

MOTHERS AND THEIR CHILDREN

One approach to reaching a battered woman is through her children. That is, when battered mothers see how the violence impacts their children, they are often motivated to make changes. Ironically children also keep women in their abusive relationships, because the mothers desire an intact family, have been threatened with losing custody of their children if they leave, or fear for their lives or their children's lives. Courts often allow abusive fathers to have unsupervised visitation. Many mothers would rather stay with the abuser, rather than allow her children to be with him without her there to protect them.

Dr. Bruce Perry, a significant researcher in the area of children and violence, freely shares his work via his Web site for the Child Trauma Academy (www.childtrauma.org). He takes Lenore Walker's theory a step further when he writes about the "vortex of violence"; he writes about how violence is a "flow of rage" that gets passed on from father, to mother, to children, to the outside world.[15] Perry describes how children not only internalize violence on a psychological level, but also how the violence actually changes their biological brain structures. Some mothers actually believe they can protect their children better if they remain in the violent relationship. For many, this belief is true because they have been threatened with losing custody of their children or fear what the batterer will do to the children if he has the opportunity to be alone with them during visitation. As a result, the courts must improve a mother's right to protect her children if she leaves a battering relationship. As previously stated, social workers can help by informing the courts about the impact of violence on children as well as advocating on behalf of family violence survivors.

INTEGRITY

One long-time social work professor tells students to follow the social work code of ethics. Also, when they make a difficult decision, she challenges them to articulate the reason they made that decision and, based on their training and experience, the reason they felt that this was the correct decision.

IPV draws on personal, basic feelings and rights. Sometimes no easy choices exist, and every decision may have potentially disastrous consequences. With their day-to-day work, social workers sometimes lose sight of clients' rights to be safe, make choices, enjoy freedom, and have basic needs met. Because social workers deal with so many emotional issues regarding personal values, they should monitor themselves to ensure that they are working from strengths and a client-centered approach. A social worker may be tempted to say inappropriate things to an abused woman if she chooses to return to a violent relationship even after the social worker has worked with her for months. Instead, the social worker should ask reality-testing questions with true compassion such as, "Well, he said that he would stop hitting you. Has he said that before? What happened?" or "How do you think he has changed?"

A battered woman must know that she can always count on her social worker. Even if the abused woman chooses to return to her batterer, all that the woman has learned from her social worker is not wasted or lost. She will use the information and, if need be, she will come back for help, especially if the social worker did not shame or humiliate her when she decided to return to the abusive relationship. There are situations in which a batterer can choose to stop using violence and control and, if he has not made such choices, the woman will return to the social worker who did not close the door on her.

CONCLUSION

Largely because of the National Association of Social Workers (NASW), social workers are trained in the same values throughout the United States. They have been taught to integrate the NASW-approved values and code of ethics into their work. Social workers hold dear the value of liberty and the freedom from oppression. In addition, they stand ready to advocate for these rights and empower individuals and groups. The fight for social justice and basic human dignity takes place on many levels—individual, family, societal, and political. The social work profession is uniquely qualified to address the intimate partner violence issue on all these fronts.

REFERENCES

1. National Association of Social Workers. *Code of Ethics of the National Association of Social Workers*. Washington, DC: National Association of Social Workers; 1999. Available at: http://www.naswdc.org/pubs/code/code.asp. Accessed August 7, 2005.

2. Dworkin A. Domestic violence: trying to flee. *Los Angeles Times*. October 8, 1995; M1.

3. Walker LE. *The Battered Women*. New York, NY: Harper & Row; 1979.

4. Dutton M. *Empowering and Healing the Battered Woman*. New York, NY: Springer Publishing; 1992.

5. Buel S. Prosecution of domestic violence cases. Presentation at: Harris County District Attorney's office; October 2004; Houston, Texas.

6. Goleman D. *Vital Lies, Simple Truths, the Psychology of Self-Deception*. New York, NY: Simon & Schuster; 1985.

7. Laing RD. In: Goleman D, ed. *The Politics of the Family*. Toronto, Canada: CBC Publications; 1969:40.

8. Campbell JC, Webster D, Koziol-McClain JK, et al. Assessing risk factors for intimate partner homicide. *NIJ J*. November 2003;250:14-19.

9. Renzetti C, Miley C. *Violence in Gay and Lesbian Domestic Partnerships*. New York, NY: The Haworth Press; 1996.

10. McFarlane J, Malecha A, Gist J, et al. An intervention to increase safety behaviors of abused women: results of a randomized clinical trial. *Nurse Res*. 2002;51:347-354.

11. Burke C, Montes C. Family court services. Presentation to demonstrate needs based upon research with the Travis County Domestic Relations Office; 2004; Austin, Texas.

12. Quindlen A. *Black and Blue*. New York, NY: Random House; 1998.

13. Brown B. *Women and Shame: Reaching Out, Speaking Truths & Building Connection*. Austin, Tex: 3C Press; 2004.

14. Bad boys. *Seventeen*. 2005;64:123.

15. Perry B. *The Vortex of Violence: How Children Adapt and Survive in a Violent World* [booklet]. Houston, Tex: Child Trauma Academy; 2002.

Chapter 10

MENTAL HEALTH ASPECTS OF INTIMATE PARTNER VIOLENCE: SURVIVORS, PROFESSIONALS, AND SYSTEMS

Sandra L. Bloom, MD

Intimate partner violence (IPV) represents a public health problem of monumental proportions, but to fully grasp the widespread nature of the problem and the innumerable implications, the issue needs to be reviewed from a life span perspective. Intimate partner violence does not just emerge "out of the blue"; rather, a relationship exists between the maltreatment of children and the violence of adults. Without gaining a perspective of the events that occurred over a person's life span, the connection between that person's exposure to childhood adversity and negative adult outcomes of all kinds (eg, being victimized by and perpetrating IPV) can easily and conveniently be missed. In overlooking these connections, the emergence of a mental health problem in adulthood can easily be seen as being solely related to genetic factors or determined by present life when, in fact, the "psychic fault line" began in childhood, thereby producing a vulnerability only unmasked in adulthood. Similarly, the violent origins of many mental health problems diagnosed in childhood can easily be overlooked because of the barriers to recognizing IPV while the abuse is occurring. Over the last few decades, many studies have connected childhood exposure to a variety of adverse experiences and negative adult outcomes; the Adverse Childhood Experiences (ACE) study has shed the most light on these interconnections.

This chapter covers the following points as related to mental health and IPV:

— The long-term mental health toll resulting from exposure to childhood adversity and the damage resulting from severe, recurrent threats

— The complex effects of IPV that map out the tasks to be completed for recovery to occur

— How the recovery process is not likely to be simple or straightforward since people progress through stages of change and find habits difficult to change

— The difficulty of overcoming the effects of violence, in part, because of the inherent barriers to the psychobiology of trauma that complicate the recovery process and because of the significant personal, professional, and organizational barriers to recovery that must be addressed

— The acronym SELF, which refers to the key domains of trauma recovery—safety, emotions, loss, and future

— That patients, family members, practitioners, and organizations can use SELF to construct the framework used to help create a trauma-informed treatment plan and guide the process of change

— The Sanctuary Model of Organizational Change, which defines the type of organizational culture most conducive to positive transformational change

— Concrete guidelines for professional activism aimed at changing not just the patients, but systems of care that hope to successfully treat them

INTIMATE PARTNER VIOLENCE AS A PUBLIC HEALTH EMERGENCY

ADVERSE CHILDHOOD EXPERIENCES STUDY

When discussing IPV, it is necessary to consider the interrelated aspects of physical, psychological, and social health in order to take into account the effects of exposure to chronic violence across the life span. Like other forms of violence, IPV rarely manifests itself in only one form, and these behaviors are rarely distinctly separate from other high-risk behaviors.

As a result of more than 20 years of research, the scientific community has learned that traumatic experiences can result in a host of chronic and often life-long physical, emotional, occupational, and social problems. The ACE study is the largest study of its kind to examine the health and social effects of adverse childhood experiences over the life span. Kaiser Permanente and the Centers for Disease Control and Prevention (CDC) collaborated on this study. Publications regarding this study began emerging in the scientific literature in 1998.

Study Description

The authors of the ACE study, Vincent Felitti and Robert Anda, asked nearly 18 000 adults who were members of a California health maintenance organization (HMO) to categorize their experiences with childhood adversity. The ACE score was calculated after asking adults whether any of these circumstances applied to conditions they had experienced growing up before the age of 18:

— Recurrent physical abuse

— Recurrent emotional abuse

— Contact sexual abuse

— An alcohol or drug abuser in the household

— An incarcerated household member

— Someone in the household who was chronically depressed, mentally ill, institutionalized, or suicidal

— Mother was treated violently

— One or no parents

— Emotional or physical neglect

The ACE score represented the simple addition of the number of categories of adverse experience in a person's life.

Study Findings

This study mainly consisted of Caucasian men and women who were older than 50 years and had some college education – a population generally considered by the researchers as middle-class. Of this population, about one-third had an ACE score of 0, 1 in 4 admitted to at least 1 category of childhood adversity, 1 in 16 had an ACE score of 4. Sixty-six percent of the women who participated in this study reported at least 1 childhood experience involving abuse, violence, or family strife. The study's researchers then analyzed the respondents' medical data and found clear and direct relationships between the ACE score and a wide variety of physical, emotional, and social diseases and disabilities. To summarize, people exposed to adverse experiences as children are at much greater risk for heart disease, chronic lung disease, liver disease, diabetes, obesity, and hypertension; adults with childhood trauma have increased teenage pregnancy rates, divorce rates, depression, suicide attempts, posttraumatic stress disorder (PTSD), alcoholism, intravenous (IV) drug abuse and dependence, failure in school, unemployment, and many other problems. In addition, as children, adolescents, and adults, people exposed to childhood adversity have a much higher probability of requiring the services of expensive public systems, including health care, special education, child protection, mental health care, and criminal justice services. Felitti and Anda concluded that the ACE study demonstrated a strong graded relationship between the breadth of exposure to abuse or household dysfunction during childhood and multiple risk factors for several of the leading causes of death in adults.[*1-3]

The greater the likelihood that children were exposed to IPV, the greater the likelihood that these children were also physically, sexually, or emotionally abused. Among women, the ACE study found a strong, graded relationship between the number of adverse childhood experiences and the risk of becoming an IPV victim. Similarly, among men the study found a strong, graded relationship between the number of these types of experiences and the risk of subsequently *perpetrating* IPV. For example, childhood physical abuse increased the risk of victimization among women as well as the risk of perpetration by men more than twofold; childhood sexual abuse increased these risks by a factor of 1.8 for both men and women; and witnessing domestic violence increased these risks approximately twofold for women and men. Compared to persons with no violent experiences, the risks for victimization among women and perpetration by men were increased by factors of 3.5 and 3.8, respectively. These results suggest that, as the number of violent experiences increases, the risks of victimization among women and perpetration by men also increase by about 60% to 70%.[3] In addition, these findings confirmed prior reports that people exposed to family aggression and violence have a substantially higher risk of becoming a victim (ie, women) or perpetrator (ie, men) of IPV as adults.[4] Several other studies found similar results, including those studies that showed a significant increase in aggressive and violent behavior among children and adults who experienced child maltreatment.[5-14]

When the researchers looked at the relationship between multiple forms of childhood maltreatment and adult mental health among more than 8000 members of the original study cohort, a dose-response relation was found between the reported number of maltreatment types and the mental health scores; the greater the number of maltreatment types, the lower the mental health scores. In addition, an emotionally abusive family environment accentuated the decrements in mental health scores.[15] When looking at the relationship between alcoholism and childhood adversity, children who grew up in alcoholic households were more likely to have had adverse experiences. The risk of alcoholism and depression in adulthood increased as the number of reported adverse experiences increased, regardless of parental alcohol

---

* *For more information about the ACE study and for a complete list of publications, visit www.acestudy.org or http://www.cdc.gov/nccdphp/ace/index.htm.*

abuse. Depression among adult children of alcoholics appeared to be largely, if not solely, due to the greater likelihood of having adverse childhood experiences in a home with alcohol-abusing parents.[16]

In looking specifically at the relationship between the ACE score and depressive disorders, the number of adverse experiences had a graded relationship to both lifetime and recent depressive disorders. The results suggest that exposure to childhood adversity is associated with an increased risk of depressive disorders even decades after the adverse events occurred.[17] A powerful, graded relationship existed between the ACE score and a risk of attempted suicide at any time during the person's life span. Such risk of suicide is mediated by alcoholism, depressed affect, and illicit drug use, which are all strongly associated with such experiences.[18]

Reasons Interpersonal Violence Is Problematic Across the Life Span

The authors of the ACE study proposed an explanatory pyramid to serve as a conceptual framework for understanding the impact of adversity across the life span (**Figure 10-1**). Exposure to violence in childhood frequently disrupts normal neurodevelopment. These disruptions of critical developmental pathways can result in a wide variety of social, emotional, and cognitive impairments in childhood and throughout adolescence. In late childhood and adolescence, these impairments put children at risk for the adoption of risky health behaviors such as drinking, drugs, smoking, and promiscuity. Over time, these behaviors, coupled with the lifestyles that support such behaviors, lead to disease, disability, social problems, and, ultimately, premature death. In the past, these linkages were overlooked because the problems were diverse in presentation, complex, and had developed over long periods of time.

Figure 10-1.
The ACE Pyramid shows how negative experiences in childhood lead to social, emotional, and cognitive impairments.

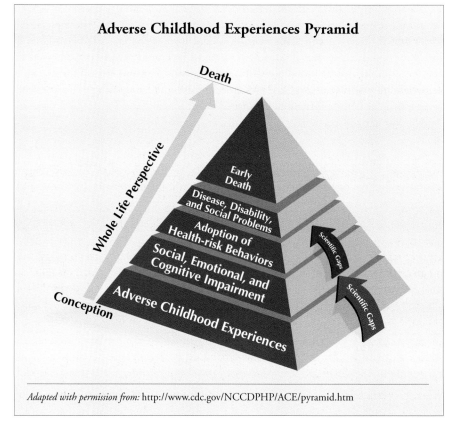

Adapted with permission from: http://www.cdc.gov/NCCDPHP/ACE/pyramid.htm

Children and adults exposed to interpersonal violence usually do not experience a single incident; rather, interpersonal violence tends to be repetitive and haunt victims' lives. The chronic nature of so many tortured life circumstances creates lifelong problems.

CHILDREN EXPOSED TO FAMILY VIOLENCE

The following provides more evidence regarding the complex mental health problems presented by so many children, adolescents, and adults who have been recurrently victimized as the result of IPV.

Incidence

Many of the studies conducted during the past 20 years confirm the findings of the ACE study. In 1973, Steinmetz and Straus called the family the *cradle of violence*.[19] Hitting children is virtually universal in the United States. A quarter of the infants between the ages of 1 and 6 months are hit; this number increases to half of all infants by the time they become 6 months to 1 year old.[20] Sibling-to-sibling violence is also the norm, in that 80% of children report experiencing peer violence.[21] According to US government statistics, more than 4 children die each day in the Untied States as a result of child abuse in the home. In 2003, an estimated 1500 children died of abuse and neglect and over three-quarters of them were younger than 4 years of age. In 2003, more than 2.9 million reports of possible maltreatment involving children were made to child protective service agencies and of those an estimated 906 000 children had substantiated cases of maltreatment.[22] It is estimated that the actual incidence of abuse and neglect is estimated to be 3 times greater than the number reported to authorities.[23] In addition, more than 60% of rape cases occur before victims reach the age of 18 years, and more than 29% of cases occur before the age of 11 years.[24]

According to another nationwide survey released by the Family Violence Prevention Fund, more than 1 in 3 Americans have witnessed an incident of IPV.[25] Many studies demonstrated that when children witness IPV, the effects are extremely detrimental and predispose male children, in particular, to the subsequent use of violence in future relationships.[26-30] Exposure to conflict and violence plays a major role in how children learn to relate to others, how they develop their self-concept and self-control, and how they interact with future dating and marital partners.

Studies demonstrate that children from violent homes exhibit higher risks for alcohol and drug abuse as well as juvenile delinquency. In addition, these children are more likely to perform poorly in school, present discipline problems in school, and have trouble getting along with other children. In understanding the problem of IPV and the effect that violence has on children, researchers highlight the ways a violent home environment negatively impacts a child's ability to succeed within a learning environment, which is usually part of a broader, interconnected problem these children face in living within a violent society.[31] Homes in which IPV occurs are perfect environments for creating bullies. Studies indicate that bullies often come from homes in which physical punishment is used, children are taught to strike back physically to handle problems, and parental involvement and warmth are lacking.[32] Such modeling of aggressive behavior may include physical and verbal aggression toward the children by their parents or the use of physical and verbal aggression by parents toward one another.[33]

Mental Health Impact on Children Who Witness Violence

Children who have witnessed violence tend to be more aggressive than children who have not witnessed violence. In essence, children who witness violence learn that violence is appropriate social behavior. One study monitored 285 inner-city children in the fourth through sixth grades. This study found that violent victimization directly correlated to negative social outcomes through the mediation of emotion dysregulation; that is, these children did not learn to manage their emotions appropriately, which left them vulnerable to many other social and academic adjustment difficulties. The results demonstrated that exposure to violence is linked to multiple levels of behavioral and social maladjustment. Additionally, these results suggested distinct patterns of risk associated with different forms of exposure to violence.[34]

Children who witness domestic violence are likely to learn destructive patterns of conflict resolution.[35] In general, childhood exposure to IPV can be associated with an increased display of aggressive behavior, increased emotional problems (eg, depression, anxiety), lower levels of social competence, and poorer academic functioning.[36]

One study showed that youths with a lot of exposure to community violence reported more fears, anxiety, internalizing behavior, and negative life experiences than those with little exposure to such violence.[37] In addition, these researchers examined the psychophysiological state of the adolescents in the study by having them watch a montage of media violence and then measuring the physical status of these adolescents. Those young people who had been exposed to high levels of community violence exhibited lower baseline heart rates than those with low exposure. Presumably, these adolescents had grown "used to" the violence and no longer had the normal physical responses associated with stress. Community violence exposure predicts both posttraumatic stress and separation anxiety symptoms, both of which increase the likelihood that a person will turn to substance abuse.[37]

One researcher wanted to find out how exposure to violence impacts the intelligence quotients (IQs) of children.[36] After controlling for confounders like a child's gender, a caregiver's IQ, the home environment, the child's socioeconomic status, and prenatal exposure to substance abuse, violence exposure was found to be related to the first-grade child's IQ and reading ability. Trauma-related distress accounted for additional variance in reading ability. A child experiencing both exposure to violence and trauma-related distress at or above the 90th percentile would be expected to have a 7.5-point decrement in IQ and a 9.8-point decrement in reading achievement.[36]

Another group of researchers wanted to determine whether young children of substance-abusing mothers witnessed more violence than children of non-substance-abusing mothers. Their study surveyed 6-year-old, inner-city children of both substance-abusing and non-substance-abusing mothers and yielded the following results[38]:

— The children of substance-abusing mothers did not witness more violence than children of non-substance-abusing mothers; however, among these children:

  — The children who had witnessed violence exhibited significantly more aggressive, anxious or depressed, and withdrawn behavior as well as attention and social problems.

  — More than half of the children had witnessed some form of violence, regardless of whether their mothers were or were not drug addicts.

One result of living within a community in which there is a high level of violence, particularly IPV, is that many of the adults who are killed are also parents. Children who lose parents often suffer long-term difficulties as a result. One study sought to measure the emotional adjustment of children. The investigators for this study compared a group of parentally bereaved children with a disaster-comparison group and with a nontraumatized control group. The parentally bereaved children reported significantly more PTSD symptoms than the other 2 groups. Among the bereaved children, the girls, younger children, and children living with a surviving parent who scored high on a measure of posttraumatic stress reported more symptoms.[39]

Violent juveniles tend to have co-occurring problems (eg, victimization, substance abuse, school failure) and can be described as "multiple-problem youths." Overall, children exposed to multiple forms of family violence reported twice the rate of youth violence as those from nonviolent families. Adolescents who were not themselves victimized but grew up in families in which partner violence occurred were 21% more likely to report violent delinquency than those not exposed to such violence.[40] In many areas of research, studies consistently find a continuous progression from childhood aggression to juvenile violence to adult violence. The onset of violence at an early age predicts a large number of violent offenses in that person's lifetime.

Risk factors for juvenile violence can be categorized as individual, family, peer, and social[41]:

— ***Individual risk factors.*** Include high impulsiveness and low intelligence, which is possibly linked to the executive functions of the brain

— ***Family risk factors.*** Include poor supervision, harsh discipline, childhood physical abuse, a violent parent, a large family, poverty, and a broken family life

— ***Peer factors.*** Include delinquent friends and gang membership

— ***Social risk factors.*** Include an urban residence in a high-crime neighborhood characterized by gangs, guns, and drugs

DATING VIOLENCE

Incidence

Dating violence is a serious problem among adolescents. According to Youth Risk Behavior Surveys performed in Massachusetts during 1997 and 1999, rates of physical and sexual violence from dating partners does not begin in adulthood; rather, such violence has roots in adolescent experience.

Adolescent responses obtained by the CDC in the Youth Dating Violence Survey indicated that approximately 1 in 5 female students reported being physically or sexually abused by a dating partner. The children reported experiencing many kinds of psychological and physical victimization within dating relationships, including the following[42]:

— Their partners did something to deliberately make them feel jealous, damaged their possessions, said things to hurt their feelings, insulted them in front of others, tried to control them, threatened them, blamed them for bad things that the dating partners did, and brought up something from the past to hurt them.

— In terms of perpetrating psychological abuse in a dating relationship, more than half of the adolescents reported that they hurt their dating partner's feelings, insulted their partner in front of others, did something just to make their partner jealous, tried to control their partner, and damaged their partner's possessions.

— Some adolescents perpetrated physical violence in dating situations by scratching, kicking, slapping, biting, choking, pushing, grabbing, or shoving their partner; hitting their partner with a fist or something hard; throwing something that hit their dating partner; physically twisting their partner's arms; slamming or holding their partner against a wall; or bending the partner's fingers.

In a Canadian study, investigators examined the relationship between child maltreatment, clinically relevant adjustment problems, and dating violence in a community sample of adolescents. For this study, adolescents from 10 high schools in Ontario completed questionnaires to assess past maltreatment, current adjustment, and dating violence. Girls who had a history of maltreatment experienced a higher risk of emotional distress when compared with girls without such histories. These girls were also at greater risk for violent and nonviolent delinquency and for carrying concealed weapons. Boys who had histories of maltreatment were 2.5 to 3.5 times more likely to report clinical levels of depression, posttraumatic stress, and overt dissociation than boys without a maltreatment history. These boys also had a significantly greater risk of using threatening behaviors or physical abuse against their dating partners.[43]

Another study examined the association between a history of dating violence and the sexual health of adolescent females. For this study, more than 500 black, adolescent females first completed a survey to assess dating violence, which was defined as having ever had a physically abusive boyfriend, and then were interviewed to assess their sexual behaviors. Dating violence was reported by 18.4% of these adolescents. Adolescents with a history of dating violence within the previous 6 months were 2.8 times more likely to have a sexually transmitted infection (STI); 2.8 times more likely to have nonmonogamous, male partners; and half as likely to use condoms consistently. Furthermore, adolescents with a history of dating violence were significantly more likely to fear the perceived consequences of negotiating condom use, fear discussing pregnancy prevention with their partners, have a higher perceived risk of acquiring an STI, perceive less control over their sexuality, have peer norms that did not support condom use, and have norms that did not support having a healthy relationship.[44]

Researchers found that girls also victimized boys. According to responses from 978 college women, 29% admitted to involvement in physical aggression against their male partners within a 5-year period. Younger women (ie, women in their 20s) were significantly more likely to exhibit physical aggression toward their partners than women who were 30 years old and older. Women stated that they expressed aggression toward their male partners partly because they wanted to engage their partner's attention, particularly emotionally. Additionally, these women did not believe that their male victims would be seriously injured or would retaliate.[45]

Another study evaluated whether perpetrators of dating violence could be differentiated from their nonviolent counterparts regarding their measures of anger and cognitive distortion. Of the 95 male and 152 female undergraduates surveyed, 27% (24 males and 43 females) reported using some form of physical aggression against their current dating partner within the past year. On a self-report measure of anger (ie, State-Trait Anger Expression Inventory), violent people reported higher levels of intense anger and lower levels of anger control when compared to nonviolent participants. While there were no differences between violent and nonviolent participants' levels of anger as a trait, the results suggested that violent individuals have difficulty controlling angry feelings when these feelings arise, which may increase the likelihood of externally directed forms of anger expression.[46] Everyone feels anger, but some people may feel anger more intensely and have more difficulty controlling anger than others.

Mental Health Effects of Dating Violence

Dating violence is associated with an increased risk for substance abuse; unhealthy weight-control behaviors (eg, using laxatives, vomiting); sexually risky behaviors (eg, first intercourse before 15 years of age); pregnancy; and suicidal tendencies.[47] Female victims of severe dating violence and forced sexual intercourse were more likely to report poor mental and physical health as well as suicide attempts than other females. Likewise, male perpetrators of severe dating violence were more likely to report poor mental and physical health, dissatisfaction with life, and suicide attempts.[48]

INTIMATE PARTNER VIOLENCE IN ADULTS

Incidence

Surveys conducted around the world indicate that between 10% and 50% of women report they have been physically abused by a male partner; in the United States, the annual estimated number of physical abuse cases ranges from about 2 to 8 million.[49] The National Violence Against Women Survey (NVAWS) and the National Crime Victimization Survey (NCVS) are generally regarded as the best sources of current data regarding violence between intimate partners. The NFVS data represent survey data collected regarding spousal and parent-child violence as well as psychological abuse in 2 national household surveys conducted in 1975 and 1985. According to the data collected, an estimated 1.8 million women were beaten by their partners annually.[50] Based on the NVAWS, which represents survey data collected during 1995 and 1996, 1.9 million women are physically assaulted each year and another 300 000 are raped; in most of these cases the perpetrators are intimate partners.[51] Between 8% and 24% of women will be stalked by someone.[51,52] Add this finding to the 25% to 35% chance that the average adult woman was sexually abused as a child, that between 15% and 25% of pregnant women are battered,[24] and that violence kills as many American women every 5 years as the total number of Americans who died in the Vietnam War,[24] and the epidemiology of IPV against women can be seen as not only a pressing social issue, but a public health emergency.[53]

Substance abuse plays a role in exacerbating, if not actually causing, situations of family violence. Between 25% and 50% of the men committing acts of IPV also have substance abuse problems. As many as 80% of child abuse cases are associated with the use of alcohol and other drugs.[54] Women who abuse alcohol or drugs are more likely to become victims of domestic violence. Victims of domestic violence are more likely to abuse alcohol and to receive prescriptions for and become dependent upon tranquilizers, sedatives, stimulants, and painkillers.[54]

Mental Health Aspects of Intimate Partner Violence in Adult Women

Many victims of family violence also suffer from mental illness. One study of 941 young adults found that half of those involved in partner violence had a psychiatric disorder and one third of those with a psychiatric disorder were involved in partner violence. Individuals involved in severe partner violence had elevated rates of a wide range of disorders.[55]

Another study was designed to determine the prevalence of domestic violence among female patients and to identify clinical characteristics associated with current domestic violence. This large study looked at 1952 female patients of varying ages and marital, educational, and economic statuses who were seen by health care personnel in a primary care setting between February and July 1993. The study determined the following[56]:

— Domestic violence was experienced by:

— 5.5% of the respondents during the year before the study was conducted

— 21.4% of respondents sometime during their adult lives

— 22% of respondents before the age of 18 years old

— 32.7% of respondents as either an adult or a child

— Compared with women who had not recently experienced domestic violence, currently abused patients were more likely to:

— Be younger than 35 years

— Be single, separated, or divorced

— Receive medical assistance or have no insurance

— Exhibit more physical symptoms

— Score higher on instruments that assess for depression, anxiety, somatization, and interpersonal sensitivity (ie, low self-esteem)

— Have a partner who abuses drugs or alcohol

— Abuse drugs or alcohol

— Have attempted suicide

— Have visited the emergency department more frequently, but have not had more hospitalizations for psychiatric disorders

Another study examined the relationship between childhood abuse and partner abuse among a sample of predominantly black and Hispanic women who were patients in methadone clinics in Harlem, NY, and the South Bronx, NY. A structured questionnaire addressing demographics, psychosocial and physical health characteristics, depression, childhood abuse, and domestic violence was given to 151 women. This study found that[57]:

— More than half of the women (60%) reported lifetime physical, life-threatening, or sexual abuse by a spouse or boyfriend.

— Women who reported childhood physical abuse were almost 9 times more likely to report having been abused by a spouse or boyfriend.

— Women who reported childhood sexual abuse were almost 4 times more likely to report having been abused by a spouse or boyfriend.

— Depression and a need for social support were significantly associated with partner abuse.

— Current heroin use was inversely associated with partner abuse.

The mentally ill frequently have a past history of victimization as children or as adults. One study looked at 331 involuntary psychiatric patients. The rate of nonviolent, criminal victimization (22.4%) was similar to that found in the general population (21.1%); the rate of violent, criminal victimization, however, was 2.5 times greater than that found in the general population (8.2% vs. 3.1%). Substance use and transient living conditions were strong predictors of criminal victimization.[58]

One study surveyed 54 adult, black, psychiatric outpatients who were previously identified as victims of sexual or physical assault. They were asked about the nature of the assaults, their relationship to the perpetrator(s), the number of assaults suffered in each relationship, and whether the assault(s) occurred before or after the onset of their mental illness. The researchers found that[59]:

— Eighty percent had experienced major physical assault as an adult.

— Fifty-nine percent had experienced major physical assault as a child.

— Thirty-seven percent reported major sexual assault as a child.

— Thirty-one percent reported major sexual assault as an adult.

— Women were more likely than men to report having been physically and sexually assaulted as an adult and as a child.

— Childhood assault most often occurred before the onset of the patient's mental illness.

— Adult sexual assault for women and physical and sexual assault for men was as likely to occur after the onset of the psychiatric disorder, thereby suggesting an increased vulnerability to victimization for the adult mentally ill.

In a series of large studies, researchers first established that exploring the temporal consistency of reports of childhood sexual abuse, adult sexual abuse, and adult physical abuse, as well as current symptoms of PTSD among 50 people with serious mental illness could yield reliable information essential to further research in this area.[60] Next, these researchers reviewed a number of studies regarding physical and sexual assault against women with serious mental illness. This review showed that, across the studies[61]:

— Between 51% and 97% of participants experienced lifetime physical or sexual assault.

— A significant proportion of participants had experienced multiple acts of victimization.

A recent, large study, which is part of a larger investigation of risky behavior and STIs in men and women with serious mental illness, found that[62]:

— Approximately one third of the women reported having been the victim of sexual assault, physical assault, or both within the past year.

— Eighty percent of women reported having been assaulted sometime since the age of 16.

— Most respondents reported a history of childhood abuse, with approximately two thirds of the women reporting being assaulted before the age of 16.

— Revictimization appears to be the norm for this population of women (87% reported having been either physically or sexually assaulted during their lifetime).

— Recent assault was associated with an alcohol use disorder, a drug use disorder, being younger, having never been married, recent homelessness, and childhood physical or sexual abuse.

— Race, poverty, and employment status were not associated with recent assault.

Posttraumatic Stress Disorder and Family Violence

Women have a higher rate of PTSD than men; in fact, some studies show that women experience PTSD at twice the rate of men.[63] Wanting to explore this difference further, investigators examined data from a community survey of trauma exposure and PTSD in Winnipeg, Canada. This study showed that after exposure to serious trauma (even when sexual trauma, which predominates in women, was excluded), women were at a significantly increased risk for PTSD. Adjusting for gender differences in the number of lifetime traumas or in the likelihood of the trauma being associated with particular reactions to or consequences of the event (eg, thinking that one would be killed or seriously injured, sustaining a serious physical injury, seeing someone else seriously injured or killed) did not result in a lessening of the PTSD risk in women. Women were found to be at increased risk for PTSD after experiencing a nonsexual assault (eg, mugging, another physical attack) but not after a trauma that did not involve an assault (eg, fire, witnessing injury to others).[64]

Another group of researchers examined potential sources of the community's gender differences regarding PTSD by reviewing data from 2181 people between the ages of 18 and 45 years old who lived in Detroit's primary metropolitan statistical area. This study concluded the following[65]:

— The lifetime prevalence of exposure and the mean number of traumas were lower in female respondents than in males.

— The overall conditional risk of PTSD (ie, the probability of PTSD among those exposed to a trauma) was approximately 2 times higher in female respondents than males, when adjusting for the gender difference in the distribution of trauma types.

— The gender difference primarily resulted from females' being at greater risk after an assault.

— The gender difference within the "avoidance and numbing symptom" group after an assault exceeded the gender differences found in other symptom groups.

Various studies showed that the rate of PTSD is very high in populations of battered women; in fact, studies indicated that PTSD in battered women ranged from 33% to 84%.[66] One group of researchers looked at battered women attending a domestic violence clinic and found the overall rate of PTSD to be 45%, while 60% of those women with high exposure to life threatening events had PTSD.[67] In another study of battered women from a shelter, 84% had PTSD.[68] Researchers studied the prevalence of PTSD in women participating in domestic violence programs and compared them to women who were not participants. The researchers found that the participants had a 60% rate of PTSD compared to nonparticipants, who had a 62% rate of PTSD.[69] In a primary care setting, 39% of the patients referred for mental health consultation met criteria for PTSD, and the most frequent traumas associated with the PTSD were domestic violence and childhood abuse.[70]

Another group of researchers wanted to explore the relationship between symptoms of PTSD and severity of abuse, so they interviewed an ethnically stratified group of 131 abused women in a primary care setting. Symptoms of PTSD, both intrusion (eg, trouble falling asleep, strong waves of feelings about the abuse) and avoidance (eg, trying not to think or talk about the abuse, staying away from reminders of the abuse) were significantly correlated to the severity of abuse regardless of ethnicity. When asked about childhood physical or sexual abuse, women who reported physical abuse had significantly higher intrusion scores, whereas those who reported sexual abuse had significantly higher avoidance scores. Sixty-five percent of the women reported dreams, flashbacks, or terror attacks regarding the abuse and had significantly higher mean results on both intrusion and avoidance.[71]

People suffering from chronic PTSD are 2 to 4 times more likely than those without PTSD to have virtually any other psychiatric disorder.[63] In addition, they are almost 8 times as likely to have 3 or more disorders. In fact, 88% of men and 79% of women with PTSD have a history of at least 1 other disorder. Women with PTSD are 4 to 5 times more likely than those without PTSD to also suffer from an affective disorder and are 2 to 4 times more likely to have another anxiety disorder.[72]

Another study showed that people with 1 or more symptoms of PTSD were more likely than those without any mental disorder to experience poor social support, marital difficulties, and occupational problems, as well as more impairment on their income and disability measures than those with a major depressive disorder. Consistent with the findings from many other studies of specific trauma groups, the study showed that people who had PTSD symptoms were also more likely to have a number of chronic illnesses. Although these patients had a disproportionate use of the health care system, they were reluctant to seek mental health treatment, a finding consistent with many other studies, as well.[63]

One group of authors proposed a model to explain the relationship between PTSD and serious mental illness. They proposed that PTSD mediates the negative effects of trauma on the course of serious mental illness by influencing both the PTSD and other psychiatric disorders directly through the effects of specific PTSD symptoms (eg, avoidance, hyperarousal, re-experiencing the trauma) as well as indirectly through the effects of common correlates of PTSD (eg, retraumatization, substance abuse, difficulties with interpersonal relationships).[73]

Posttraumatic Stress Disorder and Sexual Assault

Sexual assault is strongly associated with suicidal tendencies and other emotional problems. In one study, 22% of the women polled said that they had been forced to do sexual things against their will. Usually, an intimate partner had forced them.[74] In another study that controlled for sex, age, education, posttraumatic stress symptoms, and psychiatric disorder, the researchers associated a history of sexual assault with an increased prevalence of lifetime suicide attempts. For women, the odds of attempting suicide were 3 to 4 times greater when the first reported sexual assault occurred before the age of 16 years in comparison to a sexual assault that occurred at the age of 16 years or older.[75]

The prevalence of PTSD after rape is very high. In a review of 9 studies that investigated the prevalence of PTSD among victims of rape or other sexual violence, 4 studies showed the rate as greater than 70%.[76] In a survey of more than 2000 women who were asked about victimization experiences, rates of "nervous breakdowns," suicidal ideation, and suicide attempts were significantly higher for crime victims than for nonvictims. Victims of attempted rape, completed rape, and attempted sexual molestation had problems more frequently than victims of attempted robbery, completed robbery, aggravated assault, or completed molestation. Nearly 1 rape victim in 5 (19.2%) had attempted suicide, whereas only 2.2% of nonvictims had done so. Most sexual assault victims' mental health problems occurred after their victimization.[77]

The National Women's Study produced dramatic evidence regarding the mental health impact of rape by determining comparative rates of several mental health problems among rape victims and women who had never been victims of rape. This study found that[78]:

— Almost one third of all rape victims developed PTSD sometime during their lifetimes, and more than 1 in 10 rape victims still had PTSD at the time of assessment.

— Rape victims were 6.2 times more likely to develop PTSD than women who had never been victims of crime.

— Thirty percent of rape victims had experienced at least 1 major depressive episode in their lifetimes, and 11% of all rape victims were experiencing a major depressive episode at the time of assessment.

— Only 10% of women never victimized by violent crime had ever had a major depressive episode, and only 6% had a major depressive episode when assessed.

— Rape victims were 3 times more likely than nonvictims of crime to have ever had a major depressive episode and were 3.5 times more likely to be currently experiencing a major depressive episode.

— Rape victims were 4.1 times more likely than noncrime victims to have contemplated suicide and 13 times more likely than noncrime victims to have actually made a suicide attempt.

The fact that 13% of all rape victims had actually attempted suicide confirms the devastating and potentially life-threatening mental health impact of rape.

Stalking and Mental Health

Studies show that as many as 1 in 20 women will be stalked during their lifetimes. Most stalking victims are female, and the offenders are usually men who have been intimate partners. Stalking behaviors range from surveillance of the victim to threatening, aggressive, or violent acts toward the victim. Victims may experience anxiety, depression, guilt, helplessness, and PTSD symptoms.[79] One study looked at 35 battered women who were classified as being "relentlessly stalked" and compared them to 31 battered women who were "infrequently stalked." Compared to infrequently stalked battered women, relentlessly stalked battered women reported the following[80]:

— More severe and concurrent physical violence, sexual assault, and emotional abuse

— Increased postseparation assault and stalking

— Increased rates of depression and PTSD

— More extensive use of strategic responses to abuse

Substance Abuse and Intimate Partner Violence

People who abuse substances tend to have high rates of exposure to violence both before and after they begin using substances. Family violence and substance abuse share a number of behavioral features, which include loss of control, continuation of behavior despite adverse consequences, preoccupation or obsession, tolerance development, and family involvement. Especially when combined, both disorders predispose the next generation to both domestic violence and addictive disorders. Sexual abuse and substance abuse also have common features, and both also predispose these disorders to the next generation.[81] According to one author, the insidious process of addiction in families creates a conspiracy of silence and denial coupled with unpredictable, unavoidable stress, trauma, and deprivation. The complex interplay of isolation, inhumane treatment, inconsistency, and indoctrination within these families results in a process similar to brainwashing in which members gradually relinquish their own identity and develop robotlike patterns of adaptive behaviors. Survival role performances replace interactive relationships, thereby allowing the family member to participate in the family but avoid and hide from the painful reality of what is happening. Adaptive survival behaviors continue to operate even after a family member leaves home, and the survival maneuvers of an innocent child become the automatic behaviors of a dysfunctional adult.[82] In a study of 375 women at an inner-city clinic, researchers asked patients about intimate violence. This study learned that of the women[83]:

— 37.6% reported having experienced physical assault by an intimate partner

— 32.8% reported verbal threats of violence

— 15.5% reported at least 1 episode of physical abuse in the year preceding their participation in the study

In addition, physical violence was associated with drug use, history of sexually transmitted infection, and history of a serious medical condition.[83]

Another study assessed 105 substance abusers for family violence. This study found that[84]:

— 37% had a family history of physical violence

— 22% were adult victims of physical violence

— 14% were victims of childhood abuse

— 18% were perpetrators of physical violence

Additionally, this study found that the respondents within the group in which substance abuse was combined with family violence had significantly more self-reported and positive urine screens for cocaine use within the 2-month monitoring period, more individual therapy sessions attended, and significantly higher scores on the Michigan Alcoholism Screening Test and the Beck Depression Inventory.[84]

Studies show that women who are substance abusers are more likely than non-substance abusers to become victims of domestic violence and that pregnant women have an increased risk for forced sexual encounters than nonpregnant women. The most common perpetrators of domestic violence are boyfriends or ex-boyfriends. In one study, researchers compared a group of pregnant women who did not abuse substances with another group of pregnant women who did abuse substances. Within the non-substance-abuse group, researchers found the following[85]:

— 7% of the obstetric patients and 5% of the gynecologic patients were abused during the year preceding the study

— 1% of the obstetric patients were abused while pregnant

— 3% of the obstetric patients were forced to have a sexual encounter within the year preceding the study

Within the substance-abuse group, researchers discovered the following[85]:

— 15% of the obstetric patients were abused during the year preceding the study

— 7% were abused while pregnant

— 15% were forced to have a sexual encounter within the year preceding the study

Women who abuse substances have a significant risk of experiencing sexual trauma during their lives. In one study, researchers interviewed 60 women living in a residential treatment facility for the treatment of chemical dependency and asked them about the sexual trauma they had experienced in their lives. Of the women interviewed, 73% had been raped and 45% had been raped more than once.[86] Childhood sexual abuse is also a common problem within this population. In one study, childhood sexual abuse was reported by 13.5% of women and by 2.5% of men. There was a significant association between childhood sexual abuse and the subsequent onset of mood, anxiety, and substance-use disorders among 14 of the women. Among women, rape (versus molestation), knowing the perpetrator (versus a stranger), and chronic nature of the childhood sexual abuse (versus isolated incidents) were associated with higher odds of some disorders.[87]

The signs of substance abuse and sexual victimization sometimes overlap. Typical signs of sexual victimization within this population include vague or no memories of significant periods of time; vague memories of having been abused; promiscuous sexual relationships; avoidance of sexual relationships; unexplained or multiple gynecologic problems; significant changes over a short time in school achievement or in the person's conduct; early use of alcohol or drugs; binge eating during childhood or early adolescence; attempts made to be physically unattractive; sudden weight gain or loss; deterioration in personal grooming; dissociative experiences; abrupt personality changes; recurring nightmares with themes of victimization; inexplicable depression, anxiety, and fear; sudden changes in social, occupational, or academic functioning; running away; depression; anxiety; and irritability.[88]

As previously stated, women who abuse alcohol or drugs are more likely to become victims of domestic violence. Likewise victims of domestic violence are more likely to abuse alcohol and receive prescriptions for and become dependent upon tranquilizers, sedatives, stimulants, and painkillers.[54] A study of 91 adults seeking treatment for cocaine dependence found that[89]:

— 86% reported being physically assaulted at least once during their lifetime

— 61% reported being attacked with a weapon during their lifetime

— 56% reported being attacked without a weapon, but with the intent to kill or seriously injure

— Nearly half of respondents reported being physically assaulted by an intimate partner

— Close to half of respondents met criteria for PTSD at some point in their lives

— Women were more likely than men to be physically assaulted by an intimate partner and to report PTSD

— Those who had been physically assaulted by an intimate partner were more than 4 times as likely to meet criteria for current PTSD and more than 2 times more likely to meet criteria for lifetime PTSD

REASONS INTIMATE PARTNER VIOLENCE IS SO DAMAGING

To understand the true nature of the connections between IPV and mental health problems, both a life span perspective and the recognition that comorbidity is the rule rather than the exception are necessary. There is no one common pathway. Being battered increases the likelihood that a woman will suffer a variety of physical, emotional, and social problems. Likewise, witnessing domestic violence or being maltreated as a child leaves people vulnerable to a variety of physical, emotional, and social problems, including becoming a victim or a perpetrator of IPV.

Chronic exposure to trauma produces hypersensitivity to threat, so that even small stresses produce large and inappropriate responses.[90] Extremist thinking, which is characteristic of the acute stress response, becomes chronic in IPV victims. Chronic extremist thinking, when combined with constant attention to even the smallest threat, interferes with the person's cognitive development.[91] Aggression and poor impulse control are also normal parts of the acute stress response; under conditions of chronic stress, these may become typical responses to even mildly frustrating or aggravating life situations, thereby precipitating school, learning, and relational problems and especially affecting violence directed toward the self and others. A person's inability to manage distressing emotions further interferes with cognitive development, thereby producing even greater difficulties in the intellectual and emotional domains.

Children who exhibit such extreme levels of emotional arousal find that the usual childhood, self-soothing techniques are ineffective. In addition, when these children attempt to achieve comfort from the adults around them, their efforts backfire, which increases the likelihood that these children will turn to other means of managing distressing emotions (eg, violence, drugs, alcohol, cutting, bingeing, purging, promiscuity, risk-taking).[92] If these children find that aggressive responses help them to feel less helpless, feel more in control, and achieve a better sense of mastery, then their aggression will likely become chronic.[93-96]

Dissociative defenses, which may have been lifesaving during the traumatic events, may become chronically used. If these dissociative defenses are consistently used under less stressful conditions, then the child will not learn more positive forms of stress management.[92] If sensory flashbacks or body memories begin along the way, then the intrusive symptoms will likely create more stress, increase helplessness, and encourage the use of even more dissociation. Such a child will likely develop a negative sense of identity and trust and form skewed notions about his or her place in the world.

As is human nature, children adapt to adversity by changing their definitions of "normal"; and people naturally tend to resist changing anything that feels "normal." When a child adapts to adversity in such a manner, then the likelihood increases that the child will reenact the trauma and, in doing so, either be revictimized or victimize others.[97-101]

Moral intelligence is difficult to develop under these circumstances and the child's sense of meaning, purpose, and view of self and others will be powerfully influenced by his or her exposure to violence and the support systems' failure to protect him or her from harm.[102] Exposure to chronic childhood adversity is likely to produce profoundly disrupted attachment relationships that bode ill for future attachments, including later parenting skills.[103, 104] Children who have been exposed to the abusive use of authority are likely to have difficulty learning how to appropriately use their own personal authority with themselves and with others and are at risk for being victimized or becoming perpetrators, or both. Lacking appropriate emotional management, they may have great difficulty learning good conflict resolution skills and may be unable to grieve for the multiple losses they are likely to experience.[105] They may become addicted to stress and therefore resist efforts to help them calm down or learn to self-soothe.[106] All of this, if left untreated, is too frequently associated with continued deterioration, alienation, a foreshortened sense of future, and an inability to imagine any better alternatives. When these children become parents, they are likely to have difficulty parenting. The longer this goes on, the more normal it all may feel and, therefore, the greater the resistance to change.

If children or adults who have suffered significant adversity come together to form groups—families, gangs, organizations—new threats may make them particularly vulnerable to typical human group behavior under threat. Leaders may become bullying and willing to direct aggression at others, projecting anxiety onto any available external enemy, leading to a chronic state of conflict. Extremist thinking may become chronic and develop into a group norm and "groupthink" may supplant meaningful dialogue. Attention to repetitive threat may lead to the exclusion of other possible group goals. The increase in authoritarianism leads to a loss of critical judgment. In order to protect group unity, the group is likely to silence dissent through deception or force, increasing intragroup violence. Such a group is likely to lose transparency and become more secretive over time. Social norms develop that support the status quo, which continues to reinforce the conditions of chronic threat. In the process, democratic processes that are more flexible and responsive to complex demands are eroded and corruption increases as power becomes more centralized. The group loses a sense of shared purpose and vision and becomes increasingly fragmented; conflicts are not resolved. New and complex problems cannot be adequately addressed, and change continues to be resisted.[107-112] **Table 10-1** summarizes the impact of recurrent threats.

Table 10-1. Impact of Recurrent Threats

DISRUPTIONS	PRESENTATION
Resets the CNS	Hypersensitivity to even minor threat, hair-trigger temper, and anxiety
Hyperarousal interferes with cognitive development	Learning problems, confusion under stress, and poor problem-solving skills
Extremist thinking	Catastrophizing, oversimplifying, and loss of critical judgment becomes chronic
Attention to threat becoming chronic	Anxious, inability to relax, inability to pay attention to positive aspects of a situation, and tendency to see threat everywhere
Emotional modulation is lost or fails to develop, further interfering with cognitive development	Inability to control distressing emotional states that may overinfluence or even cloud thinking
Self-soothing skills are impaired	Inability to calm oneself down because emotions are too intense
Avoidance symptoms develop due to an inability to manage affect	Avoidance of people, places, or things that trigger distressing memories or emotions, causing a restriction of normal life activities; depressive syndromes; eating problems; and sleep problems
Aggression becomes chronic	Verbal or physical violence toward others or oneself
Dissociative defenses become chronic	Spacing out, forgetfulness, losing time, memory distortions, and amnesia
Intrusive symptoms reinforce sense of help-lessness, learned helpless-ness, failure of mastery	Flashbacks, nightmares, and body memories that are easily confused with hallucinations and misdiagnosed as psychosis
Defenses against flash-backs and highly distressing emotions develop	Attempt to manage highly distressing emotional states and stop flash-backs through use of drugs, alcohol, self-harming behavior, risk-taking behavior, and violence
Definitions of "normal" change to accommodate adversity	Abnormal circumstances, relationships, and life choices redefined as "normal"

(continued)

Table 10-1. *(continued)*

DISRUPTIONS	PRESENTATION
Ability to self-protect is lost or diminished	Inability to spot danger or respond appropriately to danger signals
Traumatic reenactment occurs	Tendency to repeat error, be revictimized, victimize others, or live a life of repetition
Sense of identity, view of self, and social relationships are affected	Demoralization, lower self-esteem, learned helplessness, and identification with the aggressor
Meaning, conscience, and view of self and others are damaged	Loss of or lack of moral intelligence
Attachments are disrupted (eg, failed trust, failed relationships)	Unfulfilling, abusive, failed relationships; inability to trust others; and trauma bonding
Problems with authority figure arise	Difficulties at school and work with respect to following orders or taking charge, bullying others, passive obedience, antisocial behavior, and increased authoritarianism
Conflict-resolving skills are impaired	Chronic, unresolved conflicts and compulsive appeasement
Ability to grieve is impaired	Chronic depression, physical problems, and displaced anger
Addiction to stress develops	Risk-taking and sensation-seeking behavior
Progressive deterioration occurs	Alienation and asocial or antisocial behavior
Sense of future is foreshortened	Failure of imagination, hopelessness, and resistance to change
Parenting practices are poor or deteriorate	Subjecting children to repetitive adversity

RECOVERY FROM INTIMATE PARTNER VIOLENCE

TASKS OF RECOVERY FROM RECURRENT THREAT

When looking at the list of disruptions that traumatized people may experience, the implications for recovery seem staggering. All helping systems need to recognize and respond to the traumatized person's chronic state of hyperarousal. Because violent acting out is always a real possibility, those who help a traumatized person must first accurately assess the degree of personal and professional threat that the child or adult poses to other people. At the same time, any threatening conditions surrounding the traumatized person must be minimized to buffer that person and provide a sense of surrounding safety.

Safety, however, is a complex subject. Adequate safety planning must include teaching the child or adult to become physically, psychologically, socially, and morally safe.[113] Medications and non-medical physical interventions (eg, massage, yoga, exercise) may help minimize physiological hyperarousal. Because no one can remain with the person all the time, each survivor must be taught self-soothing techniques. People who dissociate need to learn how to keep themselves grounded in order to stop using dissociation as a habitual behavior. Since, as the ACE study shows, chronic stress will likely already be taking a toll on the child's body, those helping the child must attend to the child's physical health, illness, and fitness.

Unfortunately, recognizing the chronic state of hyperarousal; protecting against possible personal and professional threats from the traumatized person; providing a sense of physical, psychological, social, and moral safety; teaching the traumatized person self-soothing techniques; and keeping the traumatized person grounded, so that the person does not resort to dissociative behavior, are only the beginning. People helping the traumatized person must next find methods to improve the survivor's cognitive skills, treat whatever addictive or compulsive behaviors have arisen, teach emotional management skills, and encourage the use of words instead of behavior to express feelings. Survivors must be taught conflict-resolution skills, alter negative attitudes toward authority figures, as well as address and redirect reenactment behavior. Many traumatized people require specific trauma-resolution techniques to stop flashbacks and dissociative behavior. When the time is right, trauma victims need help working through the grieving process and learning how to "let go" and "say goodbye" to the only past they may have known. This must happen within the context of learning how to make and sustain healthier relationships with peers. None of this is possible without the child or adult being pulled toward a better alternative future. This is only possible when the people surrounding the survivor have inspired the traumatized person with hope and encouraged the person's transformation of pain into what has been called a "survivor mission."[104]

STAGES OF CHANGE

Recovery from trauma, particularly chronic or repetitive trauma, can be a long and difficult journey. This is because, over time, the comorbid problems associated with prolonged exposure to trauma tend to accumulate and pose secondary and tertiary challenges to each person's recovery. For example, when a trauma survivor uses drugs or alcohol in an attempt to cope with overwhelmingly distressing emotions, that person may end up with the compounded problems of addiction; symptoms of posttraumatic stress; loss of employment, family, and social supports; learning problems; and serious medical problems. Changing just one of these problems presents difficulties, but the compounded, interactive nature of this situation, which is called ***complex PTSD***, makes recovery that much more difficult.[114]

What is so inspiring and promising is that so many survivors of IPV *do* walk the road of recovery and go on to live productive and fulfilling lives. Effective helpers must recognize the obstacles to change and assist these survivors through the stages of change.[115]

To make significant changes, research shows that people go through a series of 5 fairly distinct stages:

1. Denial that anything needs to change

2. Contemplating some change

3. Preparing for action

4. Taking action

5. Maintaining the change

At any stage, the person may relapse to an earlier stage and then move forward again. To help a person progress through these stages, helpers need to respond to the survivor in different ways depending upon the stage of change the person is in at the time of the interaction. Pushing a person toward action when that person is still in the precontemplation stage of change will simply push that person to leave the helper's office and never return. Likewise, holding back or discouraging action when a person is ready to take action may also create problems.

Because relapse can occur during any stage, the helper must be able to predict this possibility and help the person prepare to move forward again, even if the survivor must go backward first. If a person is determined to help someone who has been psychologically scarred by interpersonal violence, a number of helpful interventions exist. Many routes to recovery exist. Regardless of the helper's training or the role that person plays in the survivor's life, that person can always do something to help the survivor recover. (For more information on this topic, see Chapter 6, "Stages of Change.")

In medical, social service, mental health, and law enforcement settings, one of the most important and accessible interventions is universal psychoeducation regarding the impact of trauma in all its forms on the survivor. Pamphlets, books, videotapes, audiotapes, and DVDs are all available to provide such psychoeducation. Such sources are available through private and public sources and are appropriate for different age groups who are encountering a variety of problems.* In addition, many settings can offer emotional management tools (eg, relaxation techniques, breathing exercises, yoga, meditation training, exercise programs, wellness programs). All of these tools enable a trauma survivor to develop better emotional management skills. Offering space for self-help groups enables survivors the opportunity to build supportive social networks. Providing opportunities for trauma survivors to share their experiences to help others can provide methods for transforming personal pain into something of value to others.[116]

BARRIERS TO RECOVERY

Even under the best of circumstances, a number of barriers to recovery remain. Some of these barriers are directly related to the psychobiology of the traumatic experiences (eg, dissociation, fragmentation, amnesia, emotional numbing, intrusive re-experiencing, avoidance). Victims of domestic violence are likely to hide their symptoms for a number of reasons that range from a fear of being killed by the perpetrator to a fear of losing their children and being unable to support themselves to a fear of exposing the perpetrator to the legal system. If the survivor does reveal the IPV that is occurring, she is unlikely to make any connection between her present problems and symptoms to the previous traumatic experiences.

In the past, the mental health system has not dealt kindly with victims of domestic violence and frequently treated them as if the victim were the problem instead of the abuser. As a result, the domestic violence movement struggled *not* to pathologize women, which has frequently resulted in a split between the domestic violence

---

* *Useful educational videos have been produced by Cavalcade Productions (http://www.cavalcadeproductions.com/index.html) and Gift From Within (http://www.giftfromwithin.org/index.html#info). Useful trauma information and links to many resources can be located at http://www.trauma-pages.com*

movement and the mental health system. It is critical that health care providers situate the cause of the problem squarely at the feet of the abuser while attending to the very real needs, which include mental health needs, of the victim.

Trauma survivors are not likely to want to talk about their present or past bad experiences, because they find such experiences too painful and revealing. Instead, survivors may redirect the conversation, become angry and defensive if pressed, minimize the harm done, flee from the conversation, and even dissociate during an interview. Because of the impact of such traumatic experiences on the brain and the brain's ability to process incoming information, survivors may not remember the worst parts of their experiences. They may deny past problems simply because they have gaps in their biographical memory and may have other signs of dissociation, such as emotional numbing.

Emotional numbing can present as a failure to respond emotionally with the degree of distress that might be expected. That is, such emotional numbing may make the victim appear much less bothered by events than would be expected. Survivors may also use legal or illegal drugs or alcohol to help numb themselves from the physical and emotional pain.

Survivors of domestic violence tend to feel protective toward their family and may partially or totally deny the violence that is occurring, idealize the abusive family members, and blame themselves for whatever harm has occurred. When family issues are brought up, survivors may change the subject, tell lies that make the abusers look better than they are, and actively conceal the discovery of what is really going on in the family.

Abusers create another barrier to the process. Many abusers do not allow victims to be left alone with other adults because they fear that the victims will reveal information about the abuse.

Though survivors often create many of the barriers to obtaining help, the hesitancy of health care providers to discuss IPV with survivors provides yet another barrier. Health care providers often fail to conduct a trauma assessment, fail to remember the patient's history during later interactions, change the subject when IPV does come up in conversation, and minimize the harm that the person has experienced. In cases of IPV, health care providers frequently become angry when a victim seems to refuse to act.

In addition, the systems designed to help IPV victims have not incorporated knowledge about trauma into their policies, procedures, operations, or knowledge base. This is manifested through a lack of trauma-informed policies, a lack of mandatory trauma assessments and time to respond to these assessments, a lack of policies to address vicarious trauma with staff members, a lack of in-service training on trauma-related disorders for staff members, a lack of specific treatment approaches to address the traumatic impact, an exclusive focus on the use of medications, and an absence of a recovery framework for treatment.

Key Issues for Working With Intimate Partner Violence Victims

Warshaw outlined some of the key issues for mental health professionals in working with women who are victims of domestic violence. These include the following[117]:

— Regard the safety of victims and their children as a priority.

— Respect the right of domestic violence survivors to determine their own priorities and make their own life choices.

— Perpetrators are responsible for their abusive behavior and for stopping that behavior.

— View symptoms within the context of ongoing trauma, entrapment, and danger.

— Ensure that services are culturally sensitive and relevant.

— Advocate on behalf of survivors and their children.

Victim and Child Safety is the Priority

All treatment must begin by establishing safety for victims and their children. As long as a woman and her children remain in a dangerous relationship, the focus must be on helping her find the resources to become safe. This is *not* the time for intensive psychotherapy or trauma work. Working on resolving the traumatic effects of interpersonal violence must wait until the violence has stopped.

There are practices that a therapist or health care provider might otherwise engage in that can actually precipitate the escalation of violence in a situation of active abuse. The following practices can place survivors and their children in jeopardy[117]:

— Conducting couple's therapy within the context of ongoing violence or asking about abuse in the presence of a potential perpetrator

— Using an abusive partner as a source of collateral information

— Leaving messages at a client's home without determining whether doing so would be safe

— Sending a client home to an unsafe situation without discussing alternatives, developing a safety plan, or making referrals to a domestic violence program or hotline

— Failing to document a woman's efforts to protect and care for her children

— Making diagnoses without appropriately linking symptoms to abuse

The health professional must recognize that one of the major dynamics behind the violence used in an interpersonal context is control. As a result, the health professional must not mistake control maneuvers on the part of the perpetrator as concern for the victim.

Survivors Must Make Priorities and Life Choices

When a patient reveals ongoing exposure to violence, the health care provider's natural reaction is to rescue the person from the dangerous situation; however, when dealing with adults, the health care provider must respect the victim's priorities and not pressure her into accepting the provider's priorities. This can be extremely difficult when a provider recognizes a woman's danger before she fully recognizes the danger herself.

Only the victim can determine when the danger has reached a point of no return. Additionally, she may only be able to safely leave after laying a great deal of groundwork for the ongoing safety requirements of herself and her children. Health care providers must remember that women are in the most danger when they make the decision to separate from their abusers and then make the moves to do so. As victims come to terms with the realities of their situation, they often go through a process of denying the severity and repetitive nature of the abuse, weigh various options open to them, and consider alternatives to literal escape before formulating a plan and taking action steps.

One critical factor for victims as they make the ultimate decision to leave their abusive situations is support from friends, relatives, and health care providers. A victim can only trust such support if the support is constant, even if the victim does not do exactly what the people within their support system think should be done. Remember, an abuser undermines the victim's self-esteem, confidence in her own judgment, and abilities to accurately appraise herself and others. In the context of a caring relationship, a victim can begin to rebuild these necessary attributes that will enable her to mobilize her capacity for change. If she leaves the abusive situation because someone else tells her to do so and not because she is ready to go, her danger may increase as well as the likelihood that she will return to the abusive situation.

Perpetrators Are Responsible for Abuse and for Stopping Abuse

Though every story has 2 sides, there is no excuse for violence. As a result, no one is responsible for the abusive behavior except the abuser; however, the abusive partner will likely deny all responsibility for the abuse. Abusers believe that the abuse is always the fault of the victims (ie, the victims failed or mistreated them in some way), the alcohol he drank or drugs he took (ie, addiction rules their behavior), or the role models they had (ie, the abuser's parents settled their arguments violently). Nonetheless, violent partners, rather than their victims, must be held accountable for their dangerous behavior.

In the past, women have been chronically victimized when mental health and health care professionals labeled them as the problem and cause of their abusers' violence. Victims should not be further victimized by being made to feel that their actions caused the abuse; rather, the abusers must be held accountable for their own behavior choices.

Symptoms Are Within the Context of Ongoing Trauma, Entrapment, and Danger

Service providers who hope to assist victims of domestic violence must be informed about the findings related to the long-term effects of the victims' feelings of chronic fear, their state of hyperarousal, and their exposure to danger. As previously discussed, exposure to repetitive threat is associated with a number of symptoms. These symptoms should not be separated from the context within which they occurred. Helping IPV victims recognize that they may have sustained psychological, social, and moral injuries as well as physical injuries may also help reduce the stigma associated with the diagnostic labeling that accompanies the entry into service delivery for many clients. Professionals can play an essential role by understanding the ways victims are entrapped and then helping them find the resources necessary to escape from these traps.

Services Must Be Culturally Sensitive and Relevant

Cultural, religious, and ethnic values are likely to influence IPV experiences. Health care providers who wish to help a diverse population must become culturally competent to adequately respond to the needs of a diverse population of victims. For example, if a woman comes for care and does not speak the dominant language, efforts should be made to find a translator who is not a family member. An abuser can overcome language barriers by mistranslating what the victim says and shielding the health care provider from obtaining accurate information. Also, the abuser's presence will likely hinder the victim from revealing the abuse at all.

Survivors and Their Children Need Advocates

Advocacy involves facilitating, rather than directing, change. Service providers can do this by actively making victims aware of their options, helping them gain access to community resources, assisting them as they make choices about the best ways to reduce their exposure to ongoing violence, and helping them mitigate the impact of abuse on their lives.

SELF: A Simple, Nonlinear Framework

Knowing where to begin when confronting the great complexity of IPV can be very difficult. Especially challenging is knowing how to help trauma survivors recover within the context of a flawed and problematic system. The acronym ***SELF*** describes a simple, nonlinear, conceptual framework for managing very complex problems. As part of the

Sanctuary Model,[113,118,119] SELF provides a cognitive, behavioral, therapeutic approach for facilitating movement through the following 4 critical phases of recovery:

1. *Safety.* Attaining safety within the victim's self, other relationships, and their environment

2. *Emotional management.* Identifying levels of affect and modulating the victim's emotional responses to memories, persons, and events

3. *Loss.* Feeling grief and dealing with personal losses and resistance to change

4. *Future.* Trying out new roles and ways of relating to and behaving as a "survivor" to ensure personal safety and help others

These 4 constructs reflect the recurring themes that trauma survivors present regardless of the specific nature of the insults or traumas that they have experienced. These elements are consistent with other staged models of trauma treatment and recovery. The SELF method does not proceed in sequential stages; rather, it works as a simultaneously phased implementation tool of the Sanctuary Model.[104,120,121] This method is more like a compass that can be used as a guide while moving through the difficult recovery process. By using the SELF method, children, adults, and helpers can embrace a shared, nontechnical, and nonpejorative language, which allows them all to keep the larger recovery process in perspective. The accessible language demystifies what sometimes is seen as confusing and even insulting clinical or psychological terminology, which often confounds people, while maintaining the focus on the aspects of problematic adjustment that pose the greatest difficulties for any treatment environment. The SELF method also offers staff members and the organization as a whole a conceptual framework for thinking about and working through organizational problems that interfere with the vital work of helping the victims.

Much of the initial focus in any treatment setting must be on safety and emotions. In SELF, the definition of *safety* encompasses 4 domains: physical, psychological, social, and moral **(Table 10-2)**.[113] The development of a safety plan embraces problems as diverse as self-mutilation, running away, aggression, chronic suicidal tendencies, interpersonal abusive behavior, racial slurs, rumor-mongering, failing to follow medical directions, and inadequate self-care.

Most of the problematic behaviors and overwhelming emotions that present difficulties for children, adults, clinicians, and providers within behavioral health settings reflect

Table 10-2. Domains of Safety	
Physical Safety	— Basic needs—food, water, shelter—are met — No violence to others in any form: physical, emotional, verbal, or sexual — Absence of suicidality/self-destructive behavior — Absence of substance abuse — Healthy, safe, relational sexual behavior — Avoidance of risk-taking behavior — Good health practices — Healthy, nonviolent disciplinary practices — Able to perceive and avoid danger

(continued)

Table 10-2. *(continued)*

Psychological Safety	— Self-protection — Child protection — Attention and focus — Self-knowledge — Self-efficacy — Self-esteem — Self-empowerment — Self-control — Self-discipline
Social Safety	— Safe attachments — Safety in the group — Social responsibility — Exercise of responsible authority
Moral/Ethical Safety	— Honesty — Ethical dialogue — Tolerance — Courage — Respect for self and others — Integrity — Compassion — Commitment to human rights — Commitment to life

problems with the appropriate management of distressing emotions. Many modalities of intervention can help people better develop *emotional management* skills, allowing them to experience and cope with their emotions in healthy and productive ways.

Loss can be clinically recognized as a failure to make progress, continued acting out, reenactment behavior, chronic depressive symptoms, sudden regression, and unresolved bereavement. Mental health care providers have found that discussing "grief" instead of "depression" is more productive. Grief has sociocultural and time-limited pathways for resolution that are explicit in every culture and can be brought to bear even upon highly symbolized losses or losses that originate far in the person's past.[105]

Within the SELF acronym, *future* represents the goal and, hopefully, the vision of what the future can be as a result of recovery. In addition, this includes the willingness of the victim to engage in transformation that will lead beyond the "sick" role and require the assumption of personal and social responsibility, appropriate risk-taking, education, and a progressive change in self-image, behavior, and interpersonal relationships. Support groups based on the SELF method can be conducted in almost any setting and offer a meaningful psychoeducational framework for survivors to begin the recovery process.*

In addition, SELF can simultaneously be used in a parallel process manner to deal with problems that arise within the treatment setting among staff members, between staff members and clients, and between staff members and administration members. Applied to such issues as staff splitting, inadequate communication, poor morale, rule infraction,

---

* *For more information about SELF group curriculum, visit http://www.sanctuaryweb.com*

absenteeism, administrative withdrawal and helplessness, and misguided leadership, SELF can also assist a stressed organization to conceptualize the present dilemma and move into a better future through a course of complex decision making and conflict resolution.[122] The SELF method has proven to be of great value within many different treatment settings (eg, inpatient,[122-125] outpatient,[126] parenting programs,[127] children's residential programs,[122,128,129] domestic violence shelters,[130] substance abuse facilities[122,131]). Research funded by the National Institutes of Mental Health[132] has also supported the use of SELF as part of the implementation of The Sanctuary Model within a residential setting for children.[133-135]

Using SELF in Health Care Settings

For general health care providers, victims of interpersonal violence present a number of challenges:

— They frequently have a variety of comorbid conditions

— They do not necessarily respond to standard medical treatment

— Many may be considered "problem" or "resistant" patients

Often, their medical complaints are mysterious, inconclusive, vague, and diverse without meeting criteria for a definitive diagnosis, and yet their suffering is very apparent. It has been estimated that up to 75% of all visits to primary care providers involve the presentation of psychosocial problems through physical complaints.[136] Sometimes, though their pain is quite real, the pain's origin is found in body memories and flashbacks, which are typical responses to past trauma but unrecognized as such by the patient. In short, patients who have been exposed to chronic and recurrent trauma are likely to pose the most significant challenges to virtually any medical practice. As Dr. Lyndra Bills, Medical Director of Lancaster General Hospital Mental Health, has noted, "when care providers see someone in a clinic or an office with difficult and/or confusing constellations of complaints, they should consider the possibility of the PTSD diagnosis."[137]

A thorough medical history should include exploration of past traumatic experiences as routinely as the questions about family medical history and past surgical experiences. **Table 10-3** provides some examples of useful questions that can be included in a questionnaire or an interview. Asking such questions does not mean that the health care provider must solve every problem; rather, identifying the problem and directing someone to more information and alternative resources can be an enormous help to someone who has already survived these experiences but may still struggle with the aftermath.

Since health care providers tend to be practical and problem oriented, the SELF framework can provide a handy, goal-oriented organizing framework for complex posttraumatic problems.

Case Example

The following case provides as an example for the use of the SELF framework. In this case study, the health care provider helps develop a SELF treatment plan for the patient.

Mary is a 30-year-old diabetic woman whose diabetes has been controlled by oral medication. She sees a family physician because her diabetes is out of control. She has not been following the prescribed diet, has recently gained a great deal of weight, and, if the situation does not improve, she will have to go on insulin.

She has repeatedly been in abusive relationships and is now working on extricating herself from yet another such relationship. She has 2 children whom she loves but who seriously test her patience when she is not feeling well. She has few friends. Her mother and sister try to help her,

Table 10-3. Routine Trauma Questions Asked in a Primary Care Setting

As a child or adolescent, did you live in a household in which anyone abused drugs or alcohol?

As a child or adolescent, did you live in a household in which anyone was mentally ill or tried to commit suicide?

As a child or adolescent, did you live in a household in which anyone was imprisoned?

As a child or adolescent, did you live in a household in which anyone assaulted anyone else in the household?

As a child or adolescent, did you live with a foster family?

What is the worst thing that has ever happened to you?

What is the worst thing that has ever happened to someone in your family?

Have you ever been the victim of a crime?

Have you ever been in a natural or man-made disaster?

Have you ever been in an accident serious enough that you were medically examined?

Have you ever had excessive fear concerning medical procedures or surgery?

Have you ever served in the armed forces? If yes, were you involved in combat?

Did you suffer any form of severe physical or emotional neglect as a child?

Have you experienced psychological and/or verbal abuse as a child or as an adult?

Have you ever been physically assaulted as a child or as an adult?

Have you ever been sexually molested or assaulted as a child or as an adult?

Have you ever witnessed someone else being seriously injured or killed?

At any point during this (these) experience(s), did you think you were in danger of serious personal harm or of losing your life?

Have you ever sexually or physically assaulted someone else?

Have you been a civilian victim of war or witnessed any kind of atrocity?

Data from Bills.[137]

but Mary rejects their help, because she believes that there are always "strings" attached whenever she accepts their help.

Mary works at an unsatisfying secretarial job. She wants to attend nursing school and fulfill a childhood dream, but has been unable to mobilize her resources to do so. At work, she gets into many stressful conflicts with her boss and peers. These conflicts arise largely because she is intolerant of and impatient with people. When she comes home from work, she treats herself by eating.

Mary tends to hold back thoughts and emotions and does not speak truthfully about what she feels. She often feels like hurting other people when she is angry. During these times of anger, she is likely to take out her feelings on her children and sometimes hurts herself by secretly cutting herself. She does not feel like she really understands her own feelings. She often does things and says things impulsively and does not feel that she can control these words or feelings.

Mary has had many significant losses in her life. She has never really worked through these losses. In addition, she has a childhood history of physical and sexual abuse at the hands of her alcoholic father who is now deceased. As a child, Mary repeatedly witnessed her mother and sister being beaten by her father. Her mother was hospitalized several times for depression when Mary was very young.

An initial SELF treatment plan for Mary might look like the plan shown in **Table 10-4**. When Mary returns for follow-up visits, the practitioner can refer to the treatment plan with Mary and, in doing so, Mary will become more educated about the impact of trauma and the steps necessary to recover. Gradually, Mary will come to understand how her unsafe behavior is tied to difficulty in dealing with distressing emotions, which is tied to a history of many losses and exposure to violent abuse. This unsafe behavior and difficulty dealing with distressing emotions interferes with the achievement of possible and pleasurable future goals that she has for herself.

SELF focuses on change and not just on safety. At the same time, SELF focuses on many domains of the patient's life and not just her presenting symptoms. As a result, change becomes far more likely and the underlying causes for resistance to change can surface and be addressed. Over the course of her visits, the practitioner can give Mary reading material, suggest videos for her to watch, promote the use of support groups, and urge her to engage in creative expression, all of which, in and of themselves, provide Mary with

---

Table 10-4. Sample SELF Treatment Plan

SAFETY

Goals	Objectives
Physical	— Follow guidelines for treatment of diabetes — Recognize unsafe impulses, and use support when impulse to binge occurs — Understand and follow good nutrition guidelines — Get blood work done on schedule — Understand and properly use diabetes medications — Speak up about any side effects or concerns about medications — Determine weight weekly, and follow weight-loss diet — Take steps to avoid continuing abusive relationship — Exercise actively to remain strong and healthy as well as lose weight
Psychological	— Avoid or get out of playing a victim role with other people — Avoid or get out of playing a perpetrator role with other people — Work on building trusting relationships with family members
Social	— Recognize impulses to provoke conflict and ask for help — Develop better task schedule with children to avoid arguments — Tolerate differences that are seen as negative — Reach out to others for support — Model safe and respectful behavior toward all people
Moral	— Be honest internally — Be honest with other people — Speak up when feeling unsafe or threatened — Pursue nonviolence in relations with others

(continued)

Table 10-4. *(continued)*

Goals	Objectives
Recognize internal states, emotions, and responses of self and others	— Start to notice internal feelings and responses to situations — Express internal states using language — Express feelings in ways that allow other people to feel safe and respected — Look for a link between body language, facial expressions, and emotion internally and in others
Make connections between internal states and actions	— Name what feelings might have influenced argumentative behavior after that behavior is finished — Name what feelings might have influenced self-destructive behavior after that behavior is finished
Coping skills and strategies for managing internal states in constructive ways	— Use time away to interrupt automatic behaviors and think about outbursts and difficult situations — Create a safe space — Express feelings before they release violently — Seek help from family members or friends to stay on track and stay okay — Use relaxation techniques — Write a journal entry or poem, song, etc. — Express feelings in artistic, creative ways — Exercise — Use strategies to stay on task even when upset — Use strategies to help make better decisions even when upset — Use positive self-talk instead of falling into negative patterns

LOSS

Goals	Objectives
Recognize the painful constructive ways	— Tolerate discussion about painful realities — Use emotion management coping skills to bear the feelings instead of eating
Understand what the painful realities in life mean, that is, the implications and consequences	— Learn the facts about this loss, and how the loss can affect people in general — Learn how the losses experienced still affect life — Write about what it is like to live with this loss — Use creative expression about what it is like to live with this loss
Accept the painful realities	— Learn about how other people have come to terms with a similar loss in their lives — Write about what it is like to come to terms with these losses

(continued)

Table 10-4. *(continued)*

FUTURE

Goals	Objectives
Self-sufficiency, empowerment, and/or career	— Identify career paths and goals in nursing — Identify potential role models or mentor in nursing — Make plans for returning to school — Learn about saving money, and start to do so
Family life	— Work with family members to plan and follow routines for family life — Improve relationships with the children and adults in family — Take more responsibility for household chores and tasks
Health	— Follow health practices and recommendations — Understand and follow good nutrition guidelines — Exercise actively to remain strong and healthy
Relationships	— Reach out and build friendships in my community — Join a diabetes support group

Gus Haracopos and the treatment team at Andrus Children's Center developed this fictitious SELF treatment plan for Mary.

opportunities to invest in therapeutic change. Mary may not require a mental health provider, but as she takes a more task-oriented approach to problems that have previously felt overwhelming and impossible to resolve, she will become far more amenable to deeper therapeutic work.

The tasks, goals, and objectives in the SELF treatment plan break down the complex idea of recovery into more manageable "bites." When Mary feels less helpless and overwhelmed, she is more likely to begin chipping away at her problems. As this occurs, health care providers can use SELF on a regular basis to help guide Mary toward success. Guaranteeing that Mary has some success is critical.

Exposure to repetitive trauma robs people of the sense that they can master their own reality; instead, they feel helpless, even when they can take steps to do better. If the health care setting supplements regular medical visits with the opportunity and encouragement for Mary to join a SELF psychoeducational group as well, then progress is likely to be more rapid. Such group support will urge Mary to continue her efforts, and she will benefit from the group learning experience.

ORGANIZATIONAL COMPLEX POSTTRAUMATIC STRESS DISORDER

STRESS AS A BARRIER TO SYSTEMIC CHANGE

Larger, systemic barriers to trauma-informed change that significantly change the systemic responses to IPV exist beyond the personal barriers. Complex interactions can occur among traumatized clients, stressed staff members, pressured organizations, and social and economic environments; such conflicts hinder positive, trauma-informed change. As a result, helping systems frequently recapitulate the very experiences that have proven so toxic for the people they intend to treat.

Medical, mental health, and social service systems are experiencing significant stress caused by managed-care issues, deinstitutionalization, malpractice suits, government regulations, decreased funding, evidence-based practices, and pressures to become "trauma-informed." These stressors add to the systemic fragmentation that already affects our system of caregiving to which victims of domestic violence must turn in order to get out of the dangerous situations in which they find themselves.

As a result, this sense of tension is felt throughout many organizations so that neither the staff members nor the administrators feel particularly safe with their clients or with each other. Many helping environments are characterized by states of constant crisis that severely constrain the ability of staff members to constructively confront problems, involve all levels of staff members in decision making, engage in complex goal setting and problem solving, or, in some cases, even talk to each other. Team meetings, informal conversations, formal discussions, and shared decision making are known as important components of healthy work environments; however, without time for staff members to truly collaborate, an organization loses the capacity to manage the emotions evoked by the stress of the work.

Under the stress of time pressures and increased demands, communication networks tend to break down both within and between organizations. As this occurs, service delivery becomes increasingly fragmented. Normally, the steady flow of information and feedback causes timely and appropriate error correction. When the communication network begins to break down, this causes these normal error-correction methods to break down as well, thereby increasing the likelihood of escalating levels of systematic error.

As fewer people participate in the decision-making and problem-solving processes, decisions tend to become more shortsighted and ineffective and, worse yet, these decisions may compound the existing problems. The loss of more democratic processes within an organization results in the systemic loss of the ability to resolve difficult problems complexly; the result is a gross oversimplification of everything from staff policies to treatment decisions.

In such an environment, conflicts escalate everywhere; however, without time and resources, conflicts cannot be resolved, which leads to deterioration of trust and interpersonal relationships. Such a situation evolves insidiously. Nonetheless, as time goes by, the situation feels increasingly out of control and organizational leaders respond by becoming more controlling. As a result, the leaders institute ever more punitive measures in an attempt to forestall the impending chaos. Such an organizational climate promotes authoritarian behavior, which serves to reinforce existing hierarchies and create new ones. As this occurs, the leaders become progressively isolated, staff members feel "dumbed down," and the organization loses its overall critical judgment. Everyone within such an organization realizes that something is wrong, but no one feels able to halt the declining spiral. Helplessness begins to permeate the system so that staff members feel helpless in the face of traumatized children, adults, and families. As a result, these victims feel helpless to help themselves or each other, and administrators helplessly perceive that their best efforts are ineffective.

As the administration becomes more punitive, the staff members respond by developing a wide array of acting-out and passive-aggressive behaviors as well as escalating levels of punitive behavior directed at the children, adults, and families they are intended to serve. With funding pressures, downsizing frequently results in the loss of key staff members, leaders, affiliations, and programs; as a result, everyone left behind by the downsizing experiences multiple losses and the organization as a whole loses much of its organizational memory. As standards of care deteriorate and quality assurance standards lower, everyone becomes increasingly saddened, frustrated, and angry about the loss of former standards of care as well as their individual and shared abilities to be productive and useful.

Over time, leaders and staff members lose sight of the essential purpose of their work together and derive less satisfaction from their work. Many of the best people find this intolerable and leave; the amount of individual dysfunction becomes concentrated in the remaining people. When an organization is in this downward spiral, staff members feel increasingly angry, demoralized, burned out, helpless, and hopeless; they fail to see the almost insurmountable barriers to recovery that the system has erected. As a result, their hopelessness is projected onto the children, adults, and families who are seen as being radically different from previous generations and far less reachable. Ultimately, if this destructive sequence is not arrested, the organization can begin to look and act in uncannily similar ways to the traumatized people whom the organization should be helping. The result of this process is characterized as ***organizational complex PTSD***.[138]

THE SANCTUARY MODEL: TRANSFORMING ORGANIZATIONAL CULTURES

What happens when a victim of IPV encounters a helping system of care that appears desperately in need of help itself? When health care providers feel stressed, angry, fearful, and demoralized, they have difficulty not conveying their own emotional states onto their most sensitive patients. Despite the gadgetry and technological advances of modern medicine, healing is ultimately delivered by other human beings, so anything that interferes with the well being of staff members within any setting is bound to interfere with the delivery of vital healing services.

For many such settings, to become holistic and trauma-informed means that these settings must undergo transformation. According to Webster's 1913 dictionary, ***transformation*** means "a change in an organism which alters its general character and mode of life."[139] Children, adults, family members, and organizations represent nonlinear systems, because they are alive and capable of growth, change, and transformation; applying linear models to help them grow may be unimaginable. The solutions to our problems, whether individual, therapeutic, or social, are possible after learning to tolerate and manage complexity. Human beings and human systems are not machines. Rather their inherent ability to change must be recognized when a climate is created that promotes growth and change, which encourages the emergence of innovative and complex solutions to complex problems.

The Sanctuary Model represents a comprehensive, trauma-informed method for creating or changing an organizational culture to more effectively provide a cohesive context within which healing from psychological and social traumatic experience can be addressed. The Sanctuary Model was originally developed in a short-term, acute, inpatient, psychiatric setting for adults who were traumatized as children. This model has since been adapted by residential treatment settings for children, domestic violence shelters, homeless shelters, group homes, outpatient settings, substance abuse programs, and parenting-support programs as well as in other settings in which the method was used to promote organizational change. The Sanctuary Model is not an intervention but a full-system approach focused on helping injured children, adults, and family members recover from the damaging effects of interpersonal violence. As a full-system approach, effective implementation of the Sanctuary Model requires extensive leadership involvement in the process of change as well as staff member and client involvement at every level of the process.

The Sanctuary Model aims to guide an organization in the development of a culture through 7 dominant characteristics, all of which serve goals related to a sound treatment environment and a healthy workplace, as illustrated in **Table 10-5**. The 7 commitments include the following:

1. A commitment to nonviolence that serves to orient a program around the need to develop and model safety skills

2. A commitment to emotional intelligence emphasizing the importance of teaching and modeling emotional management skills

3. A commitment to social learning directed at building and modeling good thinking and problem-solving skills

4. A commitment to democracy ensuring an environment of civic participation that models the civic skills of self-control, self-discipline, and the administration of healthy authority

5. A commitment to open communication that encourages everyone in the environment to overcome existing barriers to healthy communication, reduce acting out, enhance self-protective and self-correcting skills, and model the skills involved in creating and maintaining healthy boundaries

6. A commitment to social responsibility that requires the learning or rebuilding of social connection skills and the establishment of healthy attachment relationships

7. A commitment to growth and change that guarantees that the environment as a whole and every individual within it will focus on the restoration of hope, meaning, and purpose.*

The impact of changing an organization in this way should be measurable. People should be able to notice the absence of violence and the presence of an environment that is physically, psychologically, socially, and morally safe. This sense of safety should be reflected in a low level of critical incidents, low staff turnover rates, low staff member and patient injuries, few patient complaints, better outcomes, and better morale.

WHAT CAN BE DONE TO HELP?

Health and mental health care providers can do a great deal to move the system to recognize and respond to child and adult victims of IPV by changing their practice in the ways described in this chapter and by challenging themselves to change in the same ways that they want their patients to change. Intimate partner violence is not just a mental health problem or a health problem, rather, such violence is a major public health problem.

The following lists many tangible ways that health care providers and citizens can contribute to systemic change:

— *Legitimatize survivors.* Support the mobilization of a survivor movement and integrate the voice of survivors into clinical settings.

— *Think outside of the box.* Disseminate notions of therapy outside of the norm and introduce that therapy into domestic violence shelters, homeless shelters, schools, childcare settings, health care settings, clinics, and so on. Integrate mental health practices and procedures into the primary care setting, and make sure these services are thoroughly trauma informed.

---

* *For more information on the* Sanctuary Model of Organizational Change, *see http://www.sanctuaryweb.com and http://www.andruschildren.org.*

Table 10-5. Creating Sanctuary

Cultural Characteristic	Trauma-Informed Goal
Culture of nonviolence	Help build safety skills and a commitment to higher goals
Culture of emotional intelligence	Help teach emotional management skills
Culture of social learning	Help build cognitive skills
Culture of democracy	Help create civic skills of self-control, self-discipline, and administration of healthy authority
Culture of open communication	Help overcome barriers to healthy communication, reduce acting out, enhance self-protective and self-correcting skills, and teach healthy boundaries
Culture of social responsibility	Help rebuild social connection skills and establish healthy attachment relationships
Culture of growth and change	Help restore hope, meaning, and purpose

— *Walk the talk.* Permeate the politics of practice settings and organizations with the implications of trauma theory.

— *Educate others.* Teach everyone who will listen and accept any opportunity that presents itself (eg, with police officers, district attorneys, family physicians, and employers as well as within courts, schools, child protection agencies, parenting programs, domestic violence programs, victims services programs, and insurance companies) to speak about domestic violence and its implications.

— *Desegregate the discourse.* Make clear connections among child abuse, family violence, criminal victimization, substance abuse, homelessness, poverty, prostitution, exploitation, physical illness, mental disorders, and the connections between abuse of human beings and abuse of the environment.

— *Penetrate academic settings.* Help get this knowledge into training programs at every level and be willing to teach from personal experience.

— *Populate the press.* Write letters to newspaper and magazine editors, make friends with journalists, write opinion-editorial articles, write a regular newspaper column, speak on news programs, or meet with and learn how to properly work with members of the press.

— *Legislate the issues.* Write letters to legislatures, visits legislatures, engage in discussions with political leaders, support candidates, and learn how to lobby.

— *Infiltrate funding streams.* Help federal, state, county, foundation, and private funders recognize the short-term and long-term economic costs of failing to respond adequately to victims of violence.

With education, patience, and support, survivors of unspeakable trauma do commit themselves to recovery, but not because someone else frightens them into doing so.

Certainly, fear may play a role in the urgency of their decision making, but ultimately survivors make changes that transform their lives because little by little they begin making different choices, fan the fires of hope, and envision a different future than the one predicted by their past behavior. Society can learn a lot from the tenacity of these survivors who transform their lives. These are treacherous times, and the exponentially increasing rate of change means that the future is perhaps less predictable than ever before in the history of humankind. People need to fan the fires of hope for one another. People must envision a different future than the solitary, deadly, and frightening future often predicted in movies and forecasted by political leaders. In 1953, Maxwell Jones, one of the founders of the democratic therapeutic community, wrote, "In the field of mental health, most attention has been given to psychotherapy; some to mental hygiene, but very little as yet, to the design of a whole culture which will foster healthy personalities."[140] This work still needs to be done; this is the work of the next generations. They must design and build a future that is worth surviving for.

REFERENCES

1. Dube SR, Anda RF, FelittiVJ, Edwards VJ, Williamson DF. Exposure to abuse, neglect, and household dysfunction among adults who witnessed intimate partner violence as children: implications for health and social services. *Violence Vict.* 2002;17:3-17.

2. Felitti VJ, Anda RF, Nordenberg D, et al. Relationship of childhood abuse and household dysfunction to many of the leading causes of death in adults: the Adverse Childhood Experiences (ACE) study. *Am J Prev Med.* 1998;14:245-258.

3. Whitfield CL, Anda RF, Dube SR, Felitti VJ. Violent childhood experiences and the risk of intimate partner violence in adults: assessment in a large health maintenance organization. *J Interpers Violence.* 2003;18:166-186.

4. Merrill LL, Thomsen CJ, Gold SR, Milner JS. Childhood abuse and premilitary sexual assault in male Navy recruits. *J Consult Clin Psychol.* 2001;69:252-261.

5. Paradise JE, Rose L, Sleeper LA, Nathanson M. Behavior, family function, school performance, and predictors of persistent disturbance in sexually abused children. *Pediatrics.* 1994;93:452-459.

6. Frothingham TE, Hobbs CJ, Wynne JM, Yee L, Goyal A, Wadsworth DJ. Follow up study eight years after diagnosis of sexual abuse. *Arch Dis Child.* 2000; 83:132-134.

7. Bagley C, Mallick K. Prediction of sexual, emotional, and physical maltreatment and mental health outcomes in a longitudinal cohort of 290 adolescent women. *Child Maltreat.* 2000;5:218-226.

8. Lewis DO, Moy E, Jackson LD, et al. Biopsychosocial characteristics of children who later murder: a prospective study. *Am J Psychiatry.* 1985;142:1161-1167.

9. Pollock VE, Briere J, Schneider L, Knop J, Mednick SA, Goodwin DW. Childhood antecedents of antisocial behavior: parental alcoholism and physical abusiveness. *Am J Psychiatry.* 1990;147:1290-1293.

10. Shields A, Cicchetti D. Parental maltreatment and emotion dysregulation as risk factors for bullying and victimization in middle childhood. *J Clin Child Psychol.* 2001;30:349-363.

11. Silverman AB, Reinherz HZ, Giaconia RM. The long-term sequelae of child and adolescent abuse: a longitudinal community study. *Child Abuse Negl.* 1996; 20:709-723.

12. Calam R, Horne L, Glasgow D, Cox A. Psychological disturbance and child sexual abuse: a follow-up study. *Child Abuse Negl.* 1998;22:901-913.

13. Herrenkohl RC, Russo MJ. Abusive early child rearing and early childhood aggression. *Child Maltreat.* 2001;6:3-16.

14. Sendi IB, Blomgren PG. A comparative study of predictive criteria in the predisposition of homicidal adolescents. *Am J Psychiatry.* 1975;132:423-427.

15. Edwards VJ, Holden GW, Felitti VJ, Anda RF. Relationship between multiple forms of childhood maltreatment and adult mental health in community respondents: results from the Adverse Childhood Experiences study. *Am J Psychiatry.* 2003;160:1453-1460.

16. Anda RF, Whitfield CL, Felitti VJ, et al. Adverse childhood experiences, alcoholic parents, and later risk of alcoholism and depression. *Psychiatr Serv.* 2002;53: 1001-1009.

17. Chapman DP, Whitfield CL, Felitti VJ, Dube SR, Edwards VJ, Anda RF. Adverse childhood experiences and the risk of depressive disorders in adulthood. *J Affect Disord.* 2004;82:217-225.

18. Dube SR, Anda RF, Felitti VJ, Chapman DP, Williamson DF, Giles WH. Childhood abuse, household dysfunction, and the risk of attempted suicide throughout the life span: findings from the Adverse Childhood Experiences study. *JAMA.* 2001;286:3089-3096.

19. Steinmetz SK, Straus MA. The family as a cradle of violence. *Society.* 1973;10(6): 50-56.

20. Straus MA. *Beating the Devil Out of Them: Corporal Punishment in American Families.* New York, NY: Lexington Books; 1994.

21. Finkelhor D, Dziuba-Leatherman J. Victimization of children. *Am Psychol.* 1994;49:173-183.

22. U.S. Department of Health and Human Services, Administration on Children, Youth and Families. *Child Maltreatment 2003.* Washington, DC: US Government Printing Office; 2005.

23. Sedlak AJ, Broadhurst DD. *Executive Summary of the Third National Incidence Study of Child Abuse and Neglect.* Washington, DC: US Dept of Health & Human Services, Administration for Children and Families, Administration on Children, Youth and Families, National Center on Child Abuse and Neglect; 1996.

24. National Center for Victims of Crime. *Crime and Victimization in America: Statistical Overview.* Arlington, Va: National Center for Victims of Crime; 1993.

25. EDK Associates, for the Family Violence Prevention Fund. *Men Beating Women: Ending Domestic Violence. A Qualitative and Quantitative Study of Public Attitudes on Violence Against Women.* New York, NY: Family Violence Prevention Fund; 1993.

26. Davies D. Intervention with male toddlers who have witnessed parental violence. *Fam Soc.* 1991;72:515-524.

27. Zuckerman B, Augustyn M, Groves BM, Parker S. Silent victims revisited: the special case of domestic violence. *Pediatrics*. 1995;96:511-513.

28. Kolbo JR, Blakely EH, Engleman D. Children who witness domestic violence: a review of empirical literature. *J Interpers Violence*. 1996;11:281-293.

29. Kolbo JR. Risk and resilience among children exposed to family violence. *Violence Vict*. 1996;11:113-128.

30. Sternberg KJ, Lamb ME, Greenbaum C, et al. Effects of domestic violence on children's behavior problems and depression. *Dev Psychol*. 1993;29:44-52.

31. Bloom SL, ed. *Final Action Plan: A Coordinated Community-Based Response to Family Violence*. Harrisburg, PA: Attorney General Mike Fisher's Task Force on Family Violence: Commonwealth of Pennsylvania; 1999.

32. Banks R. Bullying in Schools. *ERIC Digest*.1997; April.

33. Jaffe P, Wolfe D, Wilson SK, Zak L. Family violence and child adjustment: a comparative analysis of girls' and boys' behavioral symptoms. *Am J Psychiatry*. 1986;143:74-77.

34. Schwartz D, Proctor LJ. Community violence exposure and children's social adjustment in the school peer group: the mediating roles of emotion regulation and social cognition. *J Consult Clin Psychol*. 2000;68:670-683.

35. Wolfe DA, Korsch B. Witnessing domestic violence during childhood and adolescence: implication for pediatric practice. *Pediatrics*. 1994;94:594-599.

36. Delaney-Black V, Covington C, Ondersma SJ, et al. Violence exposure, trauma, and IQ and/or reading deficits among urban children. *Arch Pediatr Adolesc Med*. 2002;156:280-285.

37. Cooley-Quille M, Boyd RC, Frantz E, Walsh J. Emotional and behavioral impact of exposure to community violence in inner-city adolescents. *J Clin Child Psychol*. 2001;30:199-206.

38. Schuler ME, Nair P. Witnessing violence among inner-city children of substance-abusing and non-substance-abusing women. *Arch Pediatr Adolesc Med*. 2001; 155:342-346.

39. Stoppelbein L, Greening L. Posttraumatic stress symptoms in parentally bereaved children and adolescents. *J Am Acad Child Adolesc Psychiatry*. 2000;39:1112-1119.

40. Marans S, Berkowitz SJ, Cohen DJ. Police and mental health professionals: collaborative responses to the impact of violence on children and families. *Child Adolesc Psychiatr Clin N Am*. 1998;7:635-651.

41. Farrington DP, Loeber R. Epidemiology of juvenile violence. *Child Adolesc Psychiatr Clin N Am*. 2000;9:733-748.

42. James WH, West C, Peters KE, Armijo E. Youth dating violence. *Adolescence*. 2000;35:455-465.

43. Wolfe DA, Scott K, Wekerle C, Pittman AL. Child maltreatment: risk of adjustment problems and dating violence in adolescence. *J Am Acad Child Adolesc Psychiatry*. 2001;40:282-289.

44. Wingood GM, DiClemente RJ, McCree DH, Harrington K, Davies SL. Dating violence and the sexual health of black adolescent females. *Pediatrics*. 2001;107:72.

45. Fiebert MS, Gonzalez DM. College women who initiate assaults on their male partners and the reasons offered for such behavior. *Psychol Rep*. 1997;80:583-590.

46. Dye ML, Eckhardt CI. Anger, irrational beliefs, and dysfunctional attitudes in violent dating relationships. *Violence Vict*. 2000;15:337-350.

47. Silverman JG, Raj A, Mucci LA, Hathaway JE. Dating violence against adolescent girls and associated substance use, unhealthy weight control, sexual risk behavior, pregnancy, and suicidality. *JAMA*. 2001;286:572-579.

48. Coker AL, McKeown RE, Sanderson M, Davis KE, Valois RF, Huebner ES. Severe dating violence and quality of life among South Carolina high school students. *Am J Prev Med*. 2000;19:220-227.

49. American Medical Association Council on Scientific Affairs. *AMA Data on Violence Between Intimates*. Chicago, Ill: American Medical Association; 2000. Report 7 (1-00).

50. Straus MA, Gelles RJ. How violent are American families? Estimates from the National Family Violence Resurvey and other studies. In: Straus MA, Gelles RJ, eds. *Physical Violence in American Families: Risk Factors and Adaptations to Violence in 8,145 Families*. New Brunswick, NJ: Transaction Publishers; 1990:95-112.

51. Tjaden P, Thoennes N. *Full Report of the Prevalence, Incidence, and Consequences of Violent Against Women: Findings from the National Violence Against Women Survey*. Washington, DC: Office of Justice Programs, US Dept of Justice; November 2000.

52. Sheridan LP, Blaauw E, Davies GM. Stalking: knowns and unknowns. *Trauma Violence Abuse*. 2003;4:148-162.

53. Briere J, Jordan CE. Violence against women: outcome complexity and implications for assessment and treatment. *J Interpers Violence*. 2004;19:1252-1276.

54. Fazzone PA, Holton JK, Reed BG. *Substance abuse treatment and domestic violence*. Rockville, Md: Center for Substance Abuse Treatment, Substance Abuse and Mental Health Services Administration; 1997.

55. Danielson KK, Moffitt TE, Caspi A, Silva PA. Comorbidity between abuse of an adult and DSM-III-R mental disorders: evidence from an epidemiological study. *Am J Psychiatry*. 1998;155:131-133.

56. McCauley J, Kern DE, Kolodener K, et al. The "battering syndrome": prevalence and clinical characteristics of domestic violence in primary care internal medicine practices. Ann Intern Med. 1995;123:737-746.

57. Gilbert L, el-Bassel N, Schilling RF, Friedman E. Childhood abuse as a risk for partner abuse among women in methadone maintenance. *Am J Drug Alcohol Abuse*. 1997;23:581-595.

58. Hiday VA, Swartz MS, Swanson JW, Borum R, Wagner HR. Criminal victimization of persons with severe mental illness. *Psychiatr Serv*. 1999;50:62-68.

59. Jenkins EJ, Bell CC, Taylor J, Walker L. Circumstances of sexual and physical victimization of black psychiatric outpatients. *J Natl Med Assoc*. 1989;81:246-252.

60. Goodman LA, Thompson KM, Weinfurt K, et al. Reliability of reports of violent victimization and posttraumatic stress disorder among men and women with serious mental illness. *J Trauma Stress*. 1999;12:587-599.

61. Goodman LA, Rosenberg SD, Mueser KT, Drake RE. Physical and sexual assault history in women with serious mental illness: prevalence, correlates, treatment, and future research directions. *Schizophr Bull*. 1997;23:685-696.

62. Goodman LA, Salyers MP, Mueser KT, et al. Recent victimization in women and men with severe mental illness: prevalence and correlates. *J Trauma Stress*. 2001;14:615-632.

63. Solomon SD, Davidson JRT. Trauma: prevalence, impairment, service use, and cost. *J Clin Psychiatr*. 1997;58(suppl 9):5-11.

64. Stein MB, Walker JR, Forde DR. Gender differences in susceptibility to posttraumatic stress disorder. *Behav Res Ther*. 2000;38:619-628.

65. Breslau N, Chilcoat HD, Kessler RC, Peterson EL, Lucia VC. Vulnerability to assaultive violence: further specification of the sex difference in post-traumatic stress disorder. *Psychol Med*. 1999;29:813-821.

66. Kubany ES, McKenzie WF, Owens JA, Leisen MB, Kaplan AS, Pavich E. PTSD among women survivors of domestic violence in Hawaii. *Hawaii Med J*. 1996; 55:164-165.

67. Houskamp BM, Foy DW. The assessment of posttraumatic stress disorder in battered women. *J Interpers Violence*. 1991;6:368-376.

68. Kempe A, Rawlings J, Green B. Post-traumatic stress disorder (PTSD) in battered women: a shelter sample. *J Trauma Stress*. 1991;4:137-147.

69. Saunders DG. Posttraumatic stress symptom profiles of battered women: a comparison of survivors in two settings. *Violence Vict*. 1994;9:31-44.

70. Samson AY, Berenson S, Beck A, Price D, Nimmer C. Posttraumatic stress disorder in primary care. *J Fam Pract*. 1999;48:222-227.

71. Silva C, McFarlane J, Soeken K, Parker B, Reel S. Symptoms of post-traumatic stress disorder in abused women in a primary care setting. *J Womens Health*. 1997;6:543-552.

72. Kessler RC, Sonnega A, Bromet E, Hughes M, Nelson CB. Posttraumatic stress disorder in the National Comorbidity Survey. *Arch Gen Psychiatry*. 1995;52: 1048-1060.

73. Mueser KT, Rosenberg SD, Goodman LA, Trumbetta SL. Trauma, PTSD, and the course of severe mental illness: an interactive model. *Schizophr Res*. 2002; 53:123-143.

74. Laumann EO, Gagnon JH, Michael RT, Michaels S. *The Social Organization of Sexuality: Sexual Practices in the United States*. Chicago, Ill: University of Chicago Press; 1994.

75. Davidson JR et al. The association of sexual assault and attempted suicide within the community. *Arch Gen Psychiatry*. 1996;53:550-555.

76. De Girolamo G, McFarlane AC. Epidemiology of posttraumatic stress disorder among victims of intentional violence: a review of the literature. In: Mak FL, Nadelson CC, eds. *International Review of Psychiatry*. Vol 2. Washington, DC: American Psychiatric Press; 1996:93-119.

77. Kilpatrick DG, Best CL, Veronen LJ, Amick AE, Villeponteaux LA, Ruff GA. Mental health correlates of criminal victimization: a random community survey. *J Consult Clin Psychol.* 1985;53:866-873.

78. Kilpatrick DG, Edmunds C, Seymour A, for the National Center for Victims of Crime and Crime Victims Research Center. *Rape in America: A Report to the Nation.* Arlington, Va: National Center for Victims of Crime; 1992.

79. Abrams KM, Robinson GE. Stalking: part I: an overview of the problem. *Can J Psychiatry.* 1998;43:473-476.

80. Mechanic MB, Uhlmansiek MH, Weaver TL, Resick PA. The impact of severe stalking experienced by acutely battered women: an examination of violence, psychological symptoms and strategic responding. *Violence Vict.* 2000;15:443-458.

81. Irons R, Schneider JP. When is domestic violence a hidden face of addiction? *J Psychoactive Drugs.* 1997;29:337-344.

82. Norton JH. Addiction and family issues. *Alcohol.* 1994;11:457-460.

83. Augenbraun M, Wilson TE, Allister L. Domestic violence reported by women attending a sexually transmitted disease clinic. *Sex Transm Dis.* 2001;28:143-147.

84. Easton CJ, Swan S, Sinha R. Prevalence of family violence in clients entering substance abuse treatment. *J Subst Abuse Treat.* 2000;18:23-28.

85. Scheller TF, Berens P. Domestic violence and substance use. *Obstet Gynecol.* 2001;97(suppl 1):53.

86. Teets JM. The incidence and experience of rape among chemically dependent women. *J Psychoactive Drugs.* 1997;29:331-336.

87. Molnar BE, Buka SL, Kessler RC. Child sexual abuse and subsequent psychopathology: results from the National Comorbidity Survey. *Am J Public Health.* 2001;91:753-760.

88. Root MP. Treatment failures: the role of sexual victimization in women's addictive behavior. *Am J Orthopsychiatry.* 1989;59:542-549.

89. Dansky BS, Byrne CA, Brady KT. Intimate violence and post-traumatic stress disorder among individuals with cocaine dependence. *Am J Drug Alcohol Abuse.* 1999;25:257-258.

90. Perry BD. The neurodevelopmental impact of violence in childhood. In: Schetky D, Benedek E, eds. *Textbook of Child and Adolescent Forensic Psychiatry.* Washington, DC: American Psychiatric Press; 2001:221-238.

91. Alford JD, Mahone C, Fielstein EM. Cognitive and behavioral sequelae of combat: conceptualization and implications for treatment. *J Trauma Stress.* 1988;1:489-501.

92. van der Kolk BA, Pelcontz D, Roth S, Mandel FS, McFarlane A, Herman JL. Dissociation, somatization, and affect dysregulation: the complexity of adaptation to trauma. *Am J Psychiatry.* 1996;153:83-93.

93. Perry BD, Pollard RA, Blakely TL, Baker WL, Vigilante D. Childhood trauma, the neurobiology of adaptation and "use-dependent" development of the brain: how "states" become "traits." *Infant Mental Health J.* 1995;16:271-291.

94. Perry BD, Pollard R. Homeostasis, stress, trauma, and adaptation. A neurodevelopmental view of childhood trauma. *Child Adolesc Psychiatr Clin N Am*. 1998;7:33-51, viii.

95. Perry B. Incubated in terror: neurodevelopmental factors in the cycle of violence. In: Osofsky J, ed. *Children, Youth and Violence: Searching for Solutions*. New York, NY: Guilford Press; 1997:124-148.

96. Perry BD. Neurobiological sequelae of childhood trauma: PTSD in children. In: Murburg MM, ed. *Catecholamine Function in Posttraumatic Stress Disorders: Emerging Concepts*. Washington, DC: American Psychiatric Press; 1994:253-276. Progress in Psychiatry Series, #42.

97. van der Kolk BA. The compulsion to repeat the trauma: reenactment, revictimization, and masochism. *Psychiatr Clin North Am*. 1989;12:389-411.

98. Putnam FW. *Dissociation in Children and Adolescents: A Developmental Perspective*. New York, NY: Guilford Press; 1997.

99. Trickett P, Putnam F. Impact of child sexual abuse on females: toward a developmental, psychobiological integration. *Psychol Sci*. 1993;4:81-87.

100. van der Kolk BA. The body keeps the score: approaches to the psychobiology of posttraumatic stress disorder. In: van der Kolk BA, Weisaeth L, McFarlane AC, eds. *Traumatic Stress: The Effects of Overwhelming Experience on Mind, Body and Society*. New York, NY: Guilford Press; 1996:214-241.

101. van der Kolk BA, Ducey CP. The psychological processing of traumatic experience: Rorschach patterns in PTSD. *J Trauma Stress*. 1989;2:259-274.

102. Lennick D, Kiel F. *Moral Intelligence: Enhancing Business Performance and Leadership Success*. Upper Saddle River, NJ: Wharton School Publishing; 2005.

103. James B. *Handbook for Treatment of Attachment-Trauma Problems in Children*. New York, NY: Lexington Books; 1994.

104. Herman J. *Trauma and Recovery*. New York, NY: Basic Books; 1992.

105. Bloom SL. Beyond the beveled mirror: mourning and recovery from childhood maltreatment. In: Kauffman J, ed. *Loss of the Assumptive World: A Theory of Traumatic Loss*. New York, NY: Brunner-Routledge; 2002:139-170.

106. van der Kolk BA, Greenberg M. The psychobiology of the trauma response: hyperarousal, constriction, and addiction to traumatic reexposure. In: van der Kolk BA, ed. *Psychological Trauma*. Washington, DC: American Psychiatric Press; 1987:63-88.

107. Bloom SL. Neither liberty nor safety: the impact of fear on individuals, institutions, and societies. Part I. *Psychotherapy Politics Internat*. 2004;2:78-98.

108. Bloom SL. Neither liberty nor safety: the impact of fear on individuals, institutions, and societies. Part II. *Psychotherapy Politics Internat*. 2004;2:212-228.

109. Bloom SL. Neither liberty nor safety: the impact of trauma on individuals, institutions, and societies. Part IV. *Psychotherapy Politics Internat*. 2005;3:96-111.

110. Forsyth DR. *Group Dynamics*. 2nd ed. Pacific Grove, Calif: Brooks/Cole Publishing; 1990.

111. Janis IL. Decision making under stress. In: Goldberger L, Breznitz S, eds. *Handbook of Stress: Theoretical and Clinical Aspects*. New York, NY: Free Press; 1982:69-87.

112. Janis IL. Groupthink. *Small Groups and Social Interaction*. 1983;2:39-46.

113. Bloom SL. *Creating Sanctuary: Toward the Evolution of Sane Societies*. New York, NY: Routledge; 1997.

114. Herman JL. Complex PTSD: a syndrome in survivors of prolonged and repeated trauma. *J Trauma Stress*. 1992;5:377-391.

115. Prochaska JO, Norcross JC, Diclemente CC. *Changing for Good*. New York, NY: William Morrow; 1994.

116. Bloom SL. By the crowd they have been broken, by the crowd they shall be healed: the social transformation of trauma. In: Tedeschi R, Park C, Calhoun L, eds. *Post-Traumatic Growth: Positive Changes in the Aftermath of Crises*. Mahwah, NJ: Lawrence Erlbaum Associates; 1998.

117. Warshaw C. Women and violence. In: Stotland NL, Stewart DE, eds. *Psychological Aspects of Women's Health Care: The Interface Between Psychiatry and Obstetrics and Gynecology*. Washington, DC: American Psychiatric Press; 2001: 477-546.

118. Bloom SL. The sanctuary model: developing generic inpatient programs for the treatment of psychological trauma. In: Williams MB, Sommer JF. *Handbook of Post-Traumatic Therapy: A Practical Guide to Intervention, Treatment, and Research*. Westport, Conn: Greenwood Publishing; 1994:474-449.

119. Bloom SL. Creating sanctuary: healing from systematic abuses of power. *Therapeutic Commun*. 2000;21:67-91.

120. van der Kolk BA, van der Hart O. Pierre Janet and the breakdown of adaptation in psychological trauma. *Am J Psychiatry*. 1989;146:1530-1540.

121. van der Kolk BA, Brown P, van der Hart O. Pierre Janet on post-traumatic stress. *J Trauma Stress*. 1989;2:365-378.

122. Bloom SL, Bennington-Davis M, Farragher B, McCorkie D, Nice-Martini K, Wellbank K. Multiple opportunities for creating sanctuary. *Psychiatr Q*. 2003; 74:173-190.

123. Foderaro J, Ryan R. SAGE: mapping the course of recovery. *Therapeutic Commun*. 2000; 21(special issue):93-104.

124. Foderaro J. Creating a nonviolent environment: keeping sanctuary safe. In: Bloom S, ed. *Violence: A Public Health Menace and a Public Health Approach*. London, England: Karnac Books; 2001:57-82.

125. Bloom SL. Salem Hospital. Sanctuaryweb Web site. CommunityWorks; 2002. Available at: http://www.sanctuaryweb.com/Projects/salem_hospital.htm. Accessed February 2, 2007.

126. Bills LJ. Using trauma theory and S.A.G.E. in outpatient psychiatric practice. *Psychiatr Q*. 2003;74:191-203.

127. Bloom SL. Family Support Center. Sanctuaryweb Web site. CommunityWorks; 2003. Available at: http://www.sanctuaryweb.com/Projects/family_support_center.htm. Accessed February 2, 2007.

128. Abramovitz R, Bloom SL. Creating sanctuary in a residential treatment setting for troubled children and adolescents. *Psychiatr Q.* 2003;74:119-135.

129. Bloom SL. Andrus Memorial Children's Center. Sanctuaryweb Web site. CommunityWorks; 2002. Available at: http://www.sanctuaryweb.com/Projects/andrus_memorial_center.htm. Accessed February 2, 2007.

130. Madsen L, Blitz LV, McCorkle D, Panzer PG. Sanctuary in a domestic violence shelter: a team approach to healing. *Psychiatr Q.* 2003;74:155-171.

131. Bloom SL. Interim House. Sanctuaryweb Web site. CommunityWorks; 2003. Available at: http://www.sanctuaryweb.com/Projects/interim_house.htm. Accessed February 2, 2007.

132. Rivard JC. *Trauma Focused Intervention Targeting Risk For Violence.* Bethesda, Md: National Institutes of Health; 2000.

133. Rivard JC, Bloom SL, Abramovitz R, et al. Assessing the implementation and effects of a trauma-focused intervention for youths in residential treatment. *Psychiatr Q.* 2003;74:137-154.

134. Rivard JC McCorkle D, Duncan ME, Pasquale LE, Bloom SL, Abramovitz R. Implementing a trauma recovery framework for youths in residential treatment. *Child Adolesc Social Work J.* 2004;21:529-550.

135. Rivard JC, Bloom SL, McCorkle D, Abramovitz R. Preliminary results of a study examining the implementation and effects of a trauma recovery frame-work for youths in residential treatment. *Therapeutic Commun.* 2005;26:83-96.

136. Roberts SJ. Somatization in primary care: the common presentation of psychosocial problems through physical complaints. *Nurs Pract.* 1994;19:47, 50-56.

137. Bills L. Trauma-based psychiatry for primary care. In: Stamm BH, ed. *Secondary Traumatic Stress: Self-Care Issues for Clinicians, Researchers, and Educators.* Lutherville, Md: Sidran Press: 1995:121-148.

138. Bloom SL. *Organizational Stress as a Barrier to Trauma-Informed Change.* Alexandria, Va: National Association of State Mental Health Program Directors. Available at: http://www.nasmhpd.org/publications.cfm. Accessed February 2, 2007.

139. "Transformation." Def. 2. *Webster's Revised Unabridged Dictionary.* Springfield, MO: C. & G. Merriam Co; 1913. Available at: http://www.webster-dictionary.org/definition/transformation. Accessed March 3, 2008.

140. Jones, M., *The Therapeutic Community: A New Treatment Method in Psychiatry.* 1953, New York: Basic Books.

Chapter 11

Domestic Crimes Investigations and Law Enforcement

G.L. Isaacs, BS, Ed
Angelo Giardino, MD, PhD, MPH, FAAP

Historical Perspective

Briefly reviewing law enforcement's historical role in intimate partner violence (IPV) helps better understand the current law enforcement perspectives regarding IPV.

Clues From the Past

For centuries, men have viewed women as property. The "Rule of Thumb" adage perhaps best exemplifies this. This saying was derived from an old English law that allowed a husband to "correct" his wife by striking her with a rod, provided that the diameter of that rod was not larger than the diameter of his thumb. In the late 1800s, law enforcement officers began to move toward professional standards. During this time, Sir Robert Peel of Scotland Yard developed the notion of categorizing crimes and crime reporting. Even with Peel's genius and foresight, the "Rule of Thumb" remained the law of the land. In the early 1900s, the suffrage movement brought about the beginnings of change in women's rights, and a decline in the viewing of women as property. World War II certainly impacted traditional women's roles, as they worked in the shipyards and factories filling positions previously dominated by men. However, domestic violence continued unchecked by law enforcement, and it was not until the 1990s that we began to see movement toward any real change.

Clues From the Present

Even today, law enforcement often continues to work under this illusion of the "Rule of Thumb," because Western culture tends to view domestic violence as a private family matter. The *Family Violence Statistics* survey issued by the Bureau of Justice Statistics (BJS) in June 2005 provides interesting details regarding this "private family matter" mentality. The BJS reported the following statistics regarding family violence reported to law enforcement officers[1]:

— Between 1998 and 2002, victims reported an estimated 60% of family violence incidents to law enforcement officers. Female victims reported much more often than male victims.

— The most common reason (ie, cited by 34% of victims) given for not reporting family violence incidents was that these occurrences were a "private and personal matter."

During the past several decades, the manner in which law enforcement officers approach IPV crime has evolved considerably. As recently as the early 1990s, the response of officers assigned to "domestic" incidents was extremely limited by law.

Before 1993, domestic violence training for law enforcement officers primarily focused on officer safety. Police officers heard horror stories of victims becoming combative when an officer moved to arrest the batterer. Officer safety was and continues to be an important issue; however, at that time the older, nonspecified intimate violence laws placed responsibility for action almost entirely upon the victim. For example, for an officer to make an arrest, the assault had to occur while in the presence of an officer. The following provides an example of one law enforcement officer's response to a typical domestic violence call. His response was within the boundaries set for officers before legislation regarding domestic violence was passed during the 1990s.

Case Example: One Law Enforcement Officer's Response to a Case*

One of my earliest remembrances as a young officer is related to a domestic assault. I was assigned to a "domestic" at an apartment complex during the early evening hours. Upon arrival, I observed a young woman seated on the staircase steps that led to the second level of the complex. The front door of her ground-level apartment stood open a few feet to her left. As I approached, her head was down almost between her knees. I spoke to her. She raised her head slightly and stared at me. Blood was running from her nose and mouth, forming a sizeable puddle at her feet. What has haunted me for almost 30 years is the look of complete and utter hopelessness that I saw in her eyes.

I recall immediately asking whether she wanted an ambulance and her nodding to the negative. In fact, that was her only response to any of my questions. Beyond that gesture, I received no reply to even standard questions, such as "Who did this to you?" and "Will you press charges?" She simply stared straight ahead, never acknowledging my presence again.

As I attempted to communicate with this victim, I observed that her batterer stood bare-chested in the apartment doorway drinking beer. He watched my partner and me. Then he said something about the victim not filing any charges since he was standing on his private property, so we could not do anything about the incident. Under the then existing laws, he was correct. At that time a police officer could act only on a misdemeanor crime that the officer had observed being committed.

I approached the suspect and commented to him, "We have to keep our women in line." He looked at me, grinned, and leisurely stepped from his doorway to approach me. I, then, explained to him that he was now standing on the public sidewalk, at which time I promptly arrested him for public intoxication.

CASE EXAMPLE EVALUATION

Though this describes a typical domestic crime of the period, the response was often less successful. Usually the law enforcement officers took on the role of amateur marriage counselors and lectured the couple about the value of a good, nonviolent relationship. Frequently, the officers asked the parties to separate for the evening; the officers would then threaten that if called back, "Someone is going to jail!" If an arrest did occur, quite often both parties were arrested. The paperwork generated from these arrests did not show that one of the arrestees was actually a victim. As a result, law enforcement officers provided a quick fix to the problem and then moved along to the next service call. Little or no consideration was given to long-term solutions.

LAW ENFORCEMENT PROGRESS

Fortunately, a certain amount of enlightenment began to occur in the early 1990s. Much of the credit should be given to the women's movement for spotlighting the problem and demanding action. As a result, law enforcement officers began to recognize that domestic violence is more than a so-called "social issue"; rather, domestic violence is a crime. In addition, progressive legislation and training provided law enforcement officers with much needed tools to begin addressing crimes associated with IPV.

* All names have been changed to protect the privacy of the people involved.

PROBABLE CAUSE ARRESTS

In most states, police officers now have both the authority and a mandate to arrest batterers whenever officers encounter evidence that a domestic assault has taken place. Now, with such *probable cause* arrest scenarios, the responsibility for action lies squarely on law enforcement officers, rather than on victims.

ORDERS OF PROTECTION

The creation of court orders of protection greatly impacted law enforcement officers when addressing domestic crimes. In most states, a victim of domestic abuse, stalking, or rape may file a petition for a "protective order" with the district or tribal court within the jurisdiction in which the victim or defendant resides or within the jurisdiction in which the criminal violation occurred. The Violence Against Women Act of 1994 defines a protection order as "Any injunction or other order issued for the purpose of preventing violent or threatening acts or harassment against, contact or communication with, or physical proximity to another person."[2] These orders of protection provide specific instructions from the court requiring the defendant to cease contact with the victim as defined by the issuing court. Unlike civil restraining orders (which have restricted enforcement jurisdiction), protective orders operate under a legal primus referred to as *full faith and credit*,[3] which authorizes enforcement by any law enforcement officer operating within his or her geographic jurisdiction. This includes permanent protective orders issued by state and tribal courts, which may normally be outside the enforcing officer's jurisdiction. These orders are referred to as *foreign personal protection orders*.

In many jurisdictions, protective order offices have been established and staffed with intimate partner violence advocates and attorneys who work in partnership with law enforcement officers. Victim advocates not only assist in preparing protection order documents, but also council and assure victims that many social services are available. Most police officers working with advocates have learned to view these advocates as important tools for victims. Unfortunately, protective orders are just pieces of paper; they do not protect victims whose abusers disregard the law.

COMMUNITY POLICING MODEL

Recognizing that law enforcement is only part of the social system involved in creating change leads to the third law enforcement initiative, the community policing model, which has dramatically impacted IPV. Community policing has become or is becoming the standard for law enforcement throughout the nation. Under this model, law enforcement officers recognize that most often crime is simply a derivative of a larger social issue. As a result, officers must fully identify the source of the problem. To do so may involve using nontraditional law enforcement and multijurisdictional approaches not previously used. The overall objective is to problem solve and create long-term solutions.

For many years, police departments across the United States recognized the need for specialty units to address particular areas such as homicide and juvenile crimes. These units focus on problem solving. Likewise, under community policing, police departments began developing domestic crimes units in recent years.

Domestic crimes units have emerged in many larger police departments within the United States. These units strive to conduct the necessary follow-up investigations needed to produce a long-term impact on the IPV problem. From a police management standpoint, the creation of such units has proven an excellent investment of personnel.

STATISTICS AND RECENT TRENDS

The *Family Violence Statistics* published by the BJS showed that "Family violence accounted for 33% of all violent crimes recorded by police in 18 states and the District of Columbia in 2000. Of these, more than 207 000 family violence crimes, about half (53% or 110 000) were crimes between spouses."[1] Without even considering victimization, many police managers have recognized the potential to reduce a police department's calls for service by a significant percentage by addressing the problem at the onset of violence. Bearing in mind the recognition of IPV as a crime and the accompanying law enforcement and community response, there are a number of observable trends in victimization. The *National Crime Victimization Survey* published in 2003 specifically looked at the current problems of the victim-offender relationship and intimate violence.[4]

Victim and Offender Relationship

The *National Crime Victimization Survey* shows that men are most often violently victimized by strangers; women, however, are most often victimized by friends, acquaintances, or intimate partners.[4] Approximately 7 in 10 female rape or sexual assault victims stated that the offender was an intimate partner, relative, friend, or acquaintance. Sixty-two percent of men and 45% of women indicated that the individual who robbed them was a stranger. This survey also identified the following trends[4]:

— Between 1993 and 1998, violence against men and women by friends, acquaintances, or strangers and IPV against women fell significantly.

— Family members commit approximately 1 in 5 child murders. In fact, young children are more likely to be murdered by a family member, while older children (ie, children between the ages of 15 and 17 years) are more likely to be murdered by a friend or acquaintance.

— Approximately 40% of victims of nonfatal violence in the workplace reported that they knew their offender. In addition, victims of workplace violence identified their intimate partners as the perpetrator in about 1% of violent workplace crimes.

— In 2002, 43% of murder victims were related to or acquainted with their assailants, 14% were murdered by strangers, and 43% had an unknown relationship with their assailants.

Intimate Partner Violence

The *National Crime Victimization Survey* identified the following statistics regarding IPV[4]:

— Though dramatically down from the reported 1.1 million rapes, sexual assaults, robberies, aggravated assaults, and simple assaults perpetrated by intimate partners in 1993, women experienced an estimated 494 570 such incidents in 2002. In comparison, men were victims of violent crimes by an intimate partner 160 000 times in 1993 and 72 520 times in 2002.

— Between 1976 and 1998, the number of murders by intimate partners decreased on average by 4% per year for male victims and by 1% percent per year for female victims.

— Intimate murders of black, male victims experienced the sharpest decrease (74%) between 1976 and 1998.

— Intimate violence remains primarily a crime against women. In 1998, women were victims of 72% of intimate murders and approximately 85% of nonlethal IPV.

— Women between the ages of 16 and 24 years experienced the highest per capita rates of IPV (19.6 victimizations per 1000 women).

— Victims identified intimates partners (eg, current and former spouses, boyfriends, girlfriends) as the perpetrators of about 1% of all violent crime in the workplace.

EVIDENCE-BASED INVESTIGATIONS

Most researchers who have studied IPV subscribe to the evidence-based prosecution approach. Evidence-based prosecution occurs daily in US courts. Essentially, through the available physical evidence, prosecutors attempt to establish, beyond a reasonable doubt, that the defendant committed the crime. As a result, victim exposure during the trial process is kept to a minimum. In theft cases, the victim often has no role other than to identify the recovered stolen property. Of course, the most critical cases involving evidence-based prosecution are homicides. In such cases, dying victims rarely have the opportunity to provide a statement. By responding to IPV as a crime, the responsibility for action has moved from the victim to law enforcement, so every effort should be made to minimize the victims' involvement in the prosecution.

Case Example: A Well-Investigated Instance of Intimate Partner Violence

At approximately 3:00 AM, emergency medical technicians (EMTs) summoned local police officers to a modest, single-family residence. The EMTs had encountered what they believed to be the victim of a severe beating. The victim (Jean) was in her late 30s. She had sustained multiple head injuries and was comatose. The EMTs said that upon their arrival, they found the victim bleeding significantly and saw the victim's husband (Jim) and mother-in-law (Betty) attempting to attend to the victim. Jim told the EMTs that he believed his wife had interrupted an intruder, which resulted in the attack.

When the first officers arrived, they observed the victim being loaded into an ambulance and accompanied by her husband. Jean's 2 sons, 10-year-old Bobby and 13-year-old Tommy, and Betty were preparing to follow the ambulance. The officers requested additional police units and designated the crime scene perimeter.

As the officers entered the residence, they observed a pool of blood on the living room floor that was between 4 and 5 feet in diameter, as well as considerable blood spatter on the furniture and walls. The officers requested detectives from the scientific (ie, forensic) investigation unit (SIU) to process the scene for evidence. These original investigating officers discounted the possibility of an intruder after examining the doors and windows and finding no signs of a forced entry. Considering the likelihood that the victim had been assaulted by a family member, the domestic crimes unit (DCU) was asked to respond and lead the investigation. In addition, the DCU dispatched additional detectives to meet the ambulance at the hospital.

At the crime scene, detectives began a detailed evidentiary search. They gathered forensic evidence throughout the residence and reexamined the possible points of entry. Most of the blood evidence was located in the living room and hall bathroom. Blood spatter on the living room walls indicated multiple blunt-instrument strikes with spatter ranging from approximately 6 inches to 5 feet above the floor. No apparent weapon was located in the residence or on the surrounding properties. Uniformed officers and detectives canvassed the neighborhood in an effort to identify any potential witnesses or find any evidence of an intruder. None were found.

When the victim arrived at the hospital, health care providers examined her and described her condition as "grave." Among other injuries, the victim had sustained multiple cranial fractures and was comatose. The DCU detectives arrived at the hospital and met briefly with the victim's husband. Their objective was to obtain a brief statement from Jim and lock him into a story. Jim was somewhat vague. He stated only that a loud noise awakened him, he entered the living room and found his wife on the floor bleeding severely, then he immediately phoned his mother because she was a registered nurse and lived nearby. Betty arrived within moments. Upon observing and assessing Jean's condition, she called for an ambulance.

The DCU detectives met with Betty at the hospital and explained that they needed her to provide a statement at the detective division. When Betty arrived at the detective division, the DCU supervisor interviewed her. She displayed a genuine concern for Jean; however, she seemed very reluctant to provide details. The DCU supervisor asked Betty a series of simple, open-ended questions to establish a dialog in an effort to help Betty relax. As the questions became more specific, Betty was asked how she became involved in the incident. She quickly volunteered, "My son called, and woke me. He said, 'I think I killed....'" She stopped and attempted to recant this statement by saying, "He said she's hurt." Befuddled, Betty stopped and began explaining how she had found Jim caring for Jean on the living room floor. She continued to describe how she and her son had helped Jean into the hall bathroom in an attempt to treat Jean's injuries. Once in the bathroom, Betty observed the extent of Jean's trauma and called for an ambulance.

While Betty was being questioned, DCU detectives spoke with Bobby and Tommy at the hospital. They began by telling the boys that the detectives were there to help and reassured the boys that their mother was receiving excellent treatment. After developing a rapport with the boys, the detectives explained their mission—to find out what had happened to their mother. The detectives separated the boys during the interviews.

Bobby was more relaxed and articulate than Tommy. He spoke about baseball and told the detectives about the new bat and ball his father had given him that evening. Bobby was asked to describe the day's events leading up to his mother's injury. He began by saying that his father had just returned from being away on a job. According to Bobby, everything seemed normal until his mother announced during dinner that she wanted a divorce. Earlier that day, Jean had told her sons that she intended to tell Jim, so her announcement during dinner did not come as a surprise to Bobby. Bobby described how his father had stopped eating and simply stated there would be no divorce. Jim then resumed with his meal. Bobby indicated that the evening continued without event. In the early morning hours, a loud noise awoke Bobby. When he entered the darkened living room, Bobby saw his father standing over Jean. Jean was on the floor, and Jim held an object. Bobby could not identify the object. Bobby returned to his room and remained there until his grandmother came to get him so that they could follow the ambulance to the hospital.

The DCU detective who spoke with Tommy found him less cooperative. This detective soon discovered that Tommy was also a baseball player, so the detective mentioned the new bat that their father had given the boys before supper that evening in an effort to confirm Bobby's statement.

The detectives reported their progress to the officers working the crime scene and specifically mentioned the baseball bat as a possible weapon. The officers conducted a second comprehensive search with negative results. Based upon the information received during the interviews, as well as the absence of the baseball bat, a decision was made to take Jim into custody. He was transported to the detective division and asked to provide a statement. He refused and requested council. The District Attorney reviewed the case. Charges were quickly filed against Jim.

Jean remained in a coma for approximately 2 weeks. In addition to her skull fractures, her left leg was broken slightly above the ankle. Detectives theorized that when she was attacked, Jean was struck with such force that her weight shifted rapidly and broke the leg. The unusual masked-type bruising around both of Jeans eyes also indicated that extreme force was used. Doctors reported this bruising occurred as a result of a contrecoup concussion, in which the victim's brain pushes the eyes out of the sockets after an extraordinarily hard blow to the back of the head. Upon awakening, health care providers observed that Jean had paralysis on the left side of her body. In addition, Jean had sustained significant general memory loss, and had no recollection of the assault.

While awaiting trial, Jim spoke with his mother over the telephone daily. Although the county jail had signs posted to clearly state that telephone lines may be monitored, Jim did not expect DCU detectives to follow through and monitor his calls. About 3 weeks after his arrest, Jim telephoned his mother and begged her to place her home as a security bond for his release. During that conversation, Jim stated, "You've got to get me out. They know I did it. I've got to get away." Betty arranged for a bond later that day, and Jim was released. Jim immediately proceeded to his home and began to pack. The DCU detectives were monitoring the taped phone conversations and informed the court of Jim's plan to flee. The court revoked the bond and directed the detectives to take Jim back into custody. Jim's vehicle was packed, and he was leaving his home when he was located by the detectives and re-arrested. Jim remained in custody pending his trial.

About 6 weeks after the assault, a preliminary hearing was conducted. Preliminary hearings are designed to address 2 issues—whether probable cause exists to believe that a crime was committed and, if so, is there probable cause to believe that it was the *defendant* who committed the crime. Although these are only determinates, preliminary hearings often become mini-trials during which the defense gauges the strength of the prosecution's case.

During Jim's preliminary hearing, the prosecution reconstructed the assault using physical evidence and testimony. The prosecution believed that the evidence would prevail. Prosecutors hoped that by using experts to present their findings, Jean and her sons would not need to testify. A number of police officers testified about their observations and the collection of evidence. The prosecuting attorney introduced scene photography and photographs that highlighted Jean's injuries. Detectives testified about their follow-up investigation, the interviews they conducted, and statements they obtained. Medical experts provided graphic details of the damage inflicted on the victim and about Jean's long-term prognosis. As witnesses presented the evidence against her husband, Jean sat with her mother-in-law and repeatedly shook her head in the negative. Jean did not stop shaking her head until she heard the audiotape of Jim telling Betty, "You've got to get me out. They know I did it."

During the discovery phase of the trial, before the hearing, the defense attorney was given copies of all documents and audiotapes. The defense attorney and many other people had believed that the prosecuting attorney would present his case through the victim; however, that was not the case. The defense had little or no rebuttal evidence, so the hearing ended soon after the prosecution's presentation. Following the preceding, Jim's attorney began plea negotiations. Jim was later convicted of attempted murder, and the judge sentenced him to between 15 and 20 years in prison.

CASE EXAMPLE EVALUATION

This was an extraordinary case in several respects. Certainly, the tragedy of the victim's paralysis overshadows the victory in the courtroom. Interestingly, what stood out most to the investigators was that documented history did not exist regarding this couple and previous instances of IPV. One predictor of lethality is the frequency of episodes. Without the documentation, only Jim and Jean know how many violent episodes had actually occurred prior to this encounter. One especially telling point, however, was that when the victim's son saw his mother lying on the floor with his father standing over her, he simply returned to his room without a second thought. Experts believe that IPV is a learned behavior. In this case, hopefully the victim's sons can and will break the cycle.

Reviewing the Investigation

In reviewing the investigation, high-level training existed at all levels. That is, the police department and prosecutor's office committed the necessary resources to this case. The first-responding officers set a perimeter and called for assistance. Recognizing that evidence did not show a readily apparent forced entry, which conflicted with Jim's statement about the involvement of an intruder, these officers notified the DCU. The DCU officers and forensic investigators thoroughly processed the crime scene. As previously mentioned, experts examined the locks and windows for tool marks and found no signs of forced entry, formally discounting Jim's statement. Blood evidence and photography provided a detailed, graphic picture of the attack's savage nature. Follow-up photography of the victim displayed the continued growth of her massive bruising and the peculiar mask-type bruise surrounding her eyes.

A canvas of the neighborhood produced no witnesses to support Jim's claims. The officers who conducted the neighborhood canvas carefully recorded the names of potential witnesses in the event that a surprise witness came forth at a later date.

At the hospital, detectives made contact with the ambulance crew. The detectives obtained statements regarding the EMTs' actions. In addition, they included observations and details about what the EMTs were told by the defendant and his mother. The DCU detectives introduced themselves to hospital medical staff members and explained their presence and mission. Further, recognizing confidentiality issues, the detectives explained that subpoenas for medical records would be forthcoming. The detectives asked for a contact person regarding inquiries about the victim's condition. The victim's sons were interviewed at the hospital. After these interviews, the detectives communicated their findings to their supervising officer and to the officers at the crime scene.

The DCU supervisor assessed the physical evidence obtained from the crime scene and evaluated the witness statements obtained by the officers. After a thorough assessment, the supervisor ordered the suspect's arrest.

In the weeks following the assault, DCU detectives maintained daily contact with the hospital personnel caring for Jean and monitored the defendant's communications from prison. In preparation for the preliminary hearing, detectives met with the prosecuting attorneys and obtained subpoenas for witnesses and medical records.

The Importance of Committing the Necessary Personnel to Intimate Partner Crimes

Obviously a considerable amount of time and resources were invested in the case. Many law enforcement managers, especially those in smaller jurisdictions, may have difficulty dedicating a significant number of personnel to these investigations. However, from a strictly managerial standpoint and considering the recidivism rate associated with intimate partner crimes, committing the necessary personnel to investigating these crimes may very well prove more cost-effective in the long run.

Predicting the Lethality of an Intimate Partner Relationship

To a certain degree, lethality involving intimate partners often can be predicted by measuring increases in the following 3 components.

1. Frequency of events

2. Severity of the event(s)

3. Intensity of the event(s)

Jean had encountered both the severity and intensity of events, so her reluctance to serve as a witness during the trial was reasonable. Fortunately for Jean, Jim was convicted and cannot harm her again. Tragically, she is disabled, and she and her sons must face the considerable struggles ahead.

Reasons Victims Stay in an Abusive Relationship

Bobby's reaction when he observed his mother down and his father standing over her leads one to believe that violence in the home was not unusual. This highlights one of the most puzzling issues surrounding IPV—"Why does the victim stay in the violent relationship?" Simply put, most victims remain because they fear their partner. The victim has been conditioned to believe that she either cannot survive or will not be allowed to survive without her partner. The abuser often threatens his victim with the possibility of losing her children, being unemployed and/or having no financial support, and actual physical danger. In addition, experiences that surround even the suggestion of leaving convince the victim to stay. In fact, studies show that victims who are about to leave or have just left an abusive relationship are in the greatest danger of physical violence from their abusers. (See Chapter 5, "Intervention for Women: Why Doesn't She Just Leave?" for more information on this topic.).

Jean continually denied that her husband was her assailant. In assessing her motives, recall that the medical evidence supported Jean's assertion that she could not remember the assault. As with many victims, Jean found it impossible to believe that her husband, the father of her children, would actually kill her. In addition, Jean had undergone a degree of psychological programming, like most IPV victims. In the past, Jean had depended on Jim, but her physical condition now exacerbated her dependence upon her husband and Jim's mother. As a result, Jean fears both the known *and* the unknown.

Like most IPV victims, she wonders about the following:

— How she and her sons will survive

— Who will provide for them

— What they will do if her husband is acquitted

— What she will do if she has to testify

— What her husband is capable of doing

— Her suspicions that he has already attempted to murder her

THE VICTIMS

The *Family Violence Statistics* provides the following demographic characteristics of family violence victims according to gender, race, and age[1]:

— Gender

  — Women are more likely than men to be victims of family violence.

  — Between 1998 and 2002, women made up 51.6% of the US population aged 12 years old and older. At that time, 73.4% of the nation's family violence victims came from this population demographic.

  — Between 1998 and 2002, 84.3% of spousal abuse victims and 85.9% of abuse victims within boyfriend-girlfriend relationships were women.

  — Men are more likely than women to be victims of nonfamily violence.

  — Between 1998 and 2002, men made up 48.4% of the US population age 12 years old and older, but 58.4% of nonfamily violence victims and 68.3% of stranger violence victims.

— Race

  — White and black people were more likely to be victims of family violence than people of other ethnic backgrounds.

  — Between 1998 and 2002, white people made up 72.9% of the US population aged 12 years old and older, and 74% of family violence victims were white.

  — Between 1998 and 2002, black people made up 12.1% of the US population aged 12 years old and older, and 13.6% of family violence victims were black.

  — Between 1998 and 2002, Hispanic people made up 10.9% of the US population aged 12 years old and older, and 10.1% of family violence victims were Hispanic.

  — Between 1998 and 2002, people of other races made up 4.1% of the US population aged 12 years old and older, and 2.3% of family violence victims were people of other races.

  — American Indians and Alaska Natives have relatively high rates of family violence victimization.

  — Between 1998 and 2002, American Indians and Alaska Natives made up 0.4% of the US population aged 12 years old and older, and 1.6% of family violence victims were from these ethnic backgrounds.

  — Between 1998 and 2002, Asian Americans and Pacific Islanders made up 3.6%

of the US population aged 12 years old and older, and 0.5% of family violence victims were from these ethnic backgrounds.

— Age

— Between 1998 and 2002 the average age of the 3.5 million victims of family violence was 34 years.

— Overall, nonfamily violence victims were slightly younger between 1998 and 2002. The average age of these victims was just younger than 29 years.

— The average age for other victims between 1998 and 2002 was 35 years for people victimized by their spouses, 21 years for sons and daughters victimized by their parents, 35 years for people victimized by a family member, 27 years for victims of violence within a boyfriend-girlfriend relationship, 27 years for people victimized by a friend or acquaintance, and 30 years for victims of stranger violence.

— Adults between the ages of 25 and 54 years make up two thirds of the family violence victims.

— Between 1998 and 2002, adults between the ages of 25 and 34 years made up 16.7% of the US population and made up 24.5% of family violence victims.

— From 1998 to 2002, adults between the ages of 35 and 54 years made up 36% of the US population and made up 41.2% of family violence victims.

— Between 1998 and 2002, young adults between the ages of 18 and 24 years also represented a segment of family violence victims larger than their corresponding percentage of the US population. They made up 11.7% of the US population aged 12 years and older and made up 17.6% of family violence victims.

— Between 1998 and 2002, adults who were 55 years old or older were least likely to become victims of family violence. They made up 25% of the US population aged 12 years and older and made up 6% of family violence victims.

Researchers who study IPV do not find these statistics surprising; however, law enforcement officers working in areas highly concentrated by people of a specific ethnic or age group may a have somewhat skewed view of IPV within that culture. The analysis shows that IPV runs throughout the spectrum of gender, race, and age. Though the statistics prove enlightening, researchers realize that abuse may be underreported by victims for a variety reasons.

Though all IPV is tragic, the most troubling statistics involve people between the ages of 25 and 54, because a large number of children and teenagers are linked to this population. Despite the efforts and progress made with IPV victims, the cycle of IPV remains unbroken and a new generation of batterers awaits.

Current statistics indicate that women are the most likely victims of IPV. These women are mothers, sisters, daughters, and wives, and their batterers tend to be other family members. Though traditional male and female roles have evolved, within some cultures the notion of "male privilege" persists. Under this ideology, submission to one's partner is expected and private. As a result, some of these cultures do not understand the premise of marital rape and, in fact, view marital rape as an inconsistency. The following case study presents an extreme example of such a scenario.

Case Example: Marital Rape

In 2002, a young woman (Jane) carried her infant into the DCU. Jane was approximately 20 years old, about 5 feet 5 inches tall, and weighed less than 90 pounds. She had a gray complexion, and her eyes and cheeks appeared sunken. As she sat with the supervisor in his office, she simply said, "Help me," and then began to cry. The child she held was tiny—obviously a newborn. Uncertain of what help the victim might require, the male supervisor invited a female detective and a domestic violence advocate to join their meeting.

The detectives and advocate waited for Jane to compose herself and then asked her reason for coming to the DCU. She began by saying that she was a good wife, but she could not take it anymore. She then explained that her son was 10 days old and doing well despite a difficult pregnancy. Jane became reluctant to speak and began to ramble. She was concerned that the officers and advocate would not understand and, like her mother, say that a wife has her duties. After reassuring her that their role was not to judge, but assist her, Jane told her story.

Jane had grown up in a very traditional home in which her father was the head of the household. She was unaware of any physical abuse within her family; however, Jane's mother was clearly submissive to her husband's authority. Naturally, Jane married and carried on in a similar tradition. Upon marrying her husband, John, he had immediately exercised his authority and she had fallen into the role of submission, mirroring the model she had experienced in her childhood home. She explained to the officers and advocate that as long as she "respected" John, he was not physically abusive; however, if she was disrespectful, he would "correct" her.

Jane stated that 4 days after giving birth to their son, she returned home. Her husband had demanded intercourse. He continued to force her to have intercourse with him 3 times a day since returning home. Jane had submitted to him but was growing weak because of her continuing postpartum flow. She realized that, if she did not get away from her husband and recover, she would not be able to care for their child. Since John controlled their finances, she was forced to horde coins in order to obtain the bus fare necessary to escape and seek assistance.

Jane was transported to a local hospital emergency department. The health care providers examined and hospitalized her. Their examination produced significant evidence of rape, including trauma and fluids.

Detectives located and arrested John. He agreed to an interview after being given the *Miranda* warning. In his statement, John admitted repeatedly forcing Jane to have sex, both a few days before delivery and immediately upon her return from the hospital. John showed no signs of remorse and saw nothing wrong with his actions. He considered these actions within his right. John later pled guilty to rape after a plea negotiation. Jane and her son survived.

Case Example Evaluation

Jane's case seems almost unimaginable. Though certainly extreme, this case is actually classic with respect to the batterer's objectives—power, control, and dominance. Furthermore, Jane's conditioning throughout her upbringing led to her acceptance of John's behavior. To a large degree, she considered such behavior normal from her husband. Like so many abuse victims, protection of Jane's child became the impetus that forced her to act.

Future Trends

With changes to the traditional female role, many women compete daily with men in the workplace and often in organized sports. Such shifts have desensitized the male population, in that many men have become even less inhibited about striking a woman. Currently, female police officers are just as likely as their male counterparts to be forced to defend themselves; this was not the case in past years.

Without the commitment to thorough investigations and a multidisciplinary approach to IPV, the problem will likely grow. If law enforcement officers make IPV the priority it needs to be, then the means do exist to create change; in fact, officers can become agents of change. A number of resources provide excellent model policies for law enforcement agencies. Such resources include Office on Violence Against Women (http://www.usdoj.gov/ovw) and the International Association of Chiefs of Police (http://www.theiacp.org). Law enforcement officers owe it to the victims to strive to become these agents of change. People should not have to live in fear.

REFERENCES

1. Durose MR, Harlow CW, Langan PA, Motivans M, Rantala RR, Smith EL, for the Bureau of Justice Statistics. *Family Violence Statistics.* Washington, DC: Bureau of Justice Statistics; 2005. NCJ 207846.

2. Violence Against Women Act, 1994.

3. Sect 1, Art 4, US Constitution.

4. Bureau of Justice Statistics. *National Crime Victimization Survey.* 2003. Available at: http://www.ojp.usdoj.gov/bjs/cvict.htm. Accessed September 28, 2007.

Chapter 12

ROLE OF IPV PROFESSIONALS IN CRIMINAL PROSECUTION

Mary Graw Leary, JD
Eric Gibson, JD

The social harm caused by intimate partner violence (IPV) is difficult to adequately measure. IPV is life altering for victims on every possible level. Therefore, society's response to IPV must be multidisciplinary. A safety net woven with the threads of diverse community services must be in place to assist victims and provide them the protection and services needed to attend to their physical, psychological, and emotional safety.

One of these threads is the criminal justice system. Just as the criminal justice system cannot act in a vacuum, other disciplines cannot act without regard to the criminal justice system. Each thread must recognize the value of the other and work together. Failure to do so makes the net merely a mirage. Both locally and nationally, the criminal justice system has created several effective legal devices to benefit victims through deterrence, punishment, rehabilitation, and victims' services. Statutes, such as the reenacted Violence Against Women Act of 2006, provide important components of the societal effort to eliminate IPV and domestic violence and protect potential victims.[1]

Any professional working with potential victims of IPV must be aware of the criminal implications of the perpetrator's behavior. The professional must also understand these modern legal trends. Such knowledge is necessary, first, to avoid jeopardizing a criminal prosecution, and, second, to comprehensively serve victims. Additionally, the IPV professional should be educated on the legal process and the significant effect their work can play in a criminal prosecution and, ultimately, in securing the safety of the victim. This chapter will examine these issues.

SCOPE OF THE CRIMINAL PROBLEM

The statistics of the occurrence and reporting of these crimes dramatically demonstrates the important role IPV professionals play in supporting criminal prosecution. The US Department of Justice (Justice Department) distinguishes between "family violence" and "intimate partner violence." Family violence is defined by the Justice Department as "violent crime committed by an offender who is related to the victim either biologically or legally through marriage or adoption."[2] According to the Justice Department, family violence in America accounted for 11% of all reported and unreported violence between 1998 and 2002. Roughly 3.5 million violent crimes were committed against family members, 49% of these against spouses, 11% by a parent against a child, and 41% were committed against other family members.[2] According to Justice Department figures, family violence between 1993 and 2002 accounted for 1 in 10 violent victimizations.[2]

Intimate partner violence is defined by the Justice Department as violence between current or former spouses, boyfriends and girlfriends, or same-sex partners.[3] The

Centers for Disease Control and Prevention comports with this definition, stating that IPV includes physical, sexual, or psychological harm by current or former partners or spouses.[4] This violence includes homicides, rapes, robberies, and assaults.[3,4] Between 2001 and 2005, nonfatal IPV represented 22% of violent victimizations against females and 4% against males aged 12 and older.[3] According to its most recent figures, the Justice Department reports that the rate of family violence between 1993 and 2002 fell from an estimated 5.4 victims to 2.1 per 1000 US residents age 12 or older.[5]

The Justice Department recently announced that incidents of reported IPV declined and noted that only 23% of female victims and 9% of male victims contacted an outside agency for assistance.[3] This should concern IPV professionals because, while this serious crime is occurring at an epidemic rate, the opportunity for government intervention and protection for victims is often limited to those events of which the victims or witnesses make law enforcement aware. Therefore, often the only opportunity for a victim to disclose and obtain safety occurs with the one professional (such as a medical professional, social worker, teacher, emergency medical technician [EMT]) who encounters this victim. This person has an enormous effect on not only the quality of the prosecution, but often determines whether the crime is prosecuted at all.

A second group of statistics is relevant to our analysis, that is, not only the quantity of this crime, but the level of prosecution. As a threshold, matter statistics in this area are deceiving. While a certain outcome, such as probation, may look the same on paper from case to case, whether that is a "successful" prosecution or a failed outcome turns on the facts of each case and many other intangibles, such as the history of the offender, the safety of the victim, and so on. In addition to the low report rates of IPV mentioned above, the Justice Department reports that approximately 60% of family violence victimizations were reported to police between 1998 and 2002, and, of these, only 36% to 49% resulted in arrest.[2] A May 2000 study of state domestic violence prosecutions found that almost 50% of the felony assault defendants were released pending trial.[2] The Justice Department reports approximately 24% of state family violence cases do not go to trial because of dismissals.[2] This is consistent with federal case processing statistics, which indicate that less than 50% of offenders investigated are ultimately convicted.[6] Consequently, the criminal justice system acts as a funnel. A large number of crimes are occurring, but less than that are being reported, investigated, charged, and even brought through to disposition and conviction. Throughout this entire criminal process, however, IPV professionals play an important role in keeping the cases moving forward to the next level.

Prosecutors, like doctors, medical professionals, social workers, and others, are part of the array of professionals working toward the shared goal of ending this victimization and protecting those affected by such violence. As the safety net analogy suggests, the response of all these professionals has been increasingly coordinated over the years as jurisdictions adopt multidisciplinary approaches. This is reflected in movements such as hospital-based child abuse and domestic violence centers, forensic interviewing of child victims and witnesses, domestic violence divisions in police departments and prosecutors' offices, specialized victim witness advocates, social workers on staff at prosecutor offices, and the increased use of expert witnesses from all these disciplines in criminal trials. Overall, this provides victims with the benefit of a more comprehensive response to their crisis.[7]

CALL FOR COORDINATION

It would be a mistake for any of these disciplines to act as though they function in a vacuum. The obligation of the prosecutor is to seek justice and protect society in general, as well as protect the specific victims of the case. In spite of this important duty, the prosecutor should never proceed without considering the effect of actions on other disciplines' intervention with victims to prevent further violence. To the contrary, it is critical for the prosecutor to proceed with victim protection with an awareness of the consequences of the investigation and prosecution on other aspects of the victims' lives. Likewise, other professionals must recognize not only the tremendous value of the criminal prosecution in ending such violence, but that their actions often directly affect whether prosecution will succeed.

This chapter will explore the roles of law enforcement, prosecutors, and other IPV professionals in the multidisciplinary effort to respond to and end IPV. It will highlight some of the most common areas where the fields interconnect, and where work of the IPV professional's actions can have profound consequences on a criminal prosecution. This chapter is not a complete analysis of all of the ways interdisciplinary professionals can interface with the criminal justice system. Rather, the chapter will guide the professional on considerations to remember when working with victims, which will directly affect the success of a criminal prosecution and, therefore, the safety of the victims. This chapter is also not a suggestion that a professional should become an extension of law enforcement. The primary duty of any person working with a victim of IPV must be to the victim and to the standards of said profession. However, this duty to the victim cannot be fulfilled without an understanding of the criminal justice system and how the professional can make decisions that positively or negatively affect the pursuit of justice for this victim and her ultimate safety.

For example, let us turn to the medical professional. Accurately documenting injuries in medical records is a primary task of critical importance to the medical profession. Such a professional must also recognize that failing to do so also has significant, if not determinative, effects on a criminal prosecution, as well as medical care. When a medical professional fails to adequately document files, the effect is a lack of medical data consistent with the victim's recounting of her assault. The result is a record that calls into question the victim's credibility. Additionally, if a medical expert is needed for testimony, the records become an inadequate basis for such information that may, in turn, preclude this critical testimony. Should the author of the record need to testify, he or she is now handicapped without a clear memory of the case. Furthermore, the author will be subject to more aggressive cross-examination and his or her own credibility may be called into question.

Therefore, all IPV professionals must perform their duties with an awareness that they are working with these victims at a critical stage in the development of law enforcement's case, and the performance of their duties will directly affect the outcome of the government effort to place the victim into safety.

PRE-TRIAL ISSUES: EVALUATION OF THE CASE

The importance of all IPV professionals is evident well before a criminal case is actually tried. In fact, a well-prepared investigation, informed by the work of the other disciplines, will often not result in a trial but, rather, a guilty plea. This then ensures an increase in the victim's safety and a decrease in ongoing stress relating to a trial.

The first step for the criminal prosecutor is case evaluation. The presentation of IPV cases to prosecutors is, almost always, the result of reactive police involvement, rather than a proactive investigation. In other words, the prosecutor is presented with the case (often shortly before the first hearing), only after the victim has been victimized, the crime has been reported to the police, police have completed a preliminary investigation, and some IPV professionals have completed their work. A case of IPV may follow this typical pattern. An incident of violence occurs in the home. A neighbor, alerted by the commotion, calls the police, who respond. Upon arrival, they observe injuries on the victim and other damage consistent with an assault. They attempt to interview the victim and witnesses. If the officers find probable cause to believe a crime has been committed, they arrest the suspect and EMTs bring the victim to an emergency department for medical care, possibly within the local hospital's domestic violence program. The victim and her children may receive social work, medical, and some financial services. In the meantime, the suspect has been processed through the system and is being presented to the court for, among other legal questions, resolution of the suspect's release status. Just prior to this hearing, a prosecutor is presented a file with police investigative paperwork, which should (but often does not) include detailed interviews with the victim, witnesses (including any children in the home), medical personnel, and others who have interacted with the victim since the time of the arrest. Often this paperwork is not complete because the police investigation is in its infancy.

IMMEDIATE CONCERNS

The most immediate concern at this juncture for the prosecutor is the appropriate pretrial status for the suspect and the charges. Information received by IPV professionals, often only from the victim, is critical for this analysis. The prosecutor must assess this preliminary information to determine the level of threat the suspect poses to the victim and society as a whole. The prosecutor must ascertain whether the suspect should be released pending trial, should have bail imposed, or should have certain conditions attached to release. To assess these issues correctly, the prosecutor must have accurate and exhaustive information regarding the injuries to the victim, weapons used, threats made, the level of fear, the danger the defendant poses to the victim or other victims and witnesses, and the history between the parties. While final charges can change between arrest and trial, that in no way means that this initial assessment is not important. These initial charges remain important as they directly impact the defendant's release status. The more serious the charges, the less chance the defendant will be released with less stringent release conditions.

It is not hard to imagine the critical importance of accurate and complete information, including a way to contact the IPV professional for clarification. In the typical case example discussed above, assume that (1) this is the fifth visit to the emergency department by the victim as a result of personal violence; (2) the assault took place in the presence of children; (3) the victim is treated for old and new injuries in the hospital, as well as an evaluation for posttraumatic stress disorder and depression; and (4) while at the hospital, the staff observed the defendant calling the victim multiple times and her fearful reaction to these calls. In this scenario, if a prosecutor receives inaccurate information, such as a description of injuries as "minor," no mention of the victim's fear, and no information regarding the violent history, there are no grounds to argue against the suspect's release. The prosecutor will also not have grounds to charge his crimes as part of a continuum of conduct against the victim, which, in this scenario, could also include charges regarding endangering the welfare of the children as well. Depending on the jurisdiction, these can include exposure to IPV and psychological abuse, among others. Thus, in our scenario, it would be very possible that the defendant would be returned to the home before the victim has completed medical treatment and charged only with simple assault rather than charges allowing for his course of conduct, threats, and endangering the children.

The prosecutor also wrestles with the strength of the case and the conflicting interests of the victims. Sometimes, for example, the victim, or the entire family, is dependent upon the offender financially. The adverse consequences of incarceration, or even a conviction, can be obvious if it leads to the defendant's dismissal from employment, an inability to pay the rent or mortgage, or even cover food, utilities, and other living expenses. Is a jail sentence for a misdemeanor assault charge with "minor injuries" in the best interest of the victim? Doesn't the victim have more pressing concerns than a "successful" outcome of the criminal prosecution? How will the outcome of a prosecution affect the children in the family? In a more serious case (eg, a stabbing), the threat of increased violence and a more pronounced need to hold the defendant accountable and to protect the community will start to overwhelm these particular concerns for the prosecutor. However, the rent and the next meal may remain paramount concerns for the victim and her children, and thus affect her willingness to cooperate. The prosecutor must be aware of these concerns and balance these real pressures against the scope of the harm.

Thus, one concern of the prosecutor as the long-term movement of the case is evaluated is how to define a "successful prosecution" within the context of the case presented. While the short-term answer is whatever result will most ensure the safety of the victim, the actual answer is more complex.

LONG-TERM CONCERNS

As suggested by the aforementioned Justice Department statistics,[2,3,5,6] a large number of incidents involving some form of family violence will pass through the courts beyond that first appearance. How, then, should these cases be treated in the long term? When looking at recent trends in governmental response to IPV, two trends emerge. First, most prosecutors operate in an age of so-called "zero tolerance" policies precluding dismissing IPV cases. Second, with the advent of the multidisciplinary team (MDT) approach to IPV, there is an increased appreciation for the possible disastrous outcomes flowing from inaction. Therefore, more of these cases are being placed in front of judges and, possibly, juries at trials.

The reality is that once the incident leading to an arrest has been resolved in one fashion or another, many, if not most, of these families' lives will not be wholly disentangled. Because of this, law enforcement, in assessing how to resolve these matters, will be forced to take a realistic appraisal of the individual family situation because a "one size fits all" approach will be counterproductive. Many considerations must be evaluated as part of the case evaluation, including the parties involved, threat of the defendant, and appropriate charges.

Some of these cases can be resolved short of a criminal trial, or even a criminal conviction. Family violence can occur because of many reasons. Sometimes family violence can occur in circumstances where the family is experiencing acute stress (eg, loss of a job or income, excessive intake of intoxicants), although some professionals disagree.[8-10, 12, 13] In those instances, with victim safety remaining paramount, the source of the stress needs to be identified, and any outcome should attempt to address the underlying issue or issues. For example, conditions of sentencing, whether probationary or a period of incarceration, could include anger management therapy, drug or alcohol counseling, or marriage counseling. Where the victim refuses to cooperate with a criminal prosecution, the prosecutor may be able to insist upon a defendant's participation in such counseling prior to allowing the case to be discharged or withdrawn using the threat of continued prosecution as leverage. Such an alternative may or may not be desirable and its availability is jurisdiction specific.

Understanding the Parties Involved

A prosecutor can only begin to make an appropriate assessment of the danger risk of the suspect when in possession of complete information from investigators. This must include the specific information referenced above, as well as contact information for professionals who have worked with, or will work with, the victims.

Prosecutors must approach the case resolution within the context of the life of the victim and the world in which she lives. The type of information needed for the prosecutor to begin assessing that includes the social service needs of the victim, the level of protection needed for her, the pressures on her in other areas of her life, and the likelihood that the victim will be tampered with by the defendant or by others on his behalf. Therefore, it is critical for professionals to record information in as complete a manner as possible. Whether sharing this information with the police, including it within a business record (which will later be disclosed to the prosecution via a subpoena), or providing information to a state agency as a mandated reporter, the professional must be both detailed and thorough. Professionals must remember that every document has the potential to be blown up as an exhibit and displayed to the jury in 10 times its original size. Recalling this reality will often aid professionals to be as accurate and detailed as possible in their paperwork. Such information serves two important benefits. First, it enables the prosecutor to assess the complexities of the relationship between the parties and the level of danger the suspect presents to the victim, her children, and society. Second, by affording the prosecutor the ability to immediately contact the professional, it enables them to discuss the information when it is fresh and not several months later when memories have faded.

The IPV professional's information is essential in the criminal justice process. Within this long-term assessment, the prosecutor must understand the appropriate parties and the dynamics of the abusive relationship. IPV professionals are often witnesses to relationships where apparent dangers are present. The prosecutor must also determine the victim's perspective to understand her concerns that influence how to move forward with the case.

The prosecutor must also learn of each victim's special vulnerabilities. This inquiry often involves special scrutiny even where the victims are "on board" with the prosecution of the case. As a defense strategy, the victim's motives for reporting are often questioned and attacked. For example, where there is an ongoing divorce or child custody proceeding, the defense will often allege that the pending criminal charges are fabricated in an attempt to secure leverage for a more favorable position regarding child custody. Or, where the victim has recanted since the arrest, often the motivations for doing so are relatively obvious. A prosecutor cannot properly assess the case without cooperation from other IPV professionals, including a comprehensive assessment of the situation in which the victim finds herself.

Danger Presented by the Suspect

For a prosecutor who is used to making such evaluations, this issue often seems more in line with training and experience. An offender who presents a lengthy criminal history, particularly one involving multiple episodes of violence, should be an obvious red flag to the prosecutor. However, an individual who presents no prior convictions may be just as dangerous as he may have intimidated previous victims from testifying or simply because he has never been caught. It is imperative then for the prosecutor to collect and evaluate all of the information available; learning all there is to know about the family involved. Just like a physician, it is incumbent upon the prosecutor to obtain a detailed "history" from the family to properly evaluate the nature of the violence and how to best intervene within the family.

According to Justice Department statistics, nearly 60% of incidents of family violence were reported to police between 1998 and 2002. The Bureau of Justice Statistics reported, "Approximately a third of the 1.4 million family violence victims who did not report the incident to police stated the reason for not reporting was that it was a 'private/personal matter.' A quarter said they did not inform police for some 'other reason.' Another 12% of nonreporting family violence victims said they did not report the crime in order to 'protect the offender.'" [2] Therefore, an absence of a criminal record for either arrests or convictions for family violence does not necessarily convey an accurate picture of what is taking place within the home. A prosecutorial decision based solely upon the absence of such a record may have disastrous consequences, and IPV professionals must ensure that comprehensive information regarding the full history of abuse (or at least the first, last, and worst incidents) makes it to the fact finder.

Appropriate Charges

The decision of the appropriate charges to file is the prosecutor's alone. However, it results from all the information gathered by law enforcement and professionals who speak directly with the victims and witnesses. The importance of this evaluation cannot be underestimated, as it directly affects the safety of the victims, the release conditions of the offenders, and ultimately the verdicts and sentences. If this information provided to the prosecutor is not complete as to the number of incidents, victims, and severity of abuse, the victim will not meet a just result through no fault of her own. The prosecutor makes the initial decision very early in the process, often before being able to speak with the victim. The final decision can come several weeks after the case is initially presented. The victim may be unavailable to the prosecutor because of death, severity of injury, or loss of cooperation. Or, the victim may have had such a history of abuse that dates and details of incidents, each of which can result in different charges, are impossible to determine. Yet, the prosecutor remains duty bound to proceed forward with the most accurate and appropriate charges possible.

Because IPV professionals' information is critical to these cases, the challenge is to determine what is most relevant and useful to a criminal prosecution. To do so, a professional should have a basic understanding of what constitutes criminal activity or has other legal significance, such as a sentencing enhancement. Criminal law is a dynamic and evolving social tool. Thanks to both technology and increased social awareness, many actions today are illegal that were not recognized as crimes a generation ago. In addition to commonly understood crimes such as assault and firearms offenses, what follows are some areas of criminal activity often missed.

Many jurisdictions include a criminal charge of "domestic violence" that can include assaults against household members (eg, Idaho's Domestic Violence statute, among other aspects, includes numerous charges for abusing "a household member"[14]). Often, such statutory schemes include sentence enhancements if the perpetrator abused his victim in the presence of children (eg, the Idaho statute also doubles criminal penalties if a defendant commits an assault or battery in the presence of child[14]). Additionally, someone responsible for the care and welfare of a child who fails to protect that child from any form of abuse, or exposes him or her to witnessing abuse, may also be exposed to liability for this failure to act by statutes commonly referred to as child endangerment statutes (eg, such as that for Pennsylvania).[15]

When a sexual offense has occurred, there are many potential criminal charges as well. Those outside the lead charge often result from the relationship between the parties. For example, there may be a component to the offense suggesting prostitution occurred (see 18 USC §§ 1591, 2421-2423[16]). If the victim is a minor engaged in sexual conduct and an IPV professional learns that prior to this, a possible defendant sold the child, knowing that she would be involved in this, they may be exposed to severe criminal liability for trafficking and other federal offenses (See 18 U.S.C. § 2251[a]).[17] Without this information, often learned by the IPV professional and not necessarily the police, the prosecutor could charge inappropriately and release a defendant, enabling him to further threaten the victim.

With the advent of the Internet, a professional should routinely explore the possibility of sexual exploitation whenever he or she is working with a victim of a sexual crime. This inquiry includes an assessment of the presence of cameras, computers, telephones, and cell phones and whether any of these were used to arrange, facilitate, or exacerbate the criminal activity. This is true even if the offender's attempted sexual exploitation failed. Such action may allow the case to be charged federally, which often includes more severe penalties than on the state level. Or, the case could go to another jurisdiction with more appropriate penalties.

TRIAL CONSIDERATIONS

Intimate partner violence professionals are not only essential to a successful investigation and pretrial handling of domestic violence cases, but critical in the trial phase as well. The Rules of Evidence, although strict, provide many opportunities for information from such professionals to be presented to the jury. What follows is a discussion of some of the more common trial issues that demand the cooperation of the IPV professionals to reach a just verdict.

CORROBORATION

Often, the prosecution makes the difference between successfully isolating the offender from the victim and her continuing to live in fear. This can occur through a guilty plea or a trial. If the victim testifies, her credibility is likely the most important component of the case. To begin with, the scales are weighted against the victim. The prosecutor must not only convince the fact finder of what occurred, but they must also do so beyond a reasonable doubt. Because a jury possesses the great challenge of assessing credibility of the victim whom they do not know, they often turn to evidence from objective and neutral third parties to corroborate or inform them of the believability of the victim's accusations. This evidence is often supplied by IPV professionals, and its importance cannot be underestimated.

The value of corroboration is fourfold. First, it enhances the credibility of the victim, should she testify. Often victims enter into the trial with some issues of their own, such as failing to report, failing to leave an abusive situation, or coping with self-medication, many of which could compromise their credibility. Therefore, any information, no matter how minor, that can corroborate the victim's recollection of events is significant. Second, it changes the dynamic of the criminal trial from a "he said, she said" proceeding to one in which the victim's version of events is solidly supported by corroborating evidence. Third, it communicates to both the victim and the offender that the victim is not alone and an offense against her is one against the community—one for which it will not stand. Finally, if the victim is not present, either because it is a homicide case, or because she has been threatened, or has decided to reconcile with the offender, the case may still be able to continue. Without this evidence the prosecution may cease, and the victim may find herself in more danger, having now reported, than she was before state intervention.[18, 19, 20] "Despite proponents' arguments that mandatory prosecution makes victims safer by taking the decision out of the victim's hands, the batterer will often still hold the victim responsible for any consequences he receives." [21,22]

Because victims can often be unpredictable in terms of their ability or willingness to testify about what happened to them, it is especially critical that the prosecution obtains and uses whatever available corroboration there is to make the case. Evidence of medical treatment or injury is clearly relevant and important, as is photographic evidence (eg, photographs of the injuries or the crime scene taken by police). As with any criminal case, evidence collected at the scene (eg, bullet casings, bloody knife or clothing, broken furniture) can be particularly important to support the prosecution's theory of what took place. Additional eyewitness accounts can tip the balance in favor of the prosecution, even where the victim is now recanting or refusing to cooperate with the prosecution. Many of these items may appear in hospital records or, in the case of some physical evidence, be obtained at the hospital where the victim is being treated. Prosecutors will rely greatly upon the information collected during the course of medical treatment.

Although controversy surrounds the topic, recantation remains a special challenge in IPV cases.[23-27] One example of why this is true comes from the child abuse field: while studies have shown that as many as 72% of children initially deny sexual abuse but 96% ultimately make active disclosures,[28] others disagree.[23,28] The numbers on the extent of recantation are elusive.[23-27] The Justice Department found that victims decline to report crimes for many reasons, not the least of which is a belief that such matters are personal. Fear of the offender and a misguided desire to protect the offender and the family are also reasons why victims decline to report crimes.[3] These pressures remain even after a case is initially reported. This is true for many reasons including, but not limited to, economic constraints, conflicting loyalties, the passage of time, fear and intimidation, and pressure from others. While the research suggests that recantation can be an understandable survival mechanism, it can be devastating to a trial. Despite this fact, courts can view recantation with suspicion unless presented with expert testimony to explain its typicality ("recantation testimony is generally considered exceedingly unreliable").[29,30] In fact, some courts have concluded that "there is no less reliable form of proof, especially when it involves an admission of perjury."[31-34]

Given this rather hostile, although unrealistic, judicial reception to recanted testimony, the presence of corroborative testimony from objective professionals with no loyalty to any party in the case is very powerful. Consider the following example. Julie, a 7th-grade adolescent, runs away from home, making allegations of long-term physical abuse by her father. At the time of her disclosure, the abuse has had several negative effects, including poor performance in school, some adolescent rebellion, limited friendships, and prior denials of abuse. Were this trial to be limited to Julie's testimony against that of her father and other household members loyal to and financially dependent on him, the chances of a just result are significantly diminished. However, add to the government's case the following evidence (all of which would be provided by IPV professionals):

— Years of prior records by school nurses over several schools, all indicating suspicious old injuries following long absences from school,

— Prior reports to the Department of Social Services expressing concern, and

— School officials' documentation of an uncooperative father verbally threatening school officials after their inquiry.

When a prosecutor presents this evidence inconsistence with the time line offered by Julie, the case changes significantly. Such records and testimony transform that case into one in which the victim's previous denials and inconsistencies are now seen in the true light of behavior consistent with a violent household, rather than consistent with untruths. In short, these IPV professionals (nurses, teachers, social workers) performing their duties every day with excellence allow this child to experience a safe home for the first time in 14 years.

HISTORY OF VIOLENCE

In assessing guilt or innocence, the prosecutor, and, ultimately, the jury, must understand the history of the relationship now embroiled in violence. Often this history involves what are referred to as "prior bad acts" or "other crimes" by the defendant.[35] Such information helps to make sense out of facts that, without this information, may seem inconsistent with truth. It has become the prosecutor's duty to collect as much history as possible—like a physician obtaining a medical history—to present a complete picture to the jury. Information accumulated by medical personnel, social workers, and other professionals in the course of treatment often provides this history that may, therefore, become integral in accurately presenting the case to the jury.

As a general matter, the prosecution may not use evidence from other crimes merely to show that the defendant is a bad person or to malign his character. Such evidence is admissible if relevant for any purpose other than to show mere propensity to commit a crime.[35] Classic rationales for the admission of other crimes or bad acts evidence include using this evidence to prove identity, motive, intent, malice, absence of mistake or accident, and a common scheme or plan.[35-37] In addition to these explicit uses of such evidence, courts may create new exceptions in appropriate cases.[38,39] These will be discussed in turn.

With few exceptions, prosecutors must prove that the defendant acted with the requisite intent in order to obtain a conviction. Because defendants rarely announce their innermost thoughts, any evidence regarding what the defendant intended to do is critical. In cases of domestic violence, evidence of prior hostility between a defendant husband and victim wife has been held admissible to show the defendant's intent to kill the victim.[40,41] For example, in the murder prosecution of *Commonwealth v Rivera*,[41] evidence of prior incidents of domestic violence between the defendant and his wife that led to police intervention was admissible to show that the defendant intended to shoot his wife. Motive is admissible even when it is not an element of a crime to be proven by the prosecution, and malice is logically analogous to motive. Accordingly, evidence of prior incidents of violence between a victim and defendant are admissible to prove motive or malice (eg, *United States v Garcia-Meza*,[42] [evidence that the defendant assaulted his wife 5 months prior to her murder admissible to show the defendant's motive to murder]; *United States v Colvin*[43]; *Commonwealth v Ulatoski*[44] [evidence that defendant had previously seriously abused the son of his girlfriend was admissible as proof of malice towards the decedent child]).

Frequently in a domestic violence context, the relationship between the parties begins with threats and low-level violence but escalates into something far worse. The evidence of a defendant's prior and subsequent bad acts and assaultive behavior may be necessary and relevant to show the defendant's state of mind.[45,46] In the words of the United States Supreme Court, "Extrinsic acts evidence may be critical to the establishment of the truth as to a disputed issue, especially when the issue involves the actor's state of mind and the only means of ascertaining that mental state is by drawing inferences from conduct."[36] Thus, prosecutors will often seek admission of such evidence on the grounds specified in Rule 404(b).[35]

Additionally, other crimes or prior bad acts evidence may prove that the defendant's actions were not a mistake or accident (eg, a slip and fall, "walking into a door," self-defense) (eg, *United States v Lewis*[47] and *State v Shanahan*[48]). The 10th Circuit has held that, "when the crime is one of infanticide or child abuse, evidence of repeated incidents is especially relevant because it may be the only evidence to prove the crime."[49] For example, in *United States v Boise*,[50] the defendant was tried for the murder of his infant son. The court admitted evidence of the child's previous broken arm and 15 broken ribs to demonstrate the defendant's malice and the lack of an accidental source of the injuries to the 6-week-old child. In such a case where the victim could not state what caused his mortal injuries, this type of evidence can eliminate a claim of accident by the only other person who knows the source of the injuries, the offender.

As a general principle, evidence showing a lack of mistake or accident may be the same evidence that proves motive or intent, and thus the evidence may be admissible on either ground.[51] For example, in *United States v Harris*,[49] a defendant's prior violence against his victim was found to prove lack of mistake or accident on the part of the defendant (see also *State v Lockhart*[52]). Also, in a child abuse homicide trial, *Commonwealth v Donahue*,[53] evidence of uncharged prior abuse similar to fatal incident was admissible to show the child's death was not accidental.

Prosecutors will often argue that a defendant's prior crimes against his partner and family are admissible because the evidence is part of a chain or a sequence of acts, which is part of the history of the abuse suffered by victims. Such evidence will explain the defendant's motivations and actions as well as the reactions and behavior of the victims. A continuing escalation in the abusive behavior and violence may explain a victim's inability to extricate herself from the relationship and her state of mind during the relationship as well as the police investigation. The defendant's course of conduct is part of that natural development of the facts, and courts have concluded that such behavior is therefore admissible (eg, *U.S. v Boise*[54]; *Commonwealth v Nolen*[55]; *Commonwealth v Mayhue*[56]; *State v Yoh*[57] [in which evidence of a defendant's prior conviction for theft of wife's property is found admissible in his trial for murdering his wife "to portray the history surrounding the abusive relationship," as it "provided the needed context for the behavior in issue"]). In other words, this evidence is also admissible at times to establish "the natural history and development of the facts" (eg, *United States v Fazal-Ur-Raheman-Fazal*[58]; *State v McPherson*[59]; *Commonwealth .v Nolen*[55]; *Commonwealth v Mayhue*[56]). For example, in *McPherson*, the defendant was charged with child abuse and the court admitted evidence of sexual devices and videos the defendant placed in plain view of his daughters as relevant to the "factual setting" of the crime of child abuse.[59] Similarly, the Supreme Judicial Court in Massachusetts recently affirmed the admittance of testimony concerning "the defendant's controlling nature, the hostile relationship between the defendant and the victim, and his prior abuse of the victim… to show a pattern or course of conduct by the defendant [and] to describe the entire relationship between the defendant and the victim."[60]

Therefore, when an IPV professional encounters information regarding a history of violence, he or she should not dismiss it, but carefully record it. A professional should not only record and advise other MDT members of prior crimes, but also of crimes following the arrest as well. Evidence of both prior and subsequent bad acts is admissible. The substantive analysis is the same.[61-63] Even if the information involved old events, it should be reported (see also *Commonwealth v Odom*[64]) (in murder prosecution, defendant's attempted homicide of and alleged assaults against his decedent aunt admissible to show intent, as well as malice and absence of mistake, even though time frame of incidents exceeded 10 years). Similarly, if the prior incident seems minor, or only indirectly involves the suspect, the professional should record it and report it to the prosecutor. For example, in *State v Allen*,[65] the defendant-mother was charged with killing her infant son after calling 911 and reporting that he had broken his neck. The defendant initially claimed that his injuries were the result of a fall in the bathtub and repeated falls in his carpeted room. The child later died of a massive and recently inflicted head injury, which could have occurred only when the victim was in the sole custody of the defendant. The court admitted evidence that the defendant's husband earlier spanked the victim in the defendant's presence so severely as to cause him bruises. The court found this evidence as relevant to discount the defendant's claims the prior injuries were the result of an accident, to demonstrate that she was complicit in physically disciplining the child, and to illustrate the dynamics of the relationship between the defendant and her child.

Regardless of the government's theory of admissibility, a history of violence between the parties can be relevant at trial. Therefore, it is incumbent upon the IPV professional to record this information and communicate it within the official statement. This can often be the only way a prosecutor becomes aware of this critical evidence.

More Probative Than Prejudicial… What Does That Mean?

The public often hears mainstream media discuss evidentiary issues in terms of probative value versus prejudicial impact without a clear definition of these terms. As a threshold matter, the evidence must be "relevant evidence" in order for it to be admitted at trial. **Relevant evidence** is evidence "having any tendency to make the existence of a fact that is of consequence… more or less probable…"[66] Because our criminal justice system also is greatly concerned with protecting defendants' rights to a fair trial, the analysis does not end at that point. There are situations when relevant evidence, although probative of a fact in the trial, is also prejudicial to the defendant. For example, a defendant's prior record of IPV regarding a different victim might fall within this category.

When such a situation arises, the judge must determine whether the "probative value of the violence is substantially outweighed by the danger of unfair prejudice, confusion of issues, or misleading to the jury, or by consideration of undue delay, waste of time, or needless presentation of unnecessary evidence."[67] Therefore, in the example of prior abuse of a different victim, the prosecution would likely argue that this evidence is relevant to prove a course of conduct, *modus operandi*, absence of mistake or accident, and the defendant's state of mind. Defense counsel would assert that, because it is a different victim, the probative value of the evidence is limited and substantially outweighed by the prejudice to the defendant. The judge would then decide whether to admit or exclude the evidence because "its probative value is substantially outweighed" by its prejudicial impact on the defendant.[67]

Obstruction of Justice or Witness Tampering

Because the parties are known to each other in an IPV criminal case, it is not uncommon for the perpetrator of IPV to contact the victim or witnesses in an effort to prevent them from testifying. This is often done in violation of a court order stating that the defendant shall have no contact with the victim directly or indirectly while the case is pending. All too often, law enforcement and the prosecutor do not learn of these events because of witnesses' fear, lack of awareness of the significance of the information, or belief that nothing can be done. However, such information can enable the prosecutor to move quickly to protect the victim and obtain several other positive results. The defendant may be held in contempt for violating the court order and his conditions of release modified or even revoked. Second, the defendant can be charged with additional charges such as obstruction of justice, witness tampering, retaliation, or stalking. Third, other parties used to exert this influence can also be charged for their actions, thus removing them from a position that allows them to affect the proceeding. Fourth, when the defendant engages in wrongdoing intended to prevent the victim from testifying, and the victim does not testify as a result, the defendant has indeed forfeited his right to confront the witness.[68,69]

There are also some intangible benefits to a speedy response from the prosecution. It communicates to the victim, defendant, and third parties that the government takes the protection of victims seriously. It allows the victim to see that the government may be able to concretely increase her safety. Therefore, when a professional working with a victim of IPV hears of incidents in which the defendant has directly or indirectly attempted to contact the victim, she should immediately inform or assist the victim in informing law enforcement and insist upon expedited action from the prosecutor. This is true even if the contact seems innocuous. Such an effort can become the difference between permanent safety for the victim or continued stress and fear.

HEARSAY EXCEPTIONS

Hearsay is an out-of-court statement offered at trial for the truth of the matter asserted in the statement.[71] The person testifying about the statement is referred to as ***the witness***. The person who made the statement out of court is referred to as ***the declarant***.[72] The statement can be oral, written, or a non-verbal assertion.[73] In other words, when a witness offers testimony about something a declarant has previously said outside the courtroom, that evidence is hearsay.

A victim's statements about her injuries to a medical professional constitute hearsay. However, there are numerous exceptions to this rule that may allow the witness to testify to the out-of-court statements. This is important to the IPV professional because some statements made to him or her by the victim, defendant, or other witnesses may be necessary to admit into evidence. In fact, when a victim is unavailable at trial this evidence may be the only method available to pursuing a case to the just result.

The exceptions explicitly included in the Federal Rules of Evidence that may allow an IPV professional to testify to hearsay statements include, but are not limited to: statements by a party opponent[74] (the defendant's statements), co-conspirator statements,[75] excited utterances,[76] present sense impressions,[77] statements regarding mental, emotional, or physical condition (also known as the state of mind exception),[78] statements for purposes of medical diagnosis and treatment,[79] statements under belief of death (dying declarations),[80] statements against interest,[81] and testimony by experts.[82] Each of these exceptions is based on a specific theory of reliability. For example, dying declarations are allowed into evidence because of the belief that when a person is dying, he or she is likely to speak the truth. Statements for medical diagnosis are allowed into evidence on the theory that people are truthful with their physicians.

Each of these exceptions has certain specific requirements that must be met in order for the evidence to be admitted into evidence. In court this is referred to as "laying the foundation" for the statement. For example, an excited utterance requires the prosecutor to lay the foundation by establishing at least 3 elements: (1) that the declarant has personal knowledge of the subject of the statement; (2) that the declarant was under the influence of a startling event at the time of the statement; and (3) that the statement is about the startling event.[76] For example, assume an EMT treats a stabbing victim who tearfully discloses that her father stabbed her and her mother. The EMT may be called to testify regarding the child's statement. Prior to such testimony, the prosecutor would establish that the child was excited by eliciting testimony from the EMT regarding, among other things, the child's demeanor, notably the volume of her voice, the speed with which she was speaking, and the freshness and severity of her injuries. Then the prosecutor would establish when and where the exciting event, the stabbing, took place. Only after laying this foundation, would the prosecutor ask the EMT what the child said. This evidence could then be admitted against the father. In this scenario, the defense will often protest the admission of such a statement, arguing that at the time the statement was made the stress of the event had dissipated (eg, a statement to EMTs who arrive minutes or hours after the assault is over). Defense counsel may also argue that the statement should not qualify because it was in response to questioning and not in response to the "startling event." Thus, all of the facts and circumstances, not just about the assault itself, but about how and when the information was collected regarding the assault, will become relevant.[83] It behooves IPV professionals to record all statements by all parties in their records, in addition to the parties' demeanor. The actions and demeanor of family members in crisis are often a strong insight into roles people play in IPV and in the home. This is information not apparent once law enforcement is involved and people adjust their demeanor. Thus, the only possible source of this information is the IPV professional.

Confrontation Clause Issues

There are many obstacles to presenting hearsay evidence in a criminal case. Prior to 2004, hearsay statements of a victim to an IPV professional were often admissible. However, relatively recent Supreme Court rulings limit this, thus making the information all the more critical if admissible. Our challenge is the defendant's Sixth Amendment right to be confronted by the witness. In a criminal case hearsay that is offered against a defendant under an exception to the hearsay rule may sometimes be excluded because its admission would violate the defendant's right 'to be confronted with the witnesses against him' under the Sixth Amendment to the United States Constitution.[84-86] Thus, when hearsay is offered against the accused in a criminal case, the accused may raise at least two separate objections: first, that the statement violates the hearsay rule and, second, that it violates the Confrontation Clause.

Every defendant has a Sixth Amendment right to "be confronted by the witnesses against him." The precise meaning of this confrontation clause has been a matter of some debate over the history of our nation. This debate has become even more vigorous after the Supreme Court decision of *Crawford v Washington*,[84] which had repercussions well beyond the courtroom to all IPV professionals.

It is not difficult to see how hearsay evidence might violate the right of confrontation. The argument is that a defendant cannot be meaningfully confronted by a witness, in this case the declarant, if she does not take the stand. In the late 20th Century, such statements were often admissible if they fell within one of the "firmly rooted hearsay exceptions," or if under the specific facts of the statement possessed "particularized guarantees of trustworthiness," even if they did not fall within a specifically recognized hearsay exception.[84, 88]

After this line of cases, two trends emerged. First, prosecutors were able to proceed with IPV cases even when the victims were unable to testify for myriad reasons. This was a tremendous victory for the most vulnerable victims whose cases could continue even if they were unable to face a trial. Second, IPV professionals who work with these victims were testifying regarding such statements made to them. Thanks to the work of these dedicated professionals, cases of victims of family violence, child abuse, elder abuse, and domestic violence were moving forward.

However, all that progress was called into question when the Supreme Court ruled in *Crawford v Washington* that "testimonial statements of witnesses absent from trial [may be] admitted only where the declarant is unavailable and, only where the defendant has had a prior opportunity to cross examine."[84] The effects of this holding are both tremendous and unclear, in that *Roberts* was effectively overruled as *Crawford* requires any "testimonial" hearsay statements of an unavailable witness to have previously been the subject of cross examination before being admitted into evidence at trial. The decision is unclear in the sense that the Supreme Court has not defined what constitutes "testimonial hearsay."[84] "We leave for another day any effort to spell out a comprehensive definition of 'testimonial.'"[84,85] Therefore, the scope of this rule remains in question. The Supreme Court has offered some guidance, stating that "testimonial hearsay" includes statements made to government agents under circumstances in which the declarant reasonably expected his statements could later be used in court.[84] The Supreme Court subsequently elaborated on this language by ruling that certain 911 calls and interrogations with responding police were not testimonial if the primary purpose of the interrogation were to enable the police to assist and meet an ongoing emergency.[85] Where, however, the primary purpose of the interrogation was to investigate a past crime and prove past events relevant to a later criminal prosecution, the hearsay was testimonial.[85] The Supreme Court limited this holding to police interrogations and not necessarily interrogations by other government agents.[85] In the aftermath of *Crawford*, many professionals assumed that they could no longer testify to hearsay statements, but this has proven to be far too broad a conclusion. First, *Crawford* only applies to criminal prosecutions, as the right of confrontation is one tied to criminal trials. Therefore, such evidence may be admissible in myriad other legal proceedings, including many sentencing, probation revocation, motions to suppress, and some civil child protection hearings. Second, *Crawford* only applies when the declarant is not testifying at the trial. So, if the declarant/victim is testifying, *Crawford* does not preclude hearsay evidence offered by an IPV professional. If the scenario is a criminal trial with an unavailable witness, the parties will litigate extensively whether *Crawford* bans this testimony. The prosecutor will attempt to establish that the statement is neither one that was taken by a government agent nor one that the declarant reasonably expected to be used at trial. It should again be noted that if the defendant engaged in wrongdoing intended to procure the unavailability of the witness and the witness is not available to testify, as a result he has forfeited his Sixth Amendment confrontation right.[84, 69]

This has implications for the IPV professional both in and out of the courtroom. Because the implication of *Crawford* on all other nonlegal professional practices is a topic well beyond the scope of this chapter, what follows is only a "broad brush" guidance of issues regarding IPV professionals' role within their respective protocols and as witnesses. Prior to *Crawford*, such professional witnesses would simply have to appear in court and testify to excited utterances or other hearsay statements. This is no longer the case. While the specific facts of each case will affect the analysis, one reality is clear. Now, such a witness must testify as to why the discussion took place. The IPV professional must establish that he or she is not a government agent and that "circumstances surrounding the contested statements did not lead the declarant to reasonably believe that her disclosure would be available for use at a later trial."[89] By implication, this means that IPV professionals should consider taking action both inside and outside the courtroom to avoid conflict with their mission when subpoenaed to testify. Outside the courtroom, IPV professionals should have in their program a clear set of protocols and guidelines. This protocol is one that should not change depending upon whether they are working on a case with possible criminal court implications. Each action within the protocol should be for a purpose linked to their mission and goals. As such, they will be above reproach when their work provides them information that may later be utilized in court, as they will be free from the accusation that they were gathering evidence on behalf of the state, rather than fulfilling their obligations. Inside the courtroom witnesses should, therefore, be prepared to testify as to the purpose of all their actions, demonstrating that they are not government agents, but rather professionals fulfilling their professional obligations to their clients/patients.

For example, in *Ohio v Stahl*,[90] a nurse testified regarding statements made to her by a rape victim. The victim gave a detailed account of the rape, including the identity of the perpetrator, in the presence of a police officer at a hospital-based domestic violence program. The nurse clearly testified that there was a medically necessary reason for learning the details of the assault relating to focusing on the nurse's physical examination, creating a comfortable environment for the victim, collecting an accurate medical history, and planning an appropriate discharge plan. This testimony was enhanced by further testimony as to the purpose of the Domestic Violence program to provide the best care to the victim in a timely fashion (see contra *Medina v State*,[91] in which statements to a forensic nurse by a deceased sexual assault victim violated the Confrontation Clause because, among other reasons, the nurse described her position under oath by stating that "she gathers evidence for prosecution…"). By hearing such comprehensive testimony, the court had a basis to conclude that the nurse was asking professionally appropriate questions by demonstrating, for example, that the identity of the perpetrator was an essential component of her medical assessment.

Some professions are so disconnected from possibly being considered as government agents that *Crawford* is not implicated in their work. However, with an increase in MDT approaches to IPV, some professionals, such as sexual assault nurse examiners, forensic interviewers, and EMTs can run into difficulty trying to define their work as it relates to law enforcement or evidence gathering. Professionals should be aware that when they are performing duties independent of law enforcement, *Crawford* should have a minimal effect on their role in a trial. However, if they are working on behalf of law enforcement, or when their primary focus is to gather evidence, *Crawford* may preclude their testimony.

In the age of MDT approaches to victim interviews and investigations, the line between a government agent and an IPV professional may seem unclear. When a person does something at the direction of law enforcement, she can become a government agent. However, a professional does not necessarily become a government agent because an examination was for a diagnostic purpose and the victim's statements were a by-product of substantive medical activity.[92] Nor is the fact that one is the member of a child abuse team necessarily an indication that one is acting on behalf of the government.[89] These cases notwithstanding, the level of disclosure of protocols and purposes behind them in *Stahl* can be required of all IPV professionals. Therefore, they must develop standards and protocols to explain the purpose of their actions and prepare to testify accordingly (See *People v Vigil*,[92] in which it was found that "the fact that the doctor was a member of a child protection team [did] not, in and of itself, make him a government agent absent a more direct controlling police presence").

Expert Witnesses

The Rules of Evidence do provide an opportunity to present technical evidence designed to assist the jury in understanding a difficult area.[93] The complexities and nuances of IPV and domestic violence is one such area. As the social science field evolves and becomes more sophisticated in understanding the dynamics of victimization, these cases become ripe for the use of expert testimony to explain these phenomena.[27, 29]

While the limits of expert testimony vary greatly by jurisdiction, particularly pertaining to whether a fact witness (such as a treating physician), can also be an expert witness, some general parameters do apply. The evidence must be such that it enables the fact finder to better "understand evidence in determining [a] fact at issue." The witness can give his opinion and rely on hearsay evidence in forming the opinion.[82] An expert can never opine as to the veracity of another witness.

Intimate partner violence professionals should welcome the opportunity to share their expertise and specialized knowledge with the jury. It is often with regard to an issue that the jury will not understand without such evidence. Without this evidence, a juror may draw seemingly logical, although incorrect, conclusions. For example, the failure of a domestic violence victim to leave the offender may seem unbelievable to a juror and, not understanding this behavior, the juror may find it unbelievable and conclude the victim's testimony is unbelievable as well. However, after hearing from a social worker or psychiatrist about the dynamics of victimization in a domestic violence relationship, the juror may decide that the failure to terminate the relationship is a typical behavior of other victims.

SENTENCING

For many of the same reasons that IPV cases are difficult to try, they are difficult to sentence. Where the situation and the family relationship have deteriorated past the point of return, sometimes even minor infractions call out for severe punishments to ensure the safety of the victims.

Most courts operate within a system of sentencing guidelines. While not mandatory, these guidelines often play an important role in assisting a judge to fashion a sentence that is consistent with other similarly situated defendants. When imposing sentence, courts should consider an array of factors, including the age, propensity and character of the defendant; the rehabilitative needs of the defendant; the particular circumstances of the offense; the protection of the public; the gravity of the offense; and the impact on the victim (eg, *United States v Garner*[94]; *State v Valin*[95]; *Commonwealth v Royer*[95]). The weight to be given to the various sentencing factors is often exclusively the province of the sentencing court to determine (eg, *Covington v State*[96]; *State v Basu*[97]; *Commonwealth v Thompson*[98]). The court must apply a standard of reasonableness, considering, but not bound by, the guidelines. The court is bound only by statutory sentencing factors, which have been described as "numerous and vague, giving the judge a great deal of running room."[99] On the other hand, an increase in the types of crimes that demand mandatory minimum sentences can drastically limit a judge's discretion.

Often, the IPV professional can play an important role at the sentencing hearing of an offender. First, after a defendant is found guilty of a crime, the judge (or, in some jurisdictions, the jury) must decide the appropriate sentence that the defendant should serve. The judge usually asks for some form of psychological evaluation of the defendant before the sentencing to allow sentencing of the "whole defendant." This usually takes several weeks, and then the sentencing hearing occurs. Unlike a trial, which seeks to restrict information to just the events on the day of the offense, a sentencing hearing is focused on the defendant as a whole, and as such rules allow much more information. This means that an IPV professional may be called as an expert to educate the court on any number of issues, such as the dynamics of IPV, the significance of the injury to victim, or the "victim impact," (the harm the defendant caused the victim). Without such evidence, the prosecutor has little basis to restrain the defendant permanently, let alone obtain a basis for conditions of release. However, with such testimony the court can be educated on the true injuries and social harm created, even when the guidelines undervalue social harm (See *United States v Salinas*[100], which upheld a sentence significantly longer than recommendation because the defendant's actions "displayed not only a pattern of defying the orders of the court and his probation officer, but engaging in behavior that injured or posed a risk of injury to others,") and *Commonwealth v Leach*[101] and *State v Obojes*,[102] in which stalking was determined to be severe enough to warrant a longer sentence.

CONCLUSION

An entire book could be dedicated to the role of the IPV professional in a criminal prosecution. With the law being so dynamic, that role would alter dynamically with each important case. What is clear is that victims are reaping some benefits from the current MDT approach to protecting vulnerable victims. For that to continue, IPV professionals must become educated on the work of law enforcement and prosecutors in this area, and the massive repercussions their work will have on the criminal trials involving their victims. The criminal justice system asks a great deal from our victims. They deserve the professionals who serve them delivering as much.

REFERENCES

1. Violence Against Women Act, codified at 18 U.S.C. § 2261-2266, amended Pub. L. 109-162 (2006).

2. Durose MR, Harlow CW, Langan PA, Motivans M, Rantala RR, Schmitt EL. *Family Violence Statistics*. Washington, DC: Bureau of Justice Statistics; 2005.

3. Catalano S. Intimate Partner Violence in the United States. Washington, DC: Bureau of Justice Statistics; 2007.

4. Saltzman LE, Fanslow JL, McMahon PM, Shelley GA. *Intimate Partner Violence Surveillance: Uniform Definitions and Recommended Data Elements*. Atlanta, Ga: Centers for Disease Control and Prevention, National Center for Injury Prevention and Control; 2002.

5. Bureau of Justice Statistics Press Release. Anonymous. *Rate of Family Violence Dropped by More Than One-Half from 1993 to 2002*. Available at: http://www.ojp.usdoj.gov/bjs/pub/press/fvspr.htm. Accessed August 31, 2007.

6. Bureau of Justice Statistics. *Compendium of Federal Justice Statistics 2004*. Washington, DC: Bureau of Justice Statistics (2006).

7. *Evaluating Domestic Violence Programs*. Rockville, Md: Agency for Healthcare Research and Quality; 2002. Available at: http://www.ahrq.gov/research/domesticviol/. Accessed August 31, 2007.

8. Rhode DL. Social Research and Social Change: Meeting the Challenge of Gender Inequality and Sexual Abuse. 30 Harv. J.L. & Gender II (2007).

9. Morrison AM. Queering domestic violence to "straighten out" criminal law: what might happen when queer theory and practice meet criminal law's conventional responses to domestic violence. 13 *S. Cal. Rev. L. & Women's Stud.* 13 (2003).

10. Mateer ES. Compelling Jekyll to Ditch Hyde: how the law ought to address batterer duplicity. 48 *How. L. J.* 525 (2004).

11. Ganley AL. Domestic violence: the what, why and who, as relevant to civil court cases. In: Agtuca J, Carter J, Heisler C et al. eds. *Domestic Violence in Civil Court Cases: A National Model For Judicial Education*. San Francisco, CA: Family Violence Prevention Fund; 1992.

12. Hong KE. Parens[patriarchy]: Adoption, Eugenics, and Same-Sex Couples. 40 *Cal. W. L. Rev.* (2003).

13. National Coalition Against Domestic Violence. Why do men batter women? Available at: http://www.ncadv.org/problem/why.htm. Accessed August 31, 2007.

14. I.C. § 18-918.

15. 18 Pa. CSA § 3404.

16. 18 U.S.C. §§ 1591, 2421-2423.

17. 18 U.S.C. § 2251(a).

18. Lyon AD. Be Careful What You Wish For: An Examination of Arrest and Prosecution Patterns of Domestic Violence Cases in Two Cities in Michigan. 7 *Mich. J. Gender & L.* 181 (1999).

19. Burke AS. Rational actors, self-defense, and duress: making sense, not syndromes. 81 *N.C.L. Rev.* 211 (2002).

20. Wanless M. Mandatory arrest: a step toward eradicating domestic violence, but is it enough? 1996 v *U. Ill. L. Rev.* 533 (1996).

21. Mordini NM. Mandatory state interventions for domestic abuse cases: an examination of the effects on victim safety and autonomy. 52 *Drake L Rev.* 295 (2004).

22. McGuire L. Criminal prosecution of domestic violence. Available at: http://www.vaw.umn.edu/documents/bwjp/policev/policevhtml. Accessed Sept. 15, 2003.

23. Sorensen T, Snow B. How children tell: the process of disclosure in child sexual abuse, *Child Welfare*. Year;1:3-15.

24. Lyon T, Quas J. Filial dependency and recantation of child sexual abuse allegations. *J. Am. Acad. Adolsec.* Psychiatry 2007;46(2):162-170.

25. *State v Thomas*, 2003, WL 22429536 (Ohio Ct App 2003).

26. *People v Lafferty*, 9 P.3d 1132 (Colo. Ct. App. 1999).

27. *Odum v State*, 711 N.E.2d 71 (Ind. Ct. App. 1999).

28. Bruck M, Ceci S, Shuman, Daniel W., Disclosure of Child Sexual Abuse: What Does Research Tell Us About the Ways That Children Tell. 11 Psychol Pub Pol'y & L. 194 (2005).

29. *Allen v Woodford*, 395 F.3d 979 (9th Cir 2005).

30. 58 Am. Jur., New Trial § 345; *Archer v State*, 934 So. 2d 1187 (Fla. 2006).

31. *Commonwealth v Loner*, 836 A.2d 125, 135 (Pa. Super. Ct. 2003).

32. *Commonwealth v Wilcox*, 392 A.2d 1294, 1298 (Pa. 1978).

33. *State v Macon*, 911 P.2d 1004 (Wash. 1996).

34. *Blankenship v State*, 447 A.2d 428, 433-35 (Del. 1982).

35. FRE § 404(b).

36. *Huddleston v United States*, 485 U.S. 681 (1998).

37. *Commonwealth v Schwartz*, 615 A.2d 350 (Pa. Super. Ct. 1992).

38. *United States v Johnson*, 634 F.2d 735 (4th Cir. 1980).

39. *Commonwealth v Claypool*, 508 Pa. 198, 495 A.2d 176 (1985).

40. *Bhutto v State*, 114 P3d 1252, 1262-63 (Wyo. 2005).

41. *Commonwealth v Rivera*, 597 A.2d 690 (Pa. Super. Ct. 1991).

42. *United States v Garcia-Meza*, 403 F.3d 364 (6th Cir. 2005).

43. *United States v Colvin*, 614 F.2d 44 (5th Cir. 1980).

44. *Commonwealth v Ulatoski* 371 A.2d 186 (Pa. 1977).

45. *United States v Brand*, 467 F.3d 179 (2d Cir. 2006).

46. *United States v Zackson*, 12 F.3d 1178 (2d Cir. 1993).

47. *United States v Lewis*, 837 F.2d 415 (9th Cir. 1988).

48. *State v Shanahan*, 712 N.W. 2d 121 (Iowa 2006).

49. *United States v Harris*, 661 F.2d 138 (10th Cir. 1981).

50. *United States v Boise*, 916 F.2d 497 (9th Cir. 1990).

51. *Commonwealth v Travaglia*, 467 A.2d 288 (Pa. 1983), *cert. denied*, 467 U.S. 1256 (1984).

52. *State v Lockhart*, 830 A.2d 433 (Me. 2003).

53. *Commonwealth v Donahue*, 549 A.2d 121 (Pa. 1988).

54. *United States v Boise*, 916 F.2d 497 (9th Cir. 1990).

55. *Commonwealth v Nolen*, 634 A.2d 192 (Pa. 1993).

56. *Commonwealth v Mayhue*, 639 A.2d 421 (Pa. 1994);

57. *State v Yoh*, 910 A.2d 853 (Vt. 2006).

58. *United States v Fazal-Ur-Raheman-Fazal*, 355 F.3d (1st Cir. 2004).

59. *State v McPherson*, 668 N.W. 2d 488 (Neb. 2003).

60. *Commonwealth v Thomas*, 859 N.E. 2d 813 (Mass. 2007).

61. *Welch v Sirmons*, 451 F.3d 675 (10th Cir. 2006).

62. *United States v Gibson*, 625 F.2d 887 (9th Cir. 1980).

63. *Commonwealth v Clayton*, 483 A.2d 1345 (Pa. 1984).

64. *Commonwealth v Odom*, 584 A.2d 953 (Pa. Super. Ct. 1990).

65. *State v Allen*, 892 A.2d 447 (Me. 2006).

66. FRE 401.

67. FRE 403.

68. *Reynolds v United States*, 98 U.S. 145 (1879).

69. *Giles v. California*, 128 S. Ct. 2678 (2008).

70. *United State v Montague*, 421 F.3d 1099 (10th Cir. 2005).

71. FRE 801(c).

72. FRE 801(b).

73. FRE 801(a).

74. FRE 801(d)(2)(a).

75. FRE 801(d)(2)(e).

76. FRE 803(2).

77. FRE 803(1).

78. FRE 803(3).

79. FRE 803(4).

80. FRE 804(b)(2).

81. FRE 804(b)(3).

82. FRE 703.

83. *State v Davis*, 638 S.E. 2d 57 (SC 2006).

84. *Crawford v Washington*, 541 U.S. 36 (2004).

85. *Davis v Washington*, 126 S. Ct. (2006).

86. *California v Green*, 399 U.S. 149 (1970).

87. *Commonwealth v DiSilvio*, 335 A.2d 785 (Pa. Super. Ct. 1975).

88. *Ohio v Roberts*, 448 U.S. 56 (1980).

89. *Minnesota v Sachetti*, 690 N.W. 2d 393 (Minn. Ct. App. 2005).

90. *Ohio v Stahl*, 22261WL 602687 (Ohio Ct. App. 2005).

91. *Contra Medina v State*, 143 P.3d 471 (Nev. 2006), *cert. denied*, No. 06-8596 WL 506470 (2007).

92. *People v Vigil*, 127 P.3d 916 (Colo. 2006).

93. *State v Valin*, 724 N.W.2d 440 (Iowa 2006).

94. *United States v Garner*, 454 F.3d 743 (7th Cir. 2006).

95. *Commonwealth v Royer*, 476 A.2d 453 (Pa. Super. Ct. 1984).

96. *Covington v State*, 842 N.E.2d 345 (Ind. 2006).

97. *State v Basu*, 875 A.2d 686 (Me. 2005).

98. *Commonwealth v Thompson*, 547 A.2d 800 (1988).

99. *United States v Atencio*, 476 F.3d 1089 (10th Cir. 2007).

100. *United States v Salinas*, 365 F.3d 582 (7th Cir. 2004).

101. *Commonwealth v Leach*, 729 A.2d 608 (Pa. Super. Ct. 1999).

102. *State v Obojes*, 604 So.2d 474 (Fla. 1992).

Chapter 13

INTIMATE PARTNER VIOLENCE: IDENTIFICATION, TREATMENT, AND ASSOCIATIONS WITH MEN'S HEALTH

Peter F. Cronholm, MD, MSCE
Joseph B. Straton, MD, MSCE
Jeffrey R. Jaeger, MD

Men in the United States die an average of 5.4 years younger than women as a result of being less healthy, engaging in more high-risk and adverse health behaviors, differences in health beliefs and behaviors, and underlying biological differences.[1] The relationships between social determinants of health (eg, having a poor economic status, being part of an underserved minority population, living in relative social isolation) and the male sex have profound and negative effects on the health status of men. In addition, despite generally poorer health, men use health services at significantly lower rates than women.[2]

Violence-related deaths are responsible for a significant proportion of the potential years of life lost among men. In comparison to women, men show increased rates of death from motor vehicle–related injuries, firearm-related injuries, homicide, and suicide. When compared with white men, black men have substantially higher death rates from some violent causes such as homicide and firearm injury; however, white men have suicide rates 3 times higher black men.[3]

Intimate partner and domestic violence are sources of ongoing patterns of violence that result in negative, health-related outcomes. The Family Violence Prevention Fund defines **domestic violence** as a pattern of assaultive and coercive behaviors that may include inflicted physical injury, psychological abuse, sexual assault, progressive social isolation, stalking, deprivation, intimidation, and threats.[4] Domestic violence encompasses elder abuse, child-maltreatment, and intimate partner violence (IPV). **Intimate partner violence** is distinguished from other forms of domestic violence by the abusive behaviors perpetrated by someone who is, was, or wishes to be involved in an intimate or dating relationship with an adult or adolescent. Intimate partners include current and former spouses (eg, common-law spouses, divorced spouses, separated spouses) as well as current and former non-marital partners (eg, dating partners, boyfriends, girlfriends).

Completely differentiating victims from perpetrators in many relationships is difficult. So too is describing the nuances of IPV in a comprehensive manner. This chapter considers a **victim** to be the person who is the target of violence or abuse, and the **perpetrator** to be the person inflicting the violence or abuse (or *causing* the violence or abuse to be inflicted on the victim). In accordance with the Centers for

Disease Control and Prevention's (CDC) Uniform Definitions and recommended data elements regarding IPV surveillance, this chapter regards IPV as including the following 4 categories[5]:

1. Physical violence

2. Sexual violence

3. Threat of physical and sexual violence

4. Psychological or emotional abuse (including coercive tactics) in which there has been direct or threatened prior physical or sexual violence

The violence of IPV-related behaviors is often intended to establish control by the perpetrator over the victim. Although acknowledged as a common problem associated with a variety of health-related outcomes, IPV in the lives of men remains a complicated issue. IPV has not only proven difficult to treat in a standardized fashion, but also remains challenging to study. As a result, experts have not reached a consensus regarding what can and should be done to prevent and treat IPV. This chapter focuses on the health effects of IPV as well as the responses of health care professionals toward male victims and perpetrators of IPV.

MEN AS PERPETRATORS

THE PREVALENCE OF INTIMATE PARTNER VIOLENCE AND RELATED INJURIES

Annually within the United States, approximately 1.5 million women and more than 800 000 men are raped or physically assaulted by an intimate partner.[6] Straus and Gelles conducted one of the first national family violence surveys and estimated that 16% of couples reported episodes of IPV during the year before the study and 40% of these episodes involved actions such as punching, kicking, or weapon use.[7,8] The National Crime Victimization Survey estimates the following[9]:

— 5.8% lifetime prevalence of physical IPV for men compared to 13.3% for women

— 0.2% lifetime prevalence of sexual abuse for men compared to 4.3% for women

— 17.3% lifetime prevalence of psychological abuse for men compared to 12.1% for women

— 3% of IPV incidents result in serious physical injury

REASONS MEN ARE MOST OFTEN SEEN AS THE PERPETRATORS

It is strongly held that IPV is underreported. Men are less likely to disclose victimization because of a variety of social (eg, gender norms) and political factors (eg, a focus on female victimization) that make accurate assessments of the proportion of men as perpetrators or victims complicated. However, the data suggest that most IPV that results in injury involves violence by men against women.[10,11] Such male-to-female violence tends to be chronic and cyclical.[12,13] The National Violence Against Women Survey and the National Crime Victimization Survey found that women are more likely to report being IPV victims than men and twice as likely to report being injured in IPV incidents.[6,9] In fact, women were the victims in 95% of the episodes of IPV that lead to criminal investigation and were victims in 59% of spousal murders.[14,15]

REASONS PERPETRATORS OF INTIMATE PARTNER VIOLENCE PERPETRATE

The development of IPV perpetration behaviors and IPV victimization is likely caused by a complex combination of multiple factors. The literature suggests that one model will never explain an individual's behaviors. Studies have used normative shaping of behaviors, childhood victimization, witnessing IPV-related behaviors during childhood, depression, low self-esteem, psychopathologies (eg, antisocial personality disorder, borderline personalities), desire for power and control, social demographics (eg, age, income, employment status), stress, social isolation, drugs and alcohol, and even biological determinants to describe a person's risk of experiencing IPV. Many risk factors are associated and interdependent, and may be causal (childhood victimization leading to low self esteem). Synergy between risk factors may dominate the moderation of IPV perpetration and victimization.

THEORIES

Though many theories attempt to explain IPV perpetration, no single theory can explain the reasons perpetrators become or remain abusive.[16-20] From a health care perspective, the concepts presented in this section are critical to understanding and intervening in situations of IPV perpetration.

Conceptual Model

Harway and O'Neil propose a conceptual model of male IPV perpetration in terms of the following 4 factors[21]:

— *Macrosocial.* Patriarchal and institutional factors resulting in men's oppression and violence

— *Biological.* Hormonal and neuroendocrine factors shaping men's violent behaviors

— *Gender-role socialization.* Sexist attitudes, emotions, and behaviors learned by men that result in violence

— *Interactions.* Relational, interpersonal, and verbal interactions between partners associated with men's violence.

Cycle of Violence Theory

Studies show that children who grow up in families with IPV present are more likely to become involved in relationships affected by IPV as victims or perpetrators. The literature repeatedly demonstrates the dramatic associations between childhood victimization and increased rates for IPV perpetration and victimization.[22-24] Providers should be aware of the higher likelihood that men identified with a history of either direct or indirect exposures to IPV may experience ongoing IPV victimization or perpetration. Coker and colleagues found that men who reported being physically assaulted as children were 2.5 times more likely to report exposure to IPV as adults.[25] Interventions focusing on the trans generational impact of IPV may serve as an inroad to reach men who are perpetrating IPV, as men who may be unconcerned about the effects their abusive behavior has on either themselves or their partners may be engaged about the future negative effects such behavior will have on their children.

Feminist Theory

Feminist theory provides some important insights into understanding IPV victimization and perpetration. Feminism has provided much of the theoretical and community framework that shapes health care providers' responses to IPV situations. Feminist activism can be credited with raising society's awareness about the prevalence and impact of IPV as well as the development of national- and state-level policies and legal protection for abused women.

Feminist theory identifies societal institutions as maintaining male dominance rather than physical strength or other biological factors. As a result, IPV results from a normative, patriarchal social structure based upon gender-related power differentials that are considered a form of social control used to maintain a subordinate political status for women.[16,20,21,26]

Health care providers must understand the social constructs of behaviors when they identify controlling behaviors that may be rationalized by men in terms of strong gender roles. Addressing normative perspectives plays a key role in treating IPV perpetration. A critical component of perpetrator treatment programs is providing information regarding men's beliefs about power and control over women. Programs that include this content are usually contrasted with "anger management" programs, which primarily focus on behaviors and do not address the underlying causes of that behavior.

Exchange Theory

Gelles uses ***exchange theory*** to explain the normative process of IPV perpetration.[27] The assumptions of the exchange theory describe human behavior as driven toward rewards and away from costs or punishments. Intimate partner violence perpetration typically occurs in a social vacuum with perpetration behaviors resulting in the desired effects of coercion and control of the victim with little social sanction. In short, IPV perpetration occurs simply because it can. Offenders will use violence as long as the costs do not outweigh the rewards.

When applied to IPV, the exchange theory illustrates the need for social sanction and the promotion of strategies that favor the identification and treatment of abusive behaviors. To this end, several therapeutic interventions focus on having perpetrators process and internalize the costs of their behaviors to themselves, as well as to their partners and families.

WAYS THAT INTIMATE PARTNER VIOLENCE VICTIMIZATION AFFECTS MEN'S HEALTH

Intimate partner violence directly and indirectly affects the health of victims. Researchers have not focused on assessing the health impact of IPV on men; rather, most research has focused on the health effects of IPV victimization on women. One can reasonably conclude that health care providers can consider a parallel process is likely to occur in men who are current or former IPV victims.

Intimate partner violence victimization interacts with health in a complex fashion that affects the physical, mental, emotional, social, and financial dimensions of a person's health. Physical injuries resulting from IPV victimization include a variety of components and morbidities (eg, contusions, lacerations, broken bones, death). Health care providers should remain aware that physical injuries within the context of IPV may occur as a result of a man's direct victimization or from incidents in which the abuser's victims injure the man while defending themselves from an assault.

Exposure to violence and abusive behaviors can often result in psychological injury, which may have a greater impact than physical injuries. Victims of IPV suffer from posttraumatic stress disorder (PTSD) and are more likely than non-abused people to be depressed, attempt suicide, abuse alcohol or drugs, and transfer their aggression to their children.[28]

In a population-based study, Coker and colleagues stated that physically abused men were more likely to report poor health, depressive symptoms, or substance-use problems as well as more likely to develop a chronic disease, a chronic mental illness, or injury.[25] The men in Coker's study who reported exposure to psychological abuse were 1.8 to 2.6 times more likely to report their current health status as poor. Men who reported moderate physical or sexual IPV were twice as likely to develop a chronic disease. Men who reported high levels of physical, sexual, or psychological IPV were twice as likely to exhibit symptoms of depression.

When formulating a holistic perspective, comprehensive models that describe the effects of IPV on men's health should include the effects of this violence on the man's family members. The man's intimate partner and children are the most proximal members of his family affected by IPV. In 30% to 60% of families affected by IPV, children are also directly abused.[8,29] Children exposed to IPV have higher rates of physical and mental health problems, including depression and anxiety. These children also demonstrate higher levels of distress than children who are not exposed to IPV.[30-38] In addition, children who witness IPV are more likely to abuse drugs and alcohol, experience peer-related violence, engage in risky sexual behaviors, and experience IPV in their adult relationships.[39-43]

WAYS THE PERPETRATION OF INTIMATE PARTNER VIOLENCE AFFECTS MEN'S HEALTH

Because few studies examine health outcomes for men who perpetrate IPV, the cause and effect of this perpetration is difficult to interpret. Direct health effects resulting from IPV perpetration fall into 2 main categories: physical and mental health.

PHYSICAL EFFECTS

Physical effects of IPV perpetration include injuries incurred while carrying out the abusive behavior (eg, broken bones, abrasions, contusions), as well as injuries incurred as victims defend themselves from the assault. The use of weapons by the perpetrator increases the likelihood of injury and lethality.

Historically noted head injuries seem to be the only physical condition linked to IPV perpetration by the literature.[23,44,45] The literature also describes higher rates of drug use and alcohol consumption in perpetrators of IPV, yet the role played by drug and alcohol use in the risk for IPV remains debatable.[12,22,44,46,47-49] Some researchers assert that drug use and alcohol consumption directly increase the risk of IPV perpetration behaviors; however, others purported the use of alcohol and drugs by IPV perpetrators as a means of medicating their undesired feelings of shame, guilt, and anxiety.[50]

MENTAL HEALTH EFFECTS

Mental health outcomes associated with IPV perpetration include increased rates of depression, anxiety, and PTSD.[12,13,23,46,50,51] Many advocates for IPV victims stress the distinction between IPV perpetration and mental health issues. These advocates are concerned that IPV perpetration behaviors are *choices* made by abusive men, rather than by people who are not subject to behaviors shaped by a mental disorder.

Studies indicate that IPV perpetrators show an increased incidence of personality disorders, the most clinically significant of which may be antisocial personality disorder.[51] Men with antisocial personality disorder tend to behave indifferently to the possibility of physical pain or punishment, show no indication that they experience fear when threatened, demonstrate an apparent disregard for the consequences of their actions, and lack empathy when others suffer. Diagnostic criteria for men with antisocial personality disorder overlap significantly with IPV perpetration behaviors, which include the following[52]:

— Failure to conform to social norms with respect to lawful behaviors (as indicated by repeatedly performing acts that are grounds for arrest), deceitfulness (as indicated by repeated lying), use of aliases, or conning others for personal profit or pleasure

— Impulsivity or failure to plan ahead

— Irritability and aggressiveness (as indicated by repeated physical fights or assaults)

— Reckless disregard for the safety of themselves or others

— Consistent irresponsibility (as indicated by repeated failure to sustain steady work or honor financial obligations)

— Lack of remorse (as indicated by an indifference toward, or a rationalization of, having hurt, mistreated, or stolen from another person)

Although samples of male IPV perpetrators show an increased incidence for mental health issues, most perpetrators do not have mental health disorders.

STUDY RESULTS

Two studies examined health care use for men who are being treated for IPV perpetration. Coben and Friedman's study of health care use in a convenience sample of men enrolled in a court-mandated batterer treatment program found that 36% of visits to health care facilities were injury related, 21% were reported as "checkups," and 13% did not describe the reason for their visit.[49]

The injuries caused by IPV perpetration and comorbidities associated with IPV perpetration have been identified. Gerlock described health care use of men involved in treatment for IPV perpetration included the following[12]:

— 50% experienced musculoskeletal issues

— 14% experienced cardiovascular issues

— 13% experienced gastrointestinal issues

— 10% experienced nervous system issues

— 10% experienced dermatological issues

— 8% experienced pulmonary issues

Participants in this study ascribed a significant proportion of injuries related in part to their IPV behaviors. Approximately one third of perpetrators reported symptoms of depression and anxiety resulting from their perpetration behaviors. Gerlock's study helps support the position that IPV male offenders are aware of the connection between their behaviors and their health issues.

USE OF HEALTH SERVICES BY INTIMATE PARTNER VIOLENCE VICTIMS AND PERPETRATORS

Most studies in clinical settings have explored rates of female victimization. These studies estimate that 15% of women visiting an emergency department and 12% to 23% of women in primary care settings report having been physically abused or threatened by their partner within the last 12-month period.[53-55] Of the few studies that focus on men in a primary care setting, Oriel and colleagues reported 13% of male patients described throwing, pushing, or slapping their partners during the past 12 months. A smaller but significant percentage of these men (4.2%) reported at least one episode that they characterized as severe violence (eg, kicking, beating, threatening to use or using a knife or gun).[22] Studies about the use of health care by male IPV perpetrators suggest that half of perpetrators had sought health-related care during the 6 months before the study.[12,49] In Coben and Friedman's study, health care providers had seen 42% of male IPV perpetrators close to the time of their arrest; these perpetrators were seen for issues related to injury (36%), medical illness (30%), and "check-ups" (21%).[49]

HELP-SEEKING BEHAVIORS OF INTIMATE PARTNER VIOLENCE VICTIMS AND PERPETRATORS

Whether victims or perpetrators, before people can engage in help-seeking behaviors in a meaningful way, they must first recognize the IPV-related issues in their lives as problematic. A number of community and system-level organizations are committed to identifying and treating victims of IPV so that victims who seek help have a large group from which to obtain active and passive support. In 1983, Bowker conducted a community-based study of help-seeking strategies among self-identified IPV victims.[53] Help-seeking behaviors can take many forms, including formal (eg, police officers, social service agency personnel, lawyers and district attorneys, clergy members, members of women's groups) and informal (eg, family members, in-laws, neighbors, friends) sources.

Specific help-seeking behaviors of IPV perpetrators include self-identification and self-referral to health care providers. This may occur either with or without the perpetrator seeking the advice and support from family members and friends. As previously mentioned, perpetrators use health care services and may attend community-based, batterer-intervention programs (through professional, self, or court-mandated referral) and parenting programs (often required when custody issues affect the relationship). In Bowker's study, more than two thirds of female IPV victims reported that their male partners made contact with at least one formal or informal help source in an attempt to end the abuse.[53]

Informal sources of help (family members and friends) appear to be important factors that shape perpetrators' behaviors, supporting or preventing IPV perpetration. Bowker found that the more contact perpetrators had with their friends, the less likely they were to make efforts to address IPV within their relationships.[53] This finding suggests the existence of a "peer subculture" that normatively supports IPV and may act as a barrier to perpetrators seeking help.

Health care providers must recognize the impact of system responses and social stigma on male disclosure of IPV. For example, IPV-related training for health care providers tends to focus on men as the perpetrators and women as the victims. As a result, health care providers may not provide opportunities for men to report their IPV-related exposure, thereby leaving them feeling further isolated. Whether involved in a homosexual or heterosexual relationship, men may feel reluctant to disclose their IPV-related exposure, especially if they have been victims. Because normal gender roles and cultural ideals shape help-seeking behaviors, such roles and ideals may cause men to feel shame or guilt, thereby hindering them from describing themselves as victims or as needing support or assistance.

IDENTIFYING MALE VICTIMS AND PERPETRATORS OF INTIMATE PARTNER VIOLENCE

When discussing the appropriate health care response to IPV, health care providers rarely mention identifying male IPV victims and perpetrators in the clinical setting. Driven by concerns about victim safety and human rights violations, national policy, community-based responses, and health care systems historically focus on identifying and treating female IPV victims. As a result, health-care-system and community-level constraints have led to patterns of diagnosis, treatment, and health care delivery that do not address the root cause of IPV-perpetration. In fact, the health care system has unnecessarily and unwisely limited the focus to post-event services for victims, thereby leaving the punishment and isolation of perpetrators to the criminal justice system.

Health care providers must recognize that because primary care settings are pivotal to improving public health, they are ideally suited for identifying and referring IPV perpetrators for help in addressing their negative behaviors.

As previously mentioned, significant numbers of patients are willing to disclose IPV victimization or perpetration within the primary care setting; however, according to Sugg and colleagues, 10% of primary care providers have never identified an IPV victim and 55% have never identified an IPV perpetrator.[56]

MALE TYPOLOGIES OF INTIMATE PARTNER VIOLENCE

Though they remain controversial, male typologies of IPV do exist. Dutton is often cited for IPV characterization, which describes IPV perpetrators as falling into one of the following 3 typologies[57]:

1. *Psychopathic Wife Assaulters.* They make up approximately 20% of perpetrators. They lack emotional responsiveness, are often violent with their partners as well as other people, are frequently arrested for violent and nonviolent crimes, lack the ability to imagine another person's fear or pain, and are cool and controlled when engaging in heated arguments with their intimate partners.

2. *Over-Controlled Wife Assaulters.* They represent about 30% of perpetrators. They have a strong profile of avoidance and passive-aggressive behavior, score high on dominance and isolation scales, rigidly observe stereotypical gender roles, and are verbally and emotionally abusive

3. *Cyclical and/or Emotionally Volatile Wife Abusers.* They make up the largest number of perpetrators. They have experienced either abandonment or smothering parents regarding their expectations toward intimacy, tend to find ways to blame their partners for the abuse, hold the victims responsible for their own feelings, make impossible demands on their victims, punish their victims for inevitably failing, and have a need to shame and humiliate other people.

In their review of the literature regarding typologies, Cavanaugh and Gelles categorized IPV perpetrators as low-, moderate-, and high-risk offenders. They found that each group of offenders could be further characterized by the severity and frequency of the violence, criminal history, and the level of psychopathology exhibited in their presentations.[58]

SEPARATING MALE VICTIMS FROM PERPETRATORS

As previously mentioned, separating IPV victimization from IPV perpetration remains challenging. Men can be IPV victims, perpetrators, or both within the context of heterosexual, homosexual, or bisexual relationships.

Johnson has worked on characterizing "common couple violence" which describes mutually aggressive behaviors within relationships in which *both* partners perpetrate and are victimized.[59] As a result, health care providers need to conceptualize IPV as a complex relationship in which both partners potentially contribute to victimization and perpetration.

PREDICTORS OF INTIMATE PARTNER VIOLENCE

Although commonly cited that IPV transcends all ethnic and socio-economic barriers, IPV rates tend to be associated with younger age groups, minority ethnic groups, and lower socio-economic classes.[22,23,44] The association between race and ethnicity and men's violence is particularly difficult to isolate. Some data suggest that minority families experience disproportionate rates of lethal and nonlethal intrafamily violence, but others do not link the two because other social (especially socioeconomic) factors could contribute to the violence.

The National Family Violence Survey reported the following racial statistics when studying the self-reporting of perpetration by men: 17.1% of black men, 14.1% of Hispanic men, and 9.7% of white men.[60] In contrast, the 1992 National Crime Victimization Survey found no statistically significant differences in IPV victimization rates among ethnic groups.[9]

The driving forces behind IPV remain unclear in view of larger, contextual issues. Social disorganization characterized by resident mobility, economic disparity, social dislocation, family disruption, and population density are more consistently correlated with rates of violence than ethnicity.[61] When trying to understand the development of maladaptive behaviors related to stress, health care providers, researchers, and policymakers must not separate the disparities in destructive behaviors observed in minority populations from the context of non-minority oppression in society.

Other Characteristics

Some men affected by IPV (as either perpetrators or victims) may present with obvious injury, mental health-related issues, or symptoms of substance abuse, whereas others may appear completely asymptomatic. In fact, men exposed to IPV, especially perpetrators, appear normal compared to their partners, who have symptoms from their victimization.

Dutton described perpetrators in treatment as unexpressive, impulse driven, and traditional with rigid personalities, low self-esteem, and frequent drug and alcohol problems.[57] Other characteristics to consider include public fronts, controlling behaviors, excuses, bargaining, manipulation, and external locus of control[62]; however, no single profile can guide clinicians in identifying perpetrators.

GROUND RULES WHEN INQUIRING ABOUT INTIMATE PARTNER VIOLENCE

Ground rules do exist to help guide health care providers as they inquire about IPV-related behaviors within a clinical setting. Most importantly, victim safety must guide decisions about IPV inquiry, referral, and treatment.

Mandatory Reporting Laws

Before asking any questions about IPV, patients and health care providers must understand mandatory reporting laws within the United States regarding disclosure; that is, all states categorize health care providers as mandatory reporters in certain situations, especially with respect to child abuse and elder abuse. Mandatory reporting laws for IPV fall into the following four categories[63]:

1. States that require reporting of injuries caused by weapons

2. States that mandate reporting for injuries caused by violation of criminal laws

3. States that specifically address reporting of domestic violence exposure

4. States that have no general mandatory reporting laws

When negotiating the disclosure of sensitive information such as IPV-related behaviors, health care providers must understand the reporting laws for their state with respect to who is required to report and in what context information must be reported.

Inquiry Techniques

As in any form or inquiry into sensitive, clinical information, health care providers must develop a comfortable style for themselves that effectively obtains the necessary information from patients. Health care providers often learn "funneling" techniques when training. When using this technique, health care providers start by asking less sensitive questions and progress to more general questions. This gradually guides the conversation toward more specific and sensitive issues. Screening protocols often use these funneling techniques. No studies have been conducted to analyze the screening methods used in the primary care setting to identify IPV perpetration.

One screening method that has been suggested for identifying IPV perpetration uses an adaptation of the RADAR (ie, **R**outine inquiring; **A**sk direct questions; **D**ocument findings; **A**ssess patient safety and lethality; **R**espond, review options, and refer) instrument, which was originally designed to identify domestic violence victimization. Created by the Massachusetts Medical Society and developed into a training program by the Institute for Safe Families of Philadelphia, RADAR was designed for use in the identification and treatment of IPV within clinical settings.[64,65] This training offers health care providers suggestions for framing questions about male IPV exposure. These questions include the following:

— All people argue. How do you and your partner handle disagreements or fights?

— Do your disagreements or fights ever become physical?

— Are you in a relationship in which you are being hurt or threatened?

— Have you ever used any kind of physical force against your partner?

— Has your partner ever pushed, grabbed, slapped, choked, or hit you? Have you ever done that to her/him?

— Has your partner ever forced you to have sexual intercourse or to perform sexual acts that you did not want to do? Have you done that to her/him?

Creating a Safe Environment

When both the victim and perpetrator are patients of the same health care provider, that provider must make the safety of the victim paramount. Attempts at intervention should occur individually with both the victim and perpetrator until abusive behaviors have been controlled for at least 6 to 12 months. If a health care provider works with the victim and perpetrator individually and conducts the sessions in a comprehensive and responsible manner, then a conflict of interest does not exist.[66]

Before approaching the perpetrating patient, the health care provider should obtain the consent of the victimized patient. During such a conversation, the health care provider should assess for safety and develop a safety plan for the victim, discuss the possibility that approaching the perpetrator may increase the victim's risk, and ultimately obtain the victim's permission to discuss the IPV with the perpetrator.

Ferris demonstrated that the health care provider's relationship with the perpetrator strongly, though not always beneficially, shaped the provider's responses toward the IPV victim. For example, providers who report "good" relationships with the perpetrators were more likely to recommend high-risk behaviors (eg, couple's counseling, discussing the issue in the presence of both partners) to their patients. This finding suggests that providers are potentially influenced by their personal relationship with their patients (ie, discounting the impact of abuse in relationships) rather than objective findings suggestive of the presence of abuse.

WHAT TO DO WHEN A MAN DISCLOSES INTIMATE PARTNER VIOLENCE

Health care providers need to be prepared and have ready responses for encounters with a man who discloses a history of IPV victimization or perpetration. Not only do they need to know the appropriate words to say, but they also need to understand the next steps that must be taken. Provider responses tend to shape the patient's future disclosure of sensitive information and impact that person's ability to develop a therapeutic relationship regarding violence issues.

Responses to victimization and perpetration behaviors share the following common features:

— The provider should listen in a nonjudgmental manner, validate experiences of victimization, and reinforce the disclosure of perpetration behaviors; however, the provider should never condone abusive behaviors.

— The provider should document specific responses, quote the speaker whenever possible, and note dates and times of specific abusive events.

— The provider should assess the risk for future abusive events and provide safety planning.

Providers should assess patients' level of acceptance regarding the abusive situation and in terms of the patient's readiness to change abusive behaviors. Recent work has explored the use of the stages of change model when addressing IPV in clinical settings.[67-69] Prochaska developed the Transtheoretical Model that describes the following stages of change for behavior[70]:

— ***Precontemplation.*** When the person is unaware of issues as problems or significantly minimizes the impact of the behavior

— ***Contemplation.*** When the person acknowledges the issues as being problematic and considers changing the behavior

— ***Preparation.*** When the person makes plans to change

— ***Action.*** When the person follows through with their plans to change

— ***Maintenance.*** When the person sustains the changes to the behavior

When applying this model to patient behaviors, a common health care provider misperception is that patients who are not actively addressing their behaviors have only experienced the early stages change (ie, precontemplation and contemplation). The Transtheoretical Model is best described as a *cycle* of behavioral changes. This means that as a person proceeds through each of the five common stages, that person often reverts to earlier stages via a stage described as "relapse."

Relapse is a critical stage of behavioral change that can be used by both the patient and provider. When caring for men struggling with IPV-related issues, providers should especially consider the importance of the relapse stage. Acknowledging and deconstructing episodes of relapse frames behavioral counseling in terms of building on prior contemplation and adjustment of therapeutic strategies to increase sustained periods of behavior maintenance and determination. Health care providers should remain aware of the shame and guilt that many patients experience during periods of relapse and self-perceived failure because these feelings help reshape conditions that have lead to it.[50] Such models of the stages of change can be valuable tools for health care providers when helping men modify their behavior and promote healthy lifestyles.

As previously emphasized, safety assessments are important when IPV has been identified; however, health care providers seem to lose interest in pursuing IPV-related issues at this point during training sessions. Providers cite their time constraints and feelings of deficiency regarding the skills needed to adequately pursue such issues.

A minimum safety assessment should include the documentation of changes in the frequency or severity of violence, weapons in the house or use of weapons during assaults, abuse of drugs and/or alcohol, stalking behaviors, and prior involvement with the legal or criminal justice system. Providers should be aware and inform their victimized patients that IPV victims are at greatest risk for heightened abuse and homicide when leaving abusive relationships.[71,72]

TREATING MEN FOR INTIMATE PARTNER VIOLENCE PERPETRATION

Many associations exist between medical and mental health comorbidities and IPV victimization and perpetration; however, health care providers should isolate IPV perpetration behaviors as a condition requiring highly specialized treatment. Referral to a mental health provider who is not trained or specialized in the treatment of IPV perpetrators may not be helpful and may actually worsen certain aspects of effective treatment. Providers should familiarize themselves with local Batterer Intervention Programs (BIPs) and refer men who perpetrate to such programs. Other mental health providers can and should become involved if the health care provider is concerned about substance abuse, depression, anxiety, PTSD, or other non-IPV-related mental health conditions.

Standards for BIPs are defined at the state level; national standards do not exist. Batter Intervention Programs vary in treatment approach and provider training. Gondolf assessed the standard components of BIPs to determine which are most effective. The study revealed the following as the most effective[51]:

— Treatment models extending over a 6- to 12-month period

— Systematic monitoring and confronting of abusive behaviors for participants

— Assurance that other medical and mental health comorbidities are being addressed

— Psycho-educational curricula that incorporate common perpetration behaviors, issues of entitlement, minimization, and gender roles

— Staff members trained to work with female battering issues

— Well-developed collaborations with IPV victims' services and the criminal justice system

The clinical effectiveness of BIPs remains debatable. Most clinical BIP providers would provide anecdotal support for their practices; however, few services provided for male IPV perpetrators are based on evidence. Two recent reviews have systematically addressed the effectiveness of BIPs. In 2004, Babcock reviewed 22 studies of BIPs (5 experimental studies and 17 quasi-experimental studies) and concluded that BIPs make a small difference in rates of recidivism when compared to the rates obtained through correctional treatments with prisoners.[73] In 2003, Wathen conducted a meta-analysis of 10 studies that met strict criteria for inclusion in his systematic review of the BIP literature.[74] He noted many methodological issues that confounded the analysis of the effect of BIPs. These issues included a lack of standardization to treatment approaches with more than one approach often evaluated in a single study, more than half of the studies did not use a control group for comparison, and only 2 studies were randomized control trials. Wathen rated only one study "good." He concluded that the 3 types of interventions studied (ie, group sessions with men; group sessions with men and their partners; rigorous monitoring with monthly, individual counseling and compared with a control group) were not effective in reducing subsequent violence against women. Wathen rated the remaining studies in his review as "poor" or "fair."[74]

As mentioned earlier, sound evidence supports any medical intervention used to reduce IPV. Researchers have not used rigorous methodological approaches to adequately address IPV. In response to some of the methodological challenges previously mentioned, recent BIP outcomes investigations have included meta-analyses and reports using propensity scores. Jones and colleagues[75] and Tolman and Bennett[76] demonstrated a mild effect of BIPs in reducing IPV recidivism.

CONCLUSIONS

Since the 1970s, the response to IPV has been separated into responses to victims and responses to perpetrators. A summary of efforts targeting IPV in the 1998 National Academy of Sciences volume on Family Violence illustrates the ways that the medical response has primarily focused upon victim identification and referral without mentioning perpetration issues. The only concerted efforts directed at perpetrators have been tertiary responses of the criminal justice system with little attention paid to primary prevention. Throughout this period, efforts directed at victims have made incremental adjustments.

A shift in perspective has the potential to make a significant difference in what appears to be an intractable social issue. An improved public health approach to IPV would not ignore the role of perpetrators; however, little is known about how, when, or if perpetrators identify their behaviors as a problem or about the help-seeking behaviors that perpetrators use as they struggle with issues of violence and abuse.

One step toward primary prevention of IPV would be to identify services that could effectively identify perpetrators before their behavior negatively affects their lives. Primary care management of perpetrators is ideally suited to providing a preventive approach to the perpetration of IPV. This would involve a coordinated effort to establish community partnerships that support the prevention of IPV perpetration within the health care setting. In order to advance primary prevention, a better understanding of the social determinants of perpetration and help-seeking offenders of perpetrators is needed. Additionally, a complementary assessment is required to understand how health care providers view their roles in the prevention of perpetration. The information gained from such an assessment could be used to develop innovative changes in how communities view the role of health care providers in the treatment of perpetration and developing effective means of managing perpetration in health care settings.

REFERENCES

1. Salzman BE, Wender RC. Male sex: a major health disparity. *Prim Care*. 2006;33:1-16.

2. Hing E, Cherry DK, Woodwell DA. *National Ambulatory Medical Care Survey: 2004 Summary*. Hyattsville, Md: National Center for Health Statistics; June 2006. *Advance Data From the Vital and Health Statistics*; no 374.

3. National Center for Health Statistics. *Health, United States, 2004: With Chartbook on Trends in the Health of Americans.* Hyattsville, Md: National Center for Health Statistics; 2004.

4. The Family Violence Prevention Fund. *National Consensus Guidelines: On Identifying and Responding to Domestic Violence Victimization in Health Care Settings.* San Francisco, Calif: The Family Violence Prevention Fund; 2002.

5. Saltzman LE, Fanslow JL, McMahon JM, Shelley GA. *Intimate Partner Violence Surveillance: Uniform Definitions and Recommended Data Elements.* Atlanta, GA: Centers for Disease Control and Prevention, National Center for Injury Prevention and Control; 2002.

6. Tjaden P, Thoennes N. *Full Report of the Prevalence, Incidence, and Consequences of Violence Against Women: Findings From the National Violence Against Women Survey.* Washington, DC: US Dept of Justice, Office of Justice Programs, National Institute of Justice; 2000. NCJ 183781.

7. Straus MA, Gelles RJ, Steinmetz SK. *Behind Closed Doors: Violence in the American Family.* 1st ed. Garden City, NY: Anchor Press/Doubleday; 1980.

8. Straus MA, Gelles RJ. *Physical Violence in American Families: Risk Factors and Adaptations to Violence in 8145 Families.* New Brunswick, NJ: Transaction Publishers; 1990.

9. Bachman R. *Violence Against Women: A National Crime Victimization Survey Report.* Washington, DC: US Dept of Justice, Bureau of Justice Statistics; 1994. NCJ-145325.

10. Straus MA, Gelles RJ. Societal change and change in Family Violence from 1975 to 1986 as revealed by two national surveys. *J Marriage Fam.* 1986;48:465-479.

11. Centers for Disease Control and Prevention. Intimate partner violence among men and women—South Carolina: 1998. *MMWR Morb Mortal Wkly Rep.* 2000; 49:691-694.

12. Gerlock AA. Health impact of domestic violence. *Issues Ment Health Nurs.* 1999;20:373-385.

13. Cascardi M, Langhinrichsen J, Vivian D. Marital aggression. Impact, injury, and health correlates for husbands and wives. *Arch Intern Med.* 1992;152:1178-1184.

14. Elliott BA, Johnson MM. Domestic violence in a primary care setting. Patterns and prevalence. *Arch Fam Med.* 1995;4:113-119.

15. Dawson JM, Langan PA. *Murder in Families. Bureau of Justice Statistics Special Report.* Washington, DC: US Dept of Justice, Office of Justice Programs, Bureau of Justice Statistics; 1994. NCJ 143498.

16. Dobash RE, Dobash RP. Wives: the "appropriate" victims of marital violence. *Victimology.* 1977;2(3 suppl 4):426-442.

17. Dutton DG. *The Abusive Personality: Violence and Control in Intimate Relationships.* New York, NY: The Guilford Press; 1998.

18. Jacobson NS, Gottman JM. *When Men Batter Women: New Insights Into Ending Abusive Relationships.* New York, NY: Simon & Schuster; 1998.

19. Gelles RJ, Straus MA. *Intimate Violence: The Definitive Study of the Causes and Consequences of Abuse in the American Family*. New York, NY: Simon & Schuster; 1988.

20. McCall GJ, Shields NM. Social and structural factors in family violence. In: Lystad M. *Violence in the Home: Interdisciplinary Perspectives*. New York, NY: Brunner/Mazel; 1986:98-123.

21. Harway M, O'Neil JM. *What Causes Men's Violence Against Women?* Thousand Oaks, Calif: Sage Publications; 1999.

22. Oriel KA, Fleming MF. Screening men for partner violence in a primary care setting. A new strategy for detecting domestic violence. *J Fam Pract*. 1998;46:493-498.

23. Murphy CM. Treating perpetrators of adult domestic violence. *Md Med J*. 1994;43:877-883.

24. Fitch FJ, Papantonio A. Men who batter: some pertinent characteristics. *Compr Psychiatry*. 1992;33:411-416.

25. Coker AL, Davis KE, Arias I, et al. Physical and mental health effects of intimate partner violence for men and women. *Am J Prev Med*. 2002;23:260-268.

26. Schechter S. *Women and Male Violence: The Visions and Struggles of the Battered Women's Movement*. Boston, Mass: South End Press; 1983.

27. Gelles RJ. *Intimate Violence in Families*. 3rd ed. Thousand Oaks, Calif: Sage Publications; 1997.

28. Campbell JC. Health consequences of intimate partner violence. *Lancet*. 2002;359:1331-1336.

29. Edleson JL. The overlap between child maltreatment and woman battering. *Violence Against Women*. 1999;5:134-154.

30. Saunders BE. Understanding children exposed to violence: toward an integration of overlapping fields. *J Interpers Violence*. 2003;18:356-376.

31. Kitzmann KM, Gaylord NK, Holt AR, Kenny ED. Child witnesses to domestic violence: a meta-analytic review. *J Consult Clin Psychol*. 2003;71:339-352.

32. Fantuzzo J, Lindquist C. The effects of observing conjugal violence on children: a Review and analysis of research methodology. *J Fam Violence*. 1989;4:77-94.

33. Hughes HM, Parkinson D, Vargo M. Witnessing spouse abuse and experiencing physical abuse: a "double whammy"? *J Fam Violence*. 1989;4:197-209.

34. O'Keefe M. The differential effects of family violence on adolescent adjustment. *Child Adolesc Social Work J*. 1996;13:51-68.

35. Kolbo JR, Blakely, EH, Engelman D. Children who witness domestic violence: a review of empirical literature. *J Interpers Violence*. 1996;11:281-293.

36. Jouriles EN, Norwood WD. Physical aggression toward boys and girls in families characterized by the battering of women. *J Fam Psychol*. 1995;9:69-78.

37. McCloskey LA, Figueredo AJ, Koss MP. The effects of systemic family violence on children's mental health. *Child Dev*. 1995;66:1239-1261.

38. Holden GW. Introduction. In: Holden GW, Geffner R, Jouriles EN, eds. *Children Exposed to Marital Violence: Theory, Research, and Applied Issues*. Washington, DC: American Psychological Association; 1998:1-18.

39. Jaffe P, Sudermann M. Child witness of women abuse: research and community responses. In: Stith S, Straus M, eds. *Understanding Partner Violence: Prevalence, Causes, Consequences, and Solutions*. Minneapolis, Minn: National Council on Family Relations; 1995:213-222. Families in Focus Services; vol 2.

40. Wolfe DA, Wekerle C, Reitzel D, Gough R. Strategies to address violence in the lives of high risk youth. In: Peled E, Jaffe PG, Edleson JL, eds. *Ending the Cycle of Violence: Community Responses to Children of Battered Women*. Thousand Oaks, Calif: Sage Publications; 1995:255-274.

41. Roberts TA, Klein J. Intimate partner abuse and high-risk behavior in adolescents. *Arch Pediatr Adolesc Med*. 2003;157:375-380.

42. Whitfield CL, Anda RF, Dube SR, Felitti VJ. Violent childhood experiences and the risk of intimate partner violence in adults: assessment in a large health maintenance organization. *J Interpers Violence*. 2003;18:166-185.

43. Ehrensaft MK, Cohen P, Brown J, Smailes E, Chen H, Johnson JG. Intergenerational transmission of partner violence: a 20-year prospective study. *J Consult Clin Psychol*. 2003;71:741-753.

44. Bacaner N, Kinney TA, Biros M, Bochert S, Casuto N. The relationship among depressive and alcoholic symptoms and aggressive behavior in adult male emergency department patients. *Acad Emerg Med*. 2002;9:120-129.

45. Rosenbaum A, Hoge SK, Adelman SA, Warnken WJ, Fletcher KE, Kane RL. Head injury in partner-abusive men. *J Consult Clin Psychol*. 1994;62:1187-1193.

46. Dinwiddie SH. Psychiatric disorders among wife batterers. *Compr Psychiatry*. 1992;33:411-416.

47. Sharps PW, Campbell J, Campbell D, Gary F, Webster D. The role of alcohol use in intimate partner femicide. *Am J Addict*. 2001;10:122-135.

48. Testa M. The role of substance use in male-to-female physical and sexual violence: a brief review and recommendations for future research. *J Interpers Violence*. 2004;19:1494-1505.

49. Coben JH, Friedman DI. Health care use by perpetrators of domestic violence. *J Emerg Med*. 2002;22:313-317.

50. Mintz HA, Cornett FW. When your patient is a batterer. What you need to know before treating perpetrators of domestic violence. *Postgrad Med*. 1997;101:219-221, 225-228.

51. Gondolf EW. Identifying and assessing men who batter. In: *Assessing Woman Battering in Mental Health Services*. Thousand Oaks, Calif: Sage Publications; 1998:132-156.

52. American Psychiatric Association. *Diagnostic and Statistical Manual of Mental Disorders (DSM-IV-TR)*. 4th ed, text rev. Washington, DC: American Psychiatric Association; 2000.

53. Bowker LH. *Beating Wife-Beating*. Lexington, Mass: Lexington Books; 1983.

54. Gelles RJ, Straus MA. *Intimate Violence.* New York, NY: Simon & Schuster; 1988.

55. Abbott J, Johnson R, Koziol-McLain J, Lowenstein SR. Domestic violence against women: Incidence and prevalence in an emergency department population. *JAMA.* 1995;273:1763-1767.

56. Sugg NK, Thompson RS, Thompson DC, Maiuro R, Rivara FP. Domestic violence and primary care. Attitudes, practices, and beliefs. *Arch Fam Med.* 1999;8:301-306.

57. Dutton DG, Golant SK. *The Batterer: A Psychological Profile.* New York, NY: Basic Books; 1995.

58. Cavanaugh MM, Gelles RJ. The utility of male domestic violence offender typologies: new directions for research, policy, and practice. *J Interpers Violence.* 2005;20:155-166.

59. Johnson MP. Patriarchal terrorism and common couple violence: Two forms of violence against women. *J Marriage Fam.* 1995;57:283-294.

60. Reiss AJ, Roth JA, for the Panel on the Understanding and Control of Violent Behavior, National Research Council. *Social Influences.* Washington, DC: National Academy Press; 1994. *Understanding and Preventing Violence;* vol 3.

61. Carrillo R, Tello J, eds. *Family Violence and Men of Color: Healing the Wounded Male Spirit.* New York, NY: Springer Publishing Company; 1998.

62. Hanusa D. The next step: focusing on abusers in the health care system. *WMJ.* 1998;97:60-61.

63. Groves BM, Augustyn M, Lee D, Sawires P. *Identifying and Responding to Domestic Violence: Consensus Recommendations for Child and Adolescent Health.* San Francisco, Calif: Family Violence Prevention Fund; 2002.

64. Institute for Safe Families Web site. Available at: http://www.instituteforsafe families.org/health_care_materials.php.

65. Harwell TS, Casten RJ, Armstrong KA, Dempsey S, Coons HL, Davis M. Results of a domestic violence training program offered to the staff of urban community health centers. Evaluation Committee of the Philadelphia Family Violence Working Group. *Am J Prev Med.* 1998;15:235-242.

66. Ferris LE, Norton PG, Dunn EV, Gort EH, Degani N. Guidelines for managing domestic abuse when male and female partners are patients of the same physician. The Delphi Panel and the Consulting Group. *JAMA.* 1997;278:851-857.

67. Zink T, Elder N, Jacobson J, Klostermann B. Medical management of intimate partner violence considering the stages of change: precontemplation and contemplation. *Ann Fam Med.* 2004;2:231-239.

68. Frasier PY, Slatt L, Kowlowitz V, Glowa PT. Using the stages of change model to counsel victims of intimate partner violence. *Patient Educ Couns.* 2001;43: 211-217.

69. Scott KL, Wolfe DA. Readiness to change as a predictor of outcome in batterer treatment. *J Consult Clin Psychol.* 2003;71:879-889.

70. Prochaska JO, DiClemente CC, Norcross JC. In search of how people change. Applications to addictive behaviors. *Am Psychol.* 1992;47:1102-1114.

71. Campbell JC, Webster D, Koziol-McLain J, et al. Risk factors for femicide in abusive relationships: results from a multisite case control study. *Am J Public Health*. 2003;93:1089-1097.

72. Wilson M, Daly M. Spousal homicide risk and estrangement. *Violence Vict*. 1993;8:3-16.

73. Babcock JC, Green CE, Robie C. Does batterers' treatment work? A meta-analytic review of domestic violence treatment. *Clin Psychol Rev*. 2004;23:1023-1053.

74. Wathen CN, MacMillan HL. Interventions for violence against women: scientific review. *JAMA*. 2003;289:589-600.

75. Jones AS, D'Agostino RB Jr, Gondolf EW, Heckert A. Assessing the effect of batterer program completion on reassault using propensity scores. *J Interpers Violence*. 2004;19:1002-1020.

76. Tolman RM, Bennett LW. A review of quantitative research on men who batter. *J Interpers Violence*. 1990;5:87-118.

Chapter 14

FATHERHOOD AS A GATEWAY FOR CHANGE: INSIGHTS FROM THE FATHERING AFTER VIOLENCE INITIATIVE

Juan Carlos Areán, MM
Lonna Davis, MSW
Angelo P. Giardino, MD, PhD, MPH, FAAP*

Fathering After Violence (FAV) is a national initiative developed by the Family Violence Prevention Fund (FVPF) and its partners to enhance the safety and well being of women and children by motivating men to renounce intimate partner violence (IPV) and become better fathers (or father figures) and more supportive parenting partners. Fathering After Violence is not a program per se or a quick solution to a complex problem. Rather, it is a conceptual framework to help end violence against women by using fatherhood as a leading approach. Using this framework as a starting point, the FVPF has partnered with practitioners in the fields of batterer intervention, children's exposure to IPV, and supervised visitation to develop culturally appropriate practical tools, prevention and intervention strategies, and policy and practice recommendations.

Fathering After Violence has proposed engaging abusive fathers with an array of universal messages that may help them develop empathy for their children; thereby enabling fathers to use this empathy as a motivator to change their violent and controlling behavior. It has developed an assessment framework to help practitioners discern which fathers might be amenable to this approach. Fathering After Violence has also introduced a reparative framework for those fathers who are in the position to start healing their relationships with their children in a safe and constructive way. This framework can also be used as a guide to know whether some fathers need to stay away from their children in order for them to heal.

The Family Violence Prevention Fund, a US-based international advocacy-oriented organization that works to lessen the risk to all in society from IPV, recommends that the following principles be adopted by any practitioner who works with abusive fathers:

— The safety of the victim and the children should always be the first priority of any intervention or policy regarding men who have used violence.

— All interventions involving children who have witnessed or experienced violence should be guided by the voices of the nonabusive parents.

* Portions of this chapter are based on earlier unpublished work commissioned by the Family Violence Prevention Fund. The authors would like to gratefully acknowledge the contributions made to this work by Lucy Salcido-Carter, Betsy McAlister-Groves, and Fernando Mederos.

— Violence against women is harmful to children in multiple ways, including their safety, development, and relationships with both their violent fathers and nonoffending mothers.

— Fathers (and father figures) are important to children, and children are profoundly affected by their fathers, for better or worse.

— It is possible for some violent men to renounce violence.

— Interventions with fathers who have used violence must be implemented with awareness of the cultural context in which parenting happens.

— Relationships damaged by violence are sometimes reparable, and some men can be helped to achieve constructive and healing relationships with their children.

— Contact between the offenders and their children or parenting partners should only occur when it is safe and appropriate (eg, contact does not compromise the physical and emotional safety of mothers and children, or undermine mothers' parenting.[1]

From a review of these principles, one can see that the most important consideration for practitioners who deal with abusive fathers must be the ongoing safety of the victims, typically women and children in the perpetrator's life. This cannot be overemphasized and bears continued repetition because IPV is a complex problem, and, despite a desire for an optimistic approach, it is true that not all men can make the progress necessary to improve the relationships with their children and partners or ex-partners.

As a result of this reality, concerns have arisen over the years about the potential downside to engaging abusive fathers. These concerns include the fear of the courts overestimating the man's ability to parent, the risk of encouraging men to have more contact or seek custody when it is not appropriate, and pushing fathers to make promises they cannot fulfill. On the other hand, clinical experience and informed practice would support the notion that some men can be motivated to change and recognize the impact of their destructive actions on themselves and others. With a combination of accountability measures and appropriate supports, some men can make necessary changes to embrace and support real transformation in their thinking and in the way they relate to and treat the people around them.

This chapter will review our basic understanding of what is known about fatherhood and IPV, practice lessons from the batterer intervention and the supervised visitation contexts, and how some of these concepts may be used in other settings such as health care.

RESEARCH ON FATHERHOOD AND INTIMATE PARTNER VIOLENCE

Studies show that men who use violence with their intimate partners are also likely to use violent, controlling, and authoritarian parenting practices with their children. The limited research available on the relationship between abusive fathers and their children indicates that these fathers may be less available to their children, less likely to engage in rational discussions with their children, and less affectionate than fathers who are not violent.[2] These violent fathers are also more likely to be neglectful, self-centered and irresponsible, as well as more likely to manipulate their children and undermine the mother's parenting and authority.[3]

Not surprisingly, there is ambivalence in the domestic violence field about whether fathers who have been violent should have ongoing contact with their children.

Research shows that an abusive male's relationship to a child directly affects that child's well being, regardless of other factors such as the mental health of the mother.[4] Clinical studies have identified several risks to children of ongoing contact with perpetrators, including exposure to authoritarian parenting, risk of new exposure to violence, risk of learning beliefs that support violent behavior, and risk of being used as a tool of violence or control (**Table 14-1**).[3]

However, other studies paint a more nuanced picture, stating that the effects of violence vary significantly from one family member to another.[5] Various researchers and practitioners point out that children's perceptions of their abusive fathers are not exclusively negative; many of these children have conflicting and ambivalent feelings about their fathers and some have a strong desire to maintain contact with them.[6,7] Furthermore, qualitative research conducted by the FVPF for the FAV initiative shows that many mothers who have suffered IPV want their ex-partners to be involved in their children's lives, if it can be done safely.[8] The results of this research have been recently replicated by Tubbs and Williams.[9]

There is very little research on the use of fatherhood to engage abusers in renouncing their violence, though most practitioners agree that there is mounting anecdotal evidence and informed practice pointing in that direction. Recently, there have been interesting qualitative studies proposing that many abusive men aspire to be good fathers and see the ideal of fatherhood in a positive light.[10] Some abusive men say that they will seek and welcome help to become better fathers in order to help their children.[11] According to Litton Fox and colleagues, many men enrolled in a batterer intervention program used "the father role as a source of reentry into the moral community."[12] In a study of 546 fathers participating in batterer intervention programs, Mandel reports that most men were aware of the destructive effects of their physical and verbal abuse on their children, and three quarters of participants worried about the long-term impact of their behavior on their children.[13]

An evaluation of FAV in batterer intervention programs showed that about two thirds of the men who participated in an exercise designed to develop empathy for children were able to better understand the effects of violence on children.[14] At least one recent study has shown that some young offenders see fatherhood as a strong motivator for changing their negative behavior and create positive family relations.[15]

Aside from the few studies that focus on abusive fathers, there is a growing body of literature devoted to better understanding the role of all fathers in child development and the positive effects that fathers have on their children.[16-19] Generally, research shows that the positive involvement of a father figure in a child's life can increase that child's cognitive skills, self-esteem, self-control, empathy and social competence.[20] Recent studies also indicate that it is the quality of the fathers' involvement with their children that is most associated with positive child outcomes, not the demographic characteristics of the father or his legal relationship to the child.[21,22] Although none of these studies were conducted with families challenged by IPV, it is known that high conflict among divorcing parents is the most consistent and reliable correlate of poor outcomes for the children.[23]

All of this research lends support to an IPV intervention approach that recognizes the role fathers play in the lives of children who have witnessed violence. However, to ensure that these children and their mothers are not exposed to future maltreatment or violence, clinicians and other practitioners must always prioritize safety for all family members.

Table 14-1. Bancroft and Silverman's "Risk to Children from Batterers" Framework

RISK	DESCRIPTION
Exposure to Threats or Acts of Violence	After separation, especially when restraining orders are involved, children are at high risk of witnessing or becoming deliberately or accidentally involved in new assaults, the retraumatization or exposure, all of which are likely to impede a child's emotional recovery. During visitation, threats or revictimizations often occur, the likelihood of which is increased if the mother begins a new relationship. Evidenced more by the batterer's attempt to address causes of past behavior than his violent record alone, he is likely to repeat behavior in subsequent relationships, especially because the new partner is unlikely to disclose due to fear, the belief that he has changed or influenced opinion of his former partner.
Under-mining Mother's Relationship	The most important factor in the emotional recovery of child victims of abuse is the relationship with the non-battering parent. This relationship can be weakened by abuse, the deterioration possibly intensifying even after separation, and is therefore one of the most serious risks to children's recovery.
Physical, Sexual or Emotional Abuse	Batterers may display verbally abusive parenting, increasing after separation with visitation as the only means to control the mother, emotionally abuse children or risk parentification of children by instilling guilt. Furthermore, higher rates of child physical and sexual abuse exist among batterers, likely to increase after separation when the mother is unable to oversee the batterer's behavior. Though a batterer may not have abused his children while the family was together, there is still the possibility that the batterer will seek revenge on the mother through their children, or that children will become insubordinate with their father, placing them at a higher risk of physical abuse.
Modeling Violent or Threatening Behavior	As adults, sons and daughters of batterers have increased chances of becoming perpetrators or victims. Additionally, systemic decisions, such as granting custody to a battering parent might be perceived by the child as supporting the father's behavior and placing blame on the mother. Therefore, the batterer's effect on his children's value system needs to be addressed and his relationship with them should require limitation of his power as a role model.
Rigid Parenting	Nurturing and structured environments ease the recovery of child victims of abuse; however, the common authoritative parenting styles used by batterers impede healing. The achievement of a sense of security is crucial for recovery, but a parent's intimidation reminds the child of violence, slowing progress for a child trying to regain self-esteem while aggression is sustained.
Neglect or Irresponsible Parenting	Batterers typically focus more on themselves and are less likely to focus on their children's needs or to provide consistency, which often increases after separation. With typically more time to care for children during visitation than they have done previously, batterers are often more lenient to increase favor with the children, hindering the mother's ability to provide structure in her own home, a necessary element in children's recovery.

(continued)

Table 14-1. *(continued)*

RISK	DESCRIPTION
Neglect *(continued)*	Neglect by the visiting father can sometimes escalate to leaving children unattended or exposing them to entertainment that is frightening or inappropriate, an experience highly disturbing and influential to children who have been exposed to domestic violence.
Abduction	Many abductions take place under the circumstances of domestic violence, usually fulfilled by the father or a representative, and often having traumatizing effects on children. Typically, abductions, most commonly accomplished by failing to return a child from visitation, occur either before separation or years after the separation, instances varying little by race. Family abductions are much more likely than stranger abductions, and half of these have been threatened in some way prior to the abduction.

How to Assess Risk

DIMENSION	DESCRIPTION
Physical Danger to Childrens' Mother	The level of previous or current physical violence as well as threats of abuse during and after the relationship is an indicator of risk to children, future violence toward the mother with possible exposure to children, and likelihood of attempted or actual homicide of mother sometimes including children. Sexual assaults, violence during pregnancy and the mother's own assessment of probability of future assaults (the strongest predictor) are indicators of future incidence of violence, likelihood that children will be physically abused and possibility that the mother will be abused, the last of which varies little by race or economic class. While these situations include a history of threatened or actual high-level violence, threatened or actual homicide may occur after prior low-level violence.
Physical Abuse Towards Children	Batterers have a high risk to physically abuse children, which may continue or intensify after separation. Involved parties should question the father's disciplinary style, his reaction when angry, his use of punishments, and any child protective history. Additionally, does the father spank, leave marks, behave roughly with the children, fight with older children, or justify abusive behavior? Evaluators should be watchful of any manipulation of children to keep secrets about the father's behavior, which increases their risk of being abused.
Sexual Abuse Towards Children	While it seems that confirmed acts of sexual abuse would be handled with great concern, many professionals believe that, after disclosure, additional abuse will not occur because of the perpetrator's fear, but child sexual abuse literature is evidence to the contrary. Even boundary violations, which can be destructive, lead to future sexual abuse or signify undisclosed sexual abuse, should be scrutinized due to the higher risk of incest perpetration among batterers.

(continued)

307

Table 14-1. *(continued)*

DIMENSION	DESCRIPTION
Sexual Abuse *(continued)*	It is important to know if the batterer respects the children's and his own privacy, exposes them or allows them access to pornography, has a sexualized relationship with any of his children, pressures them to offer affection, engages in inappropriate conversation or requires them to keep secrets.
Psychological Cruelty	The extent to which a batterer is capable of being cruel to his family is a predictor of both the degree of his children's safety in his care and his desire to seek revenge against the mother. It is important for evaluators to know what his emotionally hurtful acts were toward the mother and children, which acts caused the most suffering, whether he continually justifies his behavior, and whether he has acted intentionally to harm the children emotionally.
Coercive or Manipulative Behavior	The more controlling a partner is, the greater the likelihood he will display similar parenting styles, indicating a higher risk of physical and sexual abuse in which children will likely become involved. Characteristics of a controlling partner include arrogance, prohibition of partner of being social, exclusion from financial decisions, repression of partner's voice, contempt for her opinions or close monitoring of her. As batterers are commonly manipulative, their control is not always obvious, and signifying characteristics include ability to convince or twist words, extreme change between kindness and abuse, and comfort with being dishonest.
Perpetrator's Sense of Entitlement/ Self-Center-edness	Among other sources, abuse stems from a batterer's belief that he has rights not belonging to other family members, where the greater this sense of entitlement and in some cases narcissism, the less willing to change with a tendency to use poor reasoning with children. An entitled batterer may use his children as weapons and undervalue the mother's significance, believing his relationship with the children determines their well-being. The expectation of the entitled batterer that family members should cater to his needs is linked to incest perpetration, which can be indicated by a batterer that is demanding, enraged, punishing, deserving of accommodation, possessing of family members, and maintaining of double standards.
Children Used As Weapons Against Mother	The degree to which a batterer has previously used his children as weapons or undermined their mother's authority is a good predictor of his behavior after separation. Important factors include whether the batterer has treated children differently when angry at their mother, encouraged negative beliefs about her, prevented her from attending to a child, made threats involving the children, intensified behavior when she has objected, attempted to divide the family, used children to scare her, threatened to quit his job or allowed non-permissible activities during visitation.

(continued)

Table 14-1. *(continued)*

DIMENSION	DESCRIPTION
Children Being Placed at Risk During Mother's Abuse	A batterer that does not intend to harm his children but that does so in the process is a good predictor of his future poor reasoning, which is evidence that his uncontrolled desire to abuse his victim takes priority over the children's safety and is likely to increase after separation. Important factors are whether he was abusive during the mother's pregnancies, the degree to which the children witnessed his violence, whether he placed a child in danger while throwing objects or trying to reach the mother, if he has humiliated her in front of the children or abandoned responsibilities when angry at her.
Neglectful Parenting	When the batterer's parenting pattern shows a history of neglect, placing his children in danger or minimal involvement, there is increased concern about whether he will protect his children, meet their emotional needs and his reasoning behind wanting contact with the children. When testifying in court, most batterers claim to have been highly involved; however, detailed questions about the children's history can uncover the extent to which he is knowledgeable and compassionate about his children. Batterers, who have abandoned their children in the past or do not currently use the entire time allotted for visitation, sometimes seek custody or expanded visitation, which raises the concern about his commitment and motives.
Refusal to Accept End of Relation-ship with Children's Mother	A batterer unwilling to accept the end of the relationship, especially one who is particularly jealous and possessive, is more dangerous, may be more likely to use children as weapons or expose them to violence of the mother, and is potentially lethal in his violent acts. Important factors include the degree to which the batterer desires retaliation against his victim and his perception that defense of his victim and their children is an act of abuse toward him. The batterer's parenting can also be influenced by his willingness to accept his former partner's right with new relationships, indicated by sudden custody or visitation requests, depression about the separation, threats or warnings about new partners or instilling fear or guilt in the children about the new partner.
Risk for Abduction	Domestic violence is a factor in at least half the cases in which a parent abducts a child, most of which are carried about by fathers or their representatives. Even with no existing threats, the evaluator should be attentive to signs such as passport renewal, attempts to retrieve children's passports, suspicious behavior or sudden travel plans.
Substance Abuse	While substance abusers are not necessarily batterers and most extreme physical abuse does not occur in the context of alcohol abuse, batterers have a higher rate of substance abuse and can therefore be more unpredictable and unwilling to change. More than other batterers, substance abusing batterers are more likely to physically abuse children and are linked with lethality, sexual abuse and reoffending. It is important for an evaluator to know what the batterer has done to seek recovery, how he perceives his addiction, and the details of his treatment plan.

(continued)

Table 14-1. *(continued)*	

DIMENSION	DESCRIPTION
Mental Health History	Though mental illness does not indicate domestic violence, it can cause battering to be more unpredictable and less manageable so that a batterer with mental illness may need extra supervision and require collaboration between the therapist and battering program. When mental illness is less severe, psychotherapy can distract the batterer from addressing abusive behavior and may be used as justification for violent behavior. It is important, therefore, for evaluators to understand that psychological tests are poor indicators of parenting capacity, degree of danger, and battering capability, and therefore should only be used for eliminating psychiatric concerns.

Adapted with permission from Sage Publications Inc.[3]

BACKGROUND ON BATTERER INTERVENTION PROGRAMS

Batterer intervention programs (BIPs) are a form of tertiary prevention (treatment) or intervention programs that have become an integral part of most comprehensive approaches to dealing with the perpetrators of IPV. A variety of conceptual models underpin the currently available BIPs. Many goals have been articulated for these programs, and among the most important are the perpetrator taking accountability for the violence, increased safety for the victims, and a measurable decrease in re-offense rates or recidivism.[24,25] For men who are fathers participating in BIPs, one of the major additional goals would certainly be specifically around the parenting role, and thus safeguarding the physical and emotional integrity of the mother and the children should be prominent.[24]

Through an informal survey of batterer intervention programs, the FVPF learned that though these programs often include information about the effects of violence on children, little attention is otherwise given to the issue of fatherhood. The mandated attendance creates a unique opportunity to reach fathers who have been violent and to provide them with parenting information they would not otherwise receive. This opportunity also exists with supervised visitation programs and other mandated services provided to men who have been violent.

With the recognition of IPV came a myriad of responses to this serious social malady, including the recognition of the havoc this problem inflicts on its victims, their children, and the communities in which they live, as well as the criminal nature to a number of the perpetrator's behaviors in IPV. Thus, with the increasing number of arrests and subsequent prosecutions beginning in the 1980s for the criminal aspects of IPV, perpetrators, primarily men, were being seen in criminal courts throughout the United States.[25] Many victims made it clear that they very much wanted the battering to stop, but having their partners jailed was not necessarily an ideal long-term solution. In order to have the batterer take responsibility for his actions and be held accountable for the violence that he perpetrated but also to provide a vehicle for the behavior to change, BIPs were conceived as a potentially positive or constructive response to IPV that, if successful, would move beyond just a time-limited incarceration.

The effectiveness of BIPs to actually achieve results remains an area of active study, and over time, increasingly better evaluations have emerged. Like any research that deals with complex behaviors, the answers are not crystal clear at this point. Early evaluations that were small and methodologically flawed suggested a reduction in batterer recidivism, but more recent, larger studies call these early findings into question and at best the reduction in battering appears to be small.

However, some serious research conducted by Gondolf suggests that the long-term, positive effects of BIPs can be very significant.[26] For 48 months, he studied 840 men who completed BIPs and found that 52% did not reassault their partners; however, an additional 26% reassaulted their partners once over the 4-year follow-up period.

Additionally, no specific program model appears to be superior when compared with other credible models in operation.[27] According to the National Institute of Justice, in its 2003 report entitled "Batterer Intervention Programs: Where do we go from here?" the research questions need to be refined and more focused for us to be able to answer the initial question of effectiveness[25]:

The field of batterer intervention is still in its infancy, and much remains to be learned. Rather than asking whether BIPs work, a more productive question may be which programs work best for which batterers under which circumstances, a decidedly more complex question. If this approach is adopted, improved theories of battering will need to precede new responses that will need to be tested. If differential sentencing is incorporated into the criminal justice system, procedures will need to be developed to ensure that it is carried out fairly. As BIPs are a relatively new response to a critical social problem, it is too early to abandon the concept. It is also too early to believe that we have all the answers. Research and evaluation supported by NIJ will continue to add to our growing knowledge of responses to battering, including batterer intervention programs.

In the 1998 Department of Justice report summarizing the evaluation of BIPs nationwide, one of the key actions identified for criminal justice professionals engaged with operating and overseeing BIPs was, "Be Alert to the Risks to Children in Domestically Abusive Households." Toward that end, professionals working with men who batter were warned of the danger that children may find themselves in, and these professionals were challenged to keep the needs of the children and their safety prominent in their minds as services were arranged for the entire family. This is a particularly important "alert" for all of us to keep in mind when the man who perpetrates IPV is a father and wants to stay involved in raising his children. According to research presented in this report, between 30% to 50% of men who batter share children with their victims. Thus, the care and upbringing of the children could become another area of control and manipulation such as threats of or actual violence against the children, criticism of the mother's parenting style and ability, and custody threats (in situations of joint custody, the ongoing contact may permit intimidation and actual attacks, as well as the threat of new action to attain full custody to the exclusion of the mother).[24]

FATHERING AFTER VIOLENCE AS A PART OF BATTERER INTERVENTION

The FVPF launched the FAV initiative in 2002 in a partnership with a consortium of Boston-based providers and with generous support from the Doris Duke Charitable Foundation. The goal of the project was to develop strategies and interventions to help fathers understand the impact of their behaviors on their children and on their relationship with their children. The FVPF's partners were the Dorchester Community Roundtable, the Child Witness to Violence Project at Boston Medical Center, and 3 BIPs: Common Purpose, Emerge, and Roxbury Comprehensive Community Health Services. The FVPF decided to work with batterer intervention programs because their services target men who have used violence, and with a child witness to violence program because its primary clients are the children who have been hurt by that violence. Fathering After Violence components of BIPs are fundamentally based on the belief that some men who have used violence can take responsibility for their behavior and its impact on the women and children around them and in fact become more respectful and supportive as parents and partners regardless of their level of access or type of custody.[28]

As with any intervention involving abusive men, their partners, and children, FVPF was well aware that there are risks in implementing this project. As stated earlier in this chapter, the organization's top priority is the safety of victims of family violence, and it believes that the voices of nonoffending mothers should always guide any work with abusive men trying to get access to their children. Courts, officers, and IPV experts need to responsibly assess whether contact is appropriate and under which circumstances.

It is also true that many men who use violence continue to live with their families and have uninterrupted legal or illegal contact with their children and that fathers stay present in the lives of many children even when those children never have formal contact. The FVPF is committed to finding new ways to keep men accountable and invite them to change and repair the damage they have done.

In the beginning, the FAV initiative concentrated on gathering extensive information from focus groups and interviews with mothers who have experienced IPV, fathers who have been abusive, and IPV experts and service providers. Based on all of this information, a series of exercises and policy and practice recommendations for BIPs were developed. These documents are available for downloading on the FVPF Web site (http://www.endabuse.org).

Clearly, men in batterer intervention groups are at different stages of change and some, in fact, will not stop their abuse after intervention. The FVPF wanted to be careful about not encouraging contact between fathers and their children when it would not be legal or appropriate. In the implementation guide for using the BIP exercises, it is emphasized that programs and facilitators must be at all times aware of the legal restrictions that each man of the program has and be very clear that it is never acceptable for a father to pursue contact with their children when there are orders of protection in place.

The FVPF designed the exercises described below in a way that would not involve any direct actions between fathers and their children or encourage father contact when it is not desirable. Therefore, all batterer intervention program participants can benefit from the exercises, regardless of their level of involvement with their children. In fact, the exercises can be beneficial even for fathers who have no contact with their children. Men who are not fathers can equally participate.

Exercises for Use in Batterer Intervention Groups

The FAV exercises were developed in Spanish and English and piloted in 6 groups by the 3 Boston-area batterer intervention programs. Two of the groups were primarily African American, 1 was for Spanish-speaking participants, 1 was predominantly European American, and 2 were racially mixed.

The project's intention was to provide maximum flexibility of implementation. The exercises could be used in any BIP based on an educational or psychoeducational mode of intervention. They could be utilized as a group or individually, in sequence or interspersed with other lessons. Because of the advanced nature of the materials, the FVPF made a strong recommendation that these exercises should not be implemented in the first few weeks of intervention. In Boston, they were all piloted in "second stage" groups, after participants have had a minimum of 8 sessions.

Empathy Exercise

The first exercise was designed to help participants see their abuse through their children's eyes and develop a better understanding of how children are affected by it. It is called the "Empathy Exercise." The facilitators started the exercise by showing a series of 5 overheads with actual drawings made by children about their fathers. The drawings were created by school children in Mexico, responding to the question "How do I see my father?" They were compiled as part of a project by the Men's Collective for Equal Relationships (CORIAC) in Mexico City, who generously shared them with the FVPF for this initiative. The drawings eloquently and movingly depicted both positive and negative modeling by fathers. The negative drawings included pictures of a father as a devil, a sinister figure over-shadowing a devastated mother, and Dr. Jekyll and Mr. Hyde–like cartoons. The positive ones depicted a father as a superhero and another helping his son climb the "mountain of life." **(Figures 14-1 to 14-5)**.

After having a group discussion about the drawings, the facilitators asked the participants to use paper and crayons and draw their own pictures depicting how they thought their children might

Figure 14-1 to 14-3. Images drawn by children of their fathers' roles in their lives.

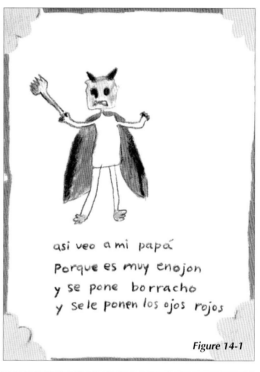

Figure 14-1

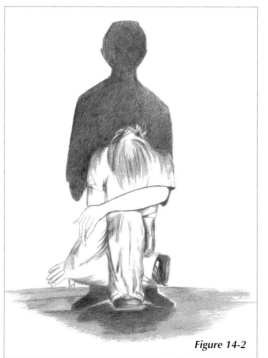

Figure 14-2

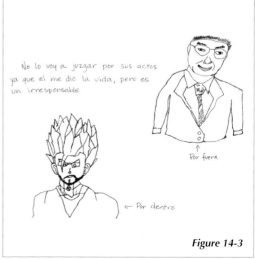

Figure 14-3

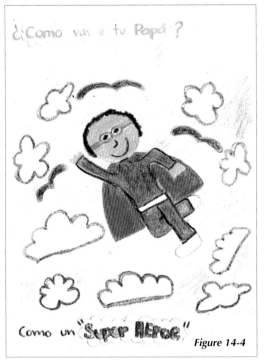

¿Como vas a tu Papá?

Como un "Super Heroe"

Figure 14-4

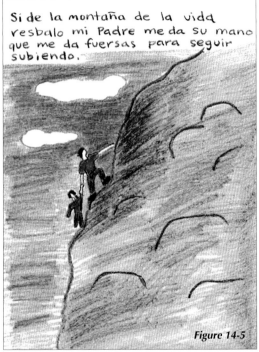

Si de la montaña de la vida resbalo mi Padre me da su mano que me da fuersas para seguir subiendo.

Figure 14-5

Figure 14-4 and 14-5. *Images drawn by children of their fathers' roles in their lives.*

see them as fathers, especially after witnessing an incident of violence. The exercise concluded with a discussion of the ways in which participants believed they might have hurt their children.

Modeling Exercise

The second exercise aimed to encourage participants to reflect on some of the positive and negative behaviors they learned from their own fathers or father figures and examine the kind of model they have been for their children. It is called the "Modeling Exercise." On implementation, men were asked to write down both bad and good examples of behaviors they witnessed from their fathers in modeling respect for their fathers' partners or ex-partners.

After sharing their examples with other men, the participants were asked to repeat the exercise, but this time thinking about ways in which they have given bad and good examples to their own children in showing respect for their children's mothers. Then they proceeded to discuss whether they thought there was a connection between their behaviors and that of their fathers. The exercise closed with a homework assignment in which the men were asked to commit to choose one act of respect towards the children's mothers that they would perform in the following 4 weeks to become a better model for their children

These actions were chosen with guidance from the facilitators to ensure that inappropriate contact was not encouraged under the guise of "respect." Furthermore, actions that did not involve any verbal or physical contact were discussed as options. Facilitators kept track of the actions each subsequent week as the men checked in to report on their progress.

Examples of the actions included fathers talking respectfully about their children's mothers, being less argumentative, being more patient, and controlling their temper.

Michael's Story Exercise

The third exercise was created to help men understand some aspects of the reparative framework between children and their fathers who have renounced the use of violence. For this exercise, the FVPF produced a compact disc recording about the story of a real man (Michael or Miguel) who was previously interviewed for the project. In the first part of the recording, Michael told about his growing up with an abusive father and not being able to ever heal the relationship because of the father's denial and continued abusive behavior. In the second part, the same man talked about his own abusive behavior, his struggle to overcome it, and the difficult journey toward repairing his relationship with his own children.

The exercise opened with the playing of the first part of the story, followed by a brainstorm by the group about what Michael's father had done wrong and about what he could have done better. The facilitators emphasized key points about the reparative framework, including the following:

— In order to start healing a relationship, the offender has to stop the abuse and begin modeling positive behaviors.

— Denial and minimization can be very damaging to children.

— Accepting the consequences of one's behavior means more than doing time in jail or being on probation. Men have to take responsibility in front of their families and communities.

The exercise ended by playing the second part of Michael's story, in which he talks about his struggles and successes in healing his relationship with his children. A facilitated discussion followed concentrating on the following ideas:

— Healing the relationship between an abusive parent and his children is a very slow and difficult process.

— The process has to take place on the children's terms and timing. The offender should not and cannot force the pace of the process.

— Victims and witnesses of family violence need to be listened to and validated for a long period of time, often over many years. The offender should not attempt to "turn the page."

Staff Training

A fundamental element for the successful implementation of the exercises was a comprehensive training for the batterer intervention program staff. The training was an opportunity to invite all staff (not only group facilitators) to discuss the program's intent and limitations. It also allowed staff to express their apprehensions, hopes, and ideas about the subject matter, understand the theoretical framework and rationale behind each exercise, and explore the cultural context in which fathering takes place.

Key training activities included an overview of the project and a brainstorm of potential benefits and challenges, an exercise to help staff understand the cultural context of fathering, a detailed presentation of the reparative framework, and a comprehensive review of each exercise. Resulting from unforeseen circumstances, the staff of the 3 batterer intervention programs received different amounts of training prior to implementing the exercises. After reviewing the evaluation data, it became clear that the sites that received more training were more successful in achieving the exercises' goals. Better trained programs tended to have a higher rate of participation in the exercises.

Cultural Context

Introducing the topic of fathering in batterer intervention programs offers an invaluable opportunity to explore issues of culture and oppression both among the program staff and with group members. Traditionally, BIPs have avoided dealing with these issues because of an understandable fear of giving participants one more chance to justify or rationalize their abuse. However, the reluctance of BIPs to deal with these topics has decreased their credibility and effectiveness in many communities. It is impractical to isolate one form of oppression (eg, sexism, gender violence) and totally ignore others (eg, racism, poverty). A skillful facilitator should be able to invite men to talk about their own experience of oppression in the context of stopping their own violence.

Batterer intervention programs have the responsibility to start understanding the role of culture in the treatment of abusive men. Racism and oppression are systematic ways to dehumanize certain populations. This dehumanization can take various forms, and one is to deprive men of their ability to protect and provide for their families. This is most obvious in the cases of slavery and genocide, but it has been perpetuated in other forms of oppression, such as colonization, discrimination, marginalization, and poverty. These injustices have had and continue to have profound consequences in the fathering abilities and styles of men of color. As Fleck-Henderson and Areán state in the FAV Implementation Guide[1]:

> [If] culture and oppression are ignored, these elements will work against the intervention. [To] stop violence in a given cultural group, the intervention has to be based on values generated by that community, rather than the dominant culture. If participants perceive that the intervention is being imposed from outside their cultural framework, they might interpret it as one more way in which the dominant culture is trying to oppress them by telling them what to do. We run the risk that they will see family violence prevention as a 'white' issue and that we just want them to be more 'white.' BIPs have to make a concerted effort to create a context worthy of the participants' trust. This necessarily involves recognition of and respect for their cultures and the structural barriers they face in establishing a constructive family life.

Examining the Impact

The evaluation component of the FAV initiative was conducted in partnership with the Dorchester Community Roundtable and Dr. Ann Fleck-Henderson and her colleagues from the Simmons College School of Social Work in Boston, Massachusetts. The evaluators employed multiple methods of data collection to explore the impact of the program. The 60 participants of the project completed evaluation forms after each group session. In-depth interviews were conducted with 3 randomly selected men and their partners (separately), 1 pair from each participating program. Short questionnaires were also used to document the reactions of women whose partners went through this curriculum (the project required that attempts be made to contact each partner in order to inform her about the new curriculum and learn how she felt about the increased attention to fatherhood). The questionnaire probed the woman's reactions to the curriculum, made inquiry to the nature of relationship between the man and her children, and informed her of local resources for herself and her children. Lastly, a debriefing session was held with the group facilitators to hear their experiences after the implementation period was completed.

Overall, the evaluation yielded positive results from the standpoint of batterer intervention group facilitators. The staff consistently reported positive experiences with the project and increased engagement with the men. The facilitators' feedback on the exercises was invaluable, allowing the training and curriculum to be modified to be more user-friendly.

Feedback from the men revealed a range of responses. While some men clearly demonstrated an increased sense of realism respective to their relationships with their children, others remained unable to see a problem or demonstrated a significant lack of understanding of what it takes to build or rebuild relationships with their children after violence. Although increased knowledge of the reparative framework was evident in only a minority of the responses from men, it appears other important lessons were learned about the effects of violence on children, particularly the intergenerational transmission of family violence, the need to change, and the value of seeking help.

Data collected on the empathy and modeling exercises suggested a continuum of acceptance of responsibility for hurting children and their role in correcting the harm. While some men referred to the need to change their own behavior, other men seem to refer to the negative effects of "fighting" without mention of their own role. The men's responses upon viewing the children's drawings from Mexico suggested that about 2 out of 3 men understood well that children had strong feelings about their father's use of violence, while the other third of men stated they were unchanged by the exercise.

Some of the comments the men made in reaction to the exercise included: "The drawings the children made show it's necessary for a father to change his ways of acting," "Makes you think about yourself and if you need to change," "I want to see how I can get my son to understand me without yelling," and "I would never want my kids to look at me in a bad way." The participants' feedback on the exercises in the pilot project gave us some important data to understand some of the differences among men who use violence. The majority of the men were most affected by the "feelings" children had and the least influenced by "the acts of violence" the children saw. Many of the men's comments also indicated some resistance to the pain illustrated in the children's pictures even when their comments indicated increased empathy for children.

Finally, although efforts were made to reach every partner of the men in the groups, only about half were contacted successfully. Of those contacted, the reaction to including child-focused exercises in men's groups was unanimously positive.

BACKGROUND ON SUPERVISED VISITATION PROGRAMS

Supervised Visitation (SV) programs are designed to provide a physical, safe space for children to have contact with parents who have been accused of perpetrating physical or sexual child abuse or IPV. Under close professional observation, the offending parent or parents can see, interact, and play with the children in a way that minimizes the possibility of creating further harm. Many SV centers also offer "safe exchanges" services, functioning as a neutral place where custodial parents can drop off their children to be picked up by noncustodial parents for off-site, unsupervised visits.

The first SV programs were created in the 1970s primarily to serve the needs of families involved in the child welfare system. The programs were originally designed to monitor family visits when there had been prior child abuse or neglect and there was a question regarding the safety of reunification. Since then, SV programs have proliferated in the United States, and some have evolved over time to include divorce cases and situations involving IPV.

Today, visitation centers across the country vary in terms of their resources, functions, and attention to IPV. On one end of the continuum, all programs work to ensure that a visiting parent and a child have a safe visit for an hour or two. As the continuum increases, programs strive to build on a foundation of safety, protect children from further harm, and enrich the quality of the child–parent relationship. At the other end of the continuum, programs practice therapeutic visitation, a modality that first came into use in the 1980s with dependency court cases. In therapeutic visitation cases, courts order both therapy and visits as a part of a family's service plan within the child protection context.

Not all SV centers have historically seen the importance of integrating the safety needs of all members of a family. Some have argued that to help victims of IPV will put them in an advocacy role and, as a consequence, they will lose their credibility as a neutral player for children. Many centers pride themselves as being on the side of children and staying out of the marital or partner dynamics. However, advocates for battered women have argued that this approach can compromise the safety of adult victims and, therefore, also put their children in danger.

In response to these concerns, the federal legislation known as the Violence Against Women Act (VAWA) directed the US Office of Violence Against Women (OVW) to establish the Safe Havens Supervised Visitation and Safe Exchange Program in 2000. This grant program supports approximately 60 SV centers across the country to "provide an opportunity for communities to support supervised visitation and safe exchange of children, by and between parents, in situations involving domestic violence, child abuse, sexual assault, or stalking."[29]

From 2002 to date, the Safe Havens Program has funded more than 100 grantee communities, with the central goal of helping the SV centers make their highest priority the safety of both the victim parent and the children. These programs see their role as ensuring that all victims of a family are safe during the visitation process. Although all SV programs have policies and procedures to ensure the safety of the children, Safe Havens Visitation Centers often have additional security measures to protect the adult victims. For example, center staff understand that some abusive men use visitation as a tool to further control the mother. Some protective measures include metal detectors to ensure that weapons are not brought into the building and separate entrances to avoid victims and their abusive ex-partners "bumping into each other" in parking lots and waiting rooms. Policies ensure that center staff member will intervene if the abuser tries to ask the child questions about the mothers life (ie, where does she live, where is she working).

There is virtually no research on the impact of supervised visitation programs on family safety and well being. Informed practice and common sense show that professional supervised visitation and safe exchanges have the capacity to be safer than informal systems in cases of significant IPV and child abuse.

To learn more about user perceptions of Safe Havens SV centers, the FVPF organized a series of focus groups in 2005. Among other findings, this qualitative research revealed that abused mothers who use the centers expressed great appreciation that both their needs and those of their children were taken into account by the centers. This approach greatly impacted the amount of trust that mothers placed in the centers.[30]

FATHERING AFTER VIOLENCE IN SUPERVISED VISITATION CENTERS

Established practices at Safe Havens visitation centers have placed great emphasis on rules and regulations for abusers to ensure the safety of both adult mothers and their children. These rules are obviously essential, but they have become almost the only structure in place to deal with abusive men in SV centers. In 2003, the Office on Violence Against Women became interested in supporting the development of other strategies for engaging abusive fathers in SV centers.

At that time, the FVPF received funding from OVW to look at the possible application of the FAV framework in the context of Supervised Visitation and to provide targeted technical assistance to 4 Safe Havens visitation centers across the United States. The 4 sites chosen were Advocates for Family Peace in Grand Rapids, Minnesota; the City of Kent Supervised Visitation Center in Washington state; the San Mateo County Family Visitation Center in California; and the Walnut Avenue Women's Center in Santa Cruz, California. The YWCA Visitation Centers in Springfield and Northampton, Massachusetts, were originally part of the collaborative and contributed important lessons to this project.

One of the early discoveries of the project was that the majority of abusive fathers who use visitation centers have neither been involved with the criminal justice system nor attended a batterer intervention program. Likewise, men who attend BIPs rarely use SV centers. This is due to the fact that BIPs receive their referrals primarily from criminal courts, while SV centers receive referrals from family or civil courts.

It became evident that visitation centers were often the only institutions available for abusers to begin a process of accountability for their behavior and to offer them the possibility to renounce their abuse. By starting to focus on the fathers' abuse and its impact on their children, the centers could create opportunities to assess their violence and control, as well as their potential for change.

The FVPF worked closely with its partners to refine the FAV principles and to design, redesign, and test innovative implementation plans for working with fathers, including the use of universal messages, orientation sessions, nonviolence groups, and a multicultural mentoring project. Some of the main lessons that emerged included the importance of always keeping the safety of victims and accountability of perpetrators in the forefront; the significance of supporting mothers who use the centers; the need to understand organizational readiness to carry out this work; the consequence of using effective assessment tools for families; the relevance of having a solid IPV and cultural analysis; and the value of undertaking community mapping and creating true collaborations with other providers.

It seemed logical that if SV centers had the opportunity to take steps toward the goal of helping abusive men become better fathers and ex-partners, they might want to explore such a possibility. Any improvement in the fathers' positive interactions with the children was likely to be welcomed by most mothers. Furthermore, a comprehensive response in conjunction with batterer intervention might assist fathers in renouncing their violence and other forms of abuse and, therefore, enhance the safety and well being of their children and ex-partners.

Program Development
Each of the Safe Havens sites was able to identify FAV implementation plans that suited their own centers and constituencies. The various implementation plans are described below.

Universal Messages
Every site was able to incorporate universal messages into their programs. These were educational materials or scripted verbal messages that could be broadly targeted for all fathers who use the centers. The messages were designed to be constructive and strengths-based and to promote models of healthy, nonoppressive fatherhood.

As part of this strategy, the FVPF produced a 15-minute DVD to be used as an educational outreach tool for non-custodial fathers who have used violence. The FVPF worked very closely with John Badalament, a filmmaker from Boston with a proven track record for creating video educational materials in the fatherhood field. The product was *Something My Father Would Do*, a documentary film that followed the stories of 3 men who grew up with violent fathers and had to wrestle with their own choices around fatherhood and intimate partnership. The first vignette was about a young African American man who became emotionally abusive with his girlfriend in college and early on made a conscious decision to renounce his violence. The second man was a European American father with a long history of abuse towards his wife and children. He told the story of how he sought treatment and began a process of healing his relationship with his partner and their children, who are also interviewed in the film. The third story was about a Latino father and firefighter who eloquently described his decision to model his fathering opposite to what he had learned from his own father. It is an inspiring tale that also involved the participation of his wife and children.

The DVD quickly became a very popular product, not only for SV centers, but also for practitioners from many different fields who want to help men stop their violence and be better role models for children. These included child welfare, batterer's intervention, criminal and civil justice, home visitation, healthy marriage, child and adult mental health, and parenting and fatherhood programs.

The FVPF also produced a series of 4 posters to complement the messages of the documentary film. Like the DVD, the posters were developed primarily for Safe Havens grantees, but they have been used in a number of professional settings that deal with men and fatherhood. The posters were designed to invite men to think about their legacies as fathers. The messages were based on a combination of open-ended questions and statements about healthy fatherhood.

All 4 posters depicted images of fathers and their children having positive interactions. There were 3 posters in English, 1 with a European American family, another with an African American family and 1 more with a Native American family, produced in collaboration with Mending the Sacred Hoop, the Native American National IPV Technical Assistance Project. The fourth poster was in Spanish, showing a Latino family.

Fathering Groups
Three of the Safe Havens sites chose to implement educational groups for fathers who use the centers to teach them about the effects of intimate partner violence on children, constructive alternatives to violence, and positive parenting skills. The groups were designed to help participants improve their parenting skills, develop empathy for their children, and think about the legacy they wanted to leave for them as fathers.

One of the sites, Advocates for Family Peace (AFP) in Minnesota, was able to implement a comprehensive program for fathers who were ordered to use the visitation center. From the beginning, AFP decided that if fathers were to participate in their new fathering groups, they needed to complete first their Intervention Group for Men (a BIP). Judges who wanted to mandate men to the fathers' group understood and agreed that the offenders had to go through a process that included a comprehensive intake, 20 sessions of batterer intervention, 1 individual aftercare session, a second intake for the fathers' group, 8 sessions on parenting, and an exit interview. As a result of this progression, the facilitators observed that most men who participated in the fathers' group had overcome the initial denial of their abusive behavior and were able to discuss the deepest fears and desires in their lives. Some were able to talk about their painful childhoods for the first time. This created an emotional opening that the facilitators could use sometimes to deepen their relationships with the men and to help them make the connection between the abuse they suffered in their own childhoods and the violence they were inflicting on their own families.

Furthermore, the group leaders were able to corroborate the FAV thesis that abusive men can be more empathetic as fathers than as intimate partners or ex-partners. In one case, one of the group participants who had been violent both with his partner and with his son was able to feel great remorse and take some important reparative steps with his child, while remaining minimally empathetic toward his partner.

Advocates for Family Peace had already integrated some of the FAV exercises in their BIP curriculum, as part of their comprehensive approach. The fathers' group built upon these exercises, covering topics such as defining healthy fatherhood, domestic violence and fatherhood, and expanding on the reparative process.

Mentoring

A multicultural mentoring program was piloted by the FPVF's project partners in California, the San Mateo County Family Visitation Center, and the Walnut Avenue Women's Center (WAWC) in Santa Cruz. Both organizations serve a significant percentage of Latino families, and the original idea behind the project was to train Latino men from the community to serve as informal mentors for the visiting fathers who use the center. The mentors would sit in the visiting parents' waiting room before and after the visit and maybe even observe some of the visits. The goal was to offer the visiting fathers role models from their own community, with whom they could develop relationships of trust and responsibility.

The implementation of this project was more complicated than originally anticipated. The initial idea was to invite men from the community as volunteers, but this proved impractical because it became clear that the mentors would need extensive training and supervision. Eventually, both agencies decided to hire men (1 each) as part-time employees who would also serve as monitors. Once both men had received extensive training on IPV, they started serving their dual function of monitors and mentors. The traditional tasks of the monitor, including making sure that the center rules are followed and observing the visits, were enhanced by the men's role of informal mentors.

As mentors, they were able to use the pre-visit and post-visit waiting times to develop supportive relationships with the visiting fathers without compromising the safety of the children and their mothers. Although neither of the men had ever worked with abusive men before, both of them were able to develop their own style of intervention that balanced supporting the fathers with challenging their negative behaviors.

Enhanced Collaboration With Other Agencies

All Safe Havens sites committed to create stronger collaborations with other agencies. In particular, they were able to partner with batterer intervention programs to provide better services to center users, including more emphasis on positive fathering, understanding the effects of violence on children, and developing empathy towards witnesses and victims of IPV.

Training

All the partner sites also embarked in intensive training about how to work with abusive fathers. The City of Kent, Washington, implemented a series of half-day trainings that included topics such as the impact of violence on children, tactics of fathers who use violence, positive engagement with men who batter, using culture to work with fathers, de-escalation of potentially dangerous situations, and motivational interviewing.

As they opened a brand new center, staff members benefited from the trainings and regular debriefings and, according to the director, "were able to be very intentional about working to build relationships with the parents using the center. They found that not all men were interested in changing, but were able to offer support and compassion for those who were."

IMPLICATIONS FOR HEALTH CARE PROVIDERS

This book proposes that health care providers can play an important role in supporting and helping victims and child witnesses of IPV. The authors of this chapter believe that clinicians can also be part of a system that engages offenders to help them change their abusive behavior while holding them accountable at the same time.

In Chapter 13, "Intimate Partner Violence: Identification, Treatment, and Associations With Men's Health," Cronholm and colleagues report that a significant number of perpetrators of IPV disclose their abuse to primary care clinicians (13% of all male patients, according to 1 study)[1]. They also emphasize the importance of informal help seeking in both victims and perpetrators.

Health care providers can use their influence and access to invite men who batter to think about the negative consequences of their behavior and, in some cases, open the door for these men to get professional help to change.

The authors of this chapter concur with the ground rules and inquiry techniques for clinicians dealing with IPV that Cronholm and colleagues propose in Chapter 13. As stated many times before, the safety of the victims and their children always has to be at the forefront of any IPV intervention. The medical principle of "first do not harm" clearly applies to cases of family violence.

Another important lesson of FAV is that anyone who has contact with men who batter can make use of universal messages to invite these men to change. The FAV has developed messages that specifically deal with fatherhood and the effects of violence on children. These messages have been used by batterer intervention practitioners, visitation center staff, child protection workers, law enforcement and judges, and fatherhood programs facilitators. Although there is not empirical evidence that they work, many professionals have reported using them successfully to engage some fathers in getting help to stop their abusive behavior. These messages can be used in the context of a medical visit.

Here are some examples of universal messages:

— Fathers are important for children. **You** are really important to your children.

— What kind of relationship do you currently have with your children?

— What kind of relationship do you want to have?

— What are you worried about?

— What do you think your children are worried about?

— How do you think violence at home affects your children?

— Your behavior has a lifelong impact on your children. It's never too late to turn it around.

— You have the power to change things for them.

— How do you want your children to remember you?

— They will carry memories of you and your actions forever.

— You are an example for your children in everything you do.

— What kind of emotional legacy do you want to leave for them?

— It's never too late to change your behavior.

— When you hurt your partner, you also hurt your children.

CONCLUSION

For men who abuse their partners, the ideal of fatherhood can be used to change their negative attitudes and behaviors. Although these men sometimes remain apathetic or negative in their views toward women, they often do care for the children and want to serve as a positive role model. The FAV initiative has worked with batterer intervention programs and supervised visitation to use fatherhood as an approach to help men make the changes they need to make in their lives to stop their abuse. Despite the appeal of father involvement, the safety and well being of the children involved and their caregivers needs to remain front and center in the ongoing discussion around BIPs. Real change is required on the part of the men involved so that the reality of ideal fatherhood can come about and children can experience the care and concern of a father in circumstances that are non-violent and safe.

REFERENCES

1. Fleck-Henderson A, Areán, JC. *Breaking the Cycle: Fathering After Violence. Curriculum Guidelines and Tools for Batterer Intervention Programs.* San Francisco, Calif: Family Violence Prevention Fund; 2004.

2. Holden GW, Ritchie KL. Linking extreme marital discord, child rearing, and child behavior problems: evidence from battered women. *Child Development.* 1991;62:311-327.

3. Bancroft L, Silverman JG. *The Batterer as Parent: Addressing the Impact of Domestic Violence on Family Dynamics.* Thousand Oaks, Calif: Sage Publications; 2002.

4. Sullivan CM, Nguyen H, Allen N, Bybee D, Juras J. Beyond searching for deficits: evidence that physically and emotionally abused women are nurturing parents. *J Emotional Abuse.* 2000;2:51-71.

5. Sternberg KJ, Lamb ME, Dawud-Noursi S. Using multiple informants to understand domestic violence and its effects. In: Holden GW, Geffner R, Jouriles EN, eds. *Children Exposed to Marital Violence: Theory, Research, and Applied Issue.* Washington, DC: American Psychological Association; 1998:121-156.

6. Peled E. Parenting by men who abuse women: issues and dilemmas. *Br J Soc Work.* 2000;30:25-36.

7. McAlister-Groves B, Van Horn P, Lieberman A. Deciding on fathers' involvement in their children's treatment after domestic violence. In: Edleson J, Williams O, eds. *Fathering by Men Who Batter.* New York: Oxford University Press; 2007:65-84.

8. Atchison G, Autry A, Davis L, Mitchell-Clark K. *Conversations with Women of Color Who Have Experienced Domestic Violence Regarding Working with Men to End Violence.* San Francisco, Calif: Family Violence Prevention Fund; 2002.

9. Tubbs C, Williams O. Shared parenting after abuse: battered mothers' perspectives on parenting after dissolution of a relationship. In: Edleson J, Williams O, eds. *Fathering by Men Who Batter.* New York: Oxford University Press; 2007:19-44.

10. Peled E, Perel G. (2007). A conceptual framework for intervening in the parenting of men who batter. In: Edleson J, Williams O, eds. *Fathering by Men Who Batter.* New York: Oxford University Press; 2007:85-101.

11. Bent-Goodle T, Williams O. Fathers voices in parenting and violence. In: Edleson J, Williams O, eds. *Fathering by Men Who Batter.* New York: Oxford University Press; 2007:32-35.

12. Litton Fox G, Sayers J, Bruce C. Beyond bravado: redemption and rehabilitation in the fathering accounts of men who batter. *Marriage Fam Rev.* 2001;32(3-4):137-163.

13. Mandel D. Highlights from National Study on Batterers' Perceptions of Their Children's Exposure to the Violence and Abuse. *Issues in Family Violence.* 2003;5. Available at: http://www.endingviolence.com/newsletters/sum2003natstudy.php. Accessed September 12, 2007.

14. Fleck-Henderson A. *The Fathering After Violence Evaluation Report.* San Francisco, Calif: Family Violence Prevention Fund; 2004.

15. Farrant F. *Out for Good: Resettlement Needs of Young Men in Prison.* London: Howard League for Penal Reform; 2006.

16. Lamb ME. Fathers and child development: an introductory overview and guide. In: Lamb ME, ed. *The Role of the Father in Child Development.* New York: Wiley; 1997: 309-313.

17. Pleck EH, Pleck JH. Fatherhood ideals in the United States: historical dimensions. In: Lamb ME, ed. *The Role of the Father in Child Development.* New York: Wiley; 1997: 1-18.

18. Sanders HA. *Daddy, We Need You Now! A Primer on African-American Male Socialization.* Lanham, Md: University Press of America; 1996.

19. Daly KJ. Reshaping fatherhood: Finding the models. In: Marsiglio W, ed. *Fatherhood: Contemporary Theory, Research, and Social Policy.* Thousand Oaks, Calif: Sage Publications; 1995: 21-40.

20. Dubowitz H, Black MM, Cox CE, et al. Father involvement and children's functioning at age 6 years: a multi-site study. *Child Maltreatment.* 2001;6:300-309.

21. Lamb ME. Male roles in families at-risk: the ecology of child maltreatment. *Child Maltreatment.* 2001;6:310-313.

22. Marshall DB, English DJ, Stewart AJ. The effects of fathers or father figures on child behavioral problems in families referred to child protective services. *Child Maltreatment.* 2001;6:290-299.

23. Kelly JB. Children's adjustment in conflicted marriage and divorce: a decade review of research. *J Acad Child Adolesc Psychiatry.* 2000;39:963-973.

24. Healey K, Smith C, O'Sullivan C. *Batterer Intervention: program approaches and criminal justice strategies.* Washington, DC: National Institute of Justice, US Department of Justice; 1998. http://www.ncjrs.gov/pdffiles/168638.pdf. Accessed June 12, 2008.

25. Jackson, S, Feder L, Frode DR, Davis RC, Maxwell CD, Taylor BG. *Batterer Intervention Programs: where do we go from here?* Washington, DC: National Institute of Justice, US Department of Justice; 2003. http://www.ncjrs.gov/pdffiles1/nij/195079.pdf. Accessed June 12, 2008.

26. Gondolf EW. *Batterers Intervention Systems.* Thousand Oaks, Calif: Sage Publications; 2002.

27. Austin J, Dankwort J. A Review of Standards for Batterer Intervention Programs. National Resource on Domestic Violence. http://new.vawnet.org/category/Main_Doc.php?docid=393. Accessed June 12, 2008.

28. Areán JC, Davis L. Working with fathers in batterer intervention programs: lessons from the Fathering After Violence project. In: Edleson J, Williams O, eds. *Fathering by Men Who Batter.* New York: Oxford University Press;2007:118-130.

29. Office of Violence Against Women, United States Department of Justice. *Safe Havens: Supervised Visitation and Safe Exchange Grant Program.* Available at: http://www.usdoj.gov/ovw/safehaven_desc.htm. Accessed September 29, 2006.

30. Family Violence Prevention Fund. *Focus Groups with Women in Visitation Centers.* Unpublished manuscript. San Francisco, Calif; 2005.

Chapter 15

Looking Ahead: The Public Health Approach to Intimate Partner Violence Prevention

Michelle Teti, DrPH
Mariana Chilton, PhD
Angelo P. Giardino, MD, PhD, MPH, FAAP*

The public health approach offers new possibilities in the effort to prevent intimate partner violence (IPV) and its deleterious consequences. Intimate partner violence has been conceptualized in various ways, and the numerous terms used to describe violence, including domestic violence, battering, and abuse, have different connotations to different readers. In this chapter, the term IPV is used to describe physical, sexual, or psychological harm inflicted by a current or former partner.[1] Intimate partner violence occurs on a continuum ranging from one hit to chronic and severe battering.[1] Violence occurs against men and in same-sex relationships,[2] but the focus in this chapter is on IPV embedded in a general pattern of relationship power and control, perpetrated by men against women.[3,4] Intimate partner violence is an extreme manifestation of gender inequity and an example of one of the numerous ways that social inequality results in concrete harm to health.

Extreme forms of IPV harm victims' immediate and long-term physical and mental health, hindering their opportunities to reach their potential throughout their lifetime. Victims of abuse are more likely to hurt others, creating a dangerous cycle of victimization and perpetration.[2] The individual and community costs of IPV are extraordinary and include billions of dollars in direct and indirect medical costs and lost productivity. Violence is pervasive and overwhelming, but it is neither acceptable nor inevitable. It is essential to use a public health approach to understand IPV, because this approach highlights the fact that IPV is a preventable behavior choice.[5]

The Institute of Medicine describes public health as "what society does collectively to [ensure] the conditions for people to be healthy."[6] Specifically, the mission of the public health system in the United States is to preserve, promote, and improve health and well being and prevent disease, injury, and disability.[7] The basic responsibilities of public health include preventing dangerous health concerns; assessing the extent of existing health problems; and designing policies and providing resources to foster community empowerment so that communities can solve health concerns once they are identified.[7] Preventing and responding to IPV is a primary public health goal, because the impact of IPV on the nation's physical and mental health is astounding.

* The authors wish to thank Mary Ann Nkansa for her assistance with the research and references for this chapter.

As an example of the impact of IPV, a sizable body of research demonstrates a link between IPV and 8 of 10 leading health indicators in *Healthy People 2010*. *Healthy People 2010* is a public health initiative that sets general prevention goals for the nation by creating objectives to reduce the harm of the most significant health problems. *Healthy People 2010* identified 10 leading health indicators to measure the health of the United States from 2000 to 2010.[8] Intimate partner violence is a significant risk factor for chronic health problems and risky health behaviors, including obesity, smoking, substance abuse, risky sexual behaviors, poor mental health, violent injuries, low immunization rates, and decreased access to health care.[9]

The public health approach to preventing IPV is characterized by 4 steps. These are outlined in **Table 15-1**[2,5,10-12] and detailed in the remainder of the chapter. The public health approach has resulted in dramatic health successes that span from the eradication of small pox to the prevention of motor vehicle crash injuries.[10] This approach to IPV prevention represents a shift in the way society views and addresses violence, from focusing on reacting to the problem to altering the conditions that *cause* violence.[12] Several key public health principles characterize this approach, including:

— An emphasis on preventing IPV before it occurs; understanding and altering the social, behavior, and environmental factors that lead to IPV[10]

— Translating scientific evidence into practical application through the implementation of evaluated programs and policies

— A commitment to collaborating across disciplines to address gaps in IPV prevention[2,5,12]

— Empowering individuals and communities to understand violence as a preventable and changeable problem[12]

In addition to presenting traditional IPV prevention approaches, this chapter presents opportunities to improve current prevention strategies, particularly at the societal level. Prevention remains frequently focused on individual-level care and support—but to stop IPV, we have to begin to think beyond individual action to alter the conditions that make women and men vulnerable to victimization and perpetration in the first place, which requires attention to social justice and human rights.

Table 15-1. The Public Health Approach to Intimate Partner Violence Prevention

STEP	DESCRIPTION	EXAMPLE ACTIVITY
1	Define and measure the extent of the problem	Collect public health surveillance data
2	Identify the risks and protective factors for IPV	Research the experiences of victims and perpetrators to learn why violence occurs
3	Develop and evaluate interventions to prevent IPV	Conduct evaluation research to identify science-based, effective programs
4	Disseminate effective IPV prevention interventions	Foster community empowerment to adopt successful programs for widespread use

STEP ONE: DEFINING AND MEASURING THE EXTENT

The first step in the public health approach focuses on defining IPV and measuring the extent of it using surveillance systems. This step is critically important to the public health approach, because the definition of a problem informs and directs prevention strategies. Surveillance data include the demographic characteristics of victims and perpetrators, the temporal and geographic characteristics of violent incidents, the relationship between victims and perpetrators, and the outcomes and severity of violent injuries.[10,11]

Common public health surveillance tools that include IPV tracking are the Behavioral Risk Factor Surveillance Survey and statewide national death reporting systems, but IPV data are collected via numerous sources.[11] These include mortality data, national probability surveys, hospital and medical data, shelter and social services data, community level data, crime data, economic data, and policy and legislation data.[2] Surveillance data form the basis of the public health approach, because these data demonstrate how IPV changes over time, capture the widespread effects of prevention efforts, and allocate services and appropriate resources.[10,12,13]

It is challenging to collect data about IPV, because it is a difficult, frightening, and shameful topic to discuss and report.[14] This is why a clear and consistent definition of IPV is important. Unfortunately, defining IPV is a complex, controversial, and value-laden task. This is especially true because there are a variety of stakeholders involved in the conceptualization, definition, and surveillance of IPV, ranging from victims and perpetrators, family violence researchers, women's rights advocates, medical and public health professionals, and criminal justice experts. Ongoing debates between the family violence and feminist perspectives on understanding IPV serve as a key example. Family violence researchers understand violence as it relates to family conflict and stress.[15] In contrast, the feminist and battered women's movement defines IPV as an act motivated by patriarchal values and males' power and control over their female partners. This conceptualization is demonstrated in **Table 15-2**, which shows how controlling behavior results in many forms of abuse against women.[16] The examples in each section of the wheel were generated from discussions with abused women about the ways their male partners were harming them.

Table 15-2. The Impact of IPV Perpetration by Men on Women

VIOLENCE (PHYSICAL, SEXUAL)

Power and Control

Using intimidation	Making her afraid by using looks, actions, gestures, smashing things, destroying her property, abusing pets, displaying weapons
Using emotional abuse	Putting her down, making her feel bad about herself, calling her names, making her think she is crazy, play mind games, humiliating her, making her feel guilty
Using isolation	Controlling what she does, who she sees and talks to, what she reads, where she goes, limiting her outside involvement, using jealousy to justify actions

(continued)

Table 15-2. *(continued)*	

VIOLENCE (PHYSICAL, SEXUAL)

Power and Control

Minimizing, denying, and blaming	Making light of the abuse and not taking her concerns about it seriously, saying the abuse did not happen, shifting responsibility for abusive behavior, saying she caused it
Using children	Making her feel guilty about the children, using the children to relay messages
Using male privilege	Treating her like a servant, making all the big decisions, acting like the "master of the castle," being the one to define men's and women's roles
Using economy abuse	Preventing her from getting or keeping a job, making her ask for money, giving her an allowance, taking her money, not letting her know about or have access to family income
Using coercion and threats	Making threats to do something to hurt her, threatening to leave her, to commit suicide, to report her to welfare, making her drop charges, making her do illegal things

Recreated with permission from the Domestic Abuse Intervention Project; *202 E. Superior Street Duluth, MN 55802; 218-722-2781; http://duluth-model.org*

Michael Johnson distinguishes between various types of IPV, describing chronic control-motivated battering as "intimate terrorism," which differs from "common couple violence," or arguments\or violence that result from everyday family stress.[3,4] He argued that the family and feminist perspectives disagreed about the definitions of violence and the corresponding different violence statistics because they were analyzing 2 different types of violence.[3] He described various types of IPV and contended that the feminist researchers were really describing mostly male perpetrated control-motivated violence (intimate terrorism) and that the family violence researchers were really describing common couple violence, such as situational or everyday conflicts.[17] Johnson suggested that multiple common names for IPV and violence against women contribute to a false concept of a domestic violence "prototype" that does not exist in practical terms and argued that it is extremely important to distinguish between the different types of violence, because they require different research questions, interventions, and policy responses.[3,4,17,18] While the distinctions between different types of violence are critical to defining, measuring, and understanding IPV, these distinctions are not always made by IPV researchers.

In addition to terminology debates, IPV researchers disagree about several key IPV measurement issues, such as using broad or narrow definitions; lifetime or shorter measurement time frames; men, women, couples, victims, and perpetrators to gather information; specific measurement collection tools; and which data sources should be prioritized to understand and respond to IPV.[19] Defining violence requires value judgments about acceptable and unacceptable behaviors.[2] One victim may perceive a slap as minor, while another victim might consider it to be dangerous. Judging the seriousness of abusive acts is also complex, given that some women describe psychological and verbal aggression to be as hurtful as physical abuse.[20] Work groups continue to meet and discuss IPV measurement and monitoring. In 1998, a data system, monitoring, and response working group comprised of participants from government, university, and violence prevention agencies convened and made numerous IPV measurement recommendations. These included using open-ended violence measurements to capture diverse violent experiences, pretesting questions and data elements, coordinating existing violence data sources, supporting collaborations between different disciplines to understand violence, using both quantitative and qualitative methods to understand violence, and ensuring that data collection instruments and surveys include descriptions of the context of surveys to facilitate appropriate interpretation of findings.[21]

The Centers for Disease Control and Prevention (CDC) is one of the federal government's leading public health agencies. The CDC developed uniform IPV definition recommendations to promote and improve the consistency of IPV surveillance, but the agency reminds users that the definitions are general to increase their value for a wide range of researchers and practitioners, and may require further refinement. The CDC's definition of IPV describes violence as multifaceted and occurring on a continuum. According to the CDC Intimate Partner Violence Surveillance uniform definitions report, IPV includes 4 main components[14]:

— **Physical violence.** The intentional use of physical force to inflict harm, injury, disability, or death, including hitting, pushing, shoving, burning, using weapons, and restraint is termed *physical violence.*

— **Sexual violence.** *Sexual violence* includes the use of force to engage in attempted or completed sex with another person against their will or when he/she is not able to understand, decline participation, or communicate about the act because of illness, disability or drugs and alcohol, or abuse.

— **Threats of physical or sexual violence.** Words, gestures, or weapons to communicate the intent to cause injury, harm, disability, or death are referred to as *threats of physical or sexual violence.*

— **Psychological or emotional violence.** Harm caused by acts or threats, such as humiliating the victim, controlling the victim, withholding information, embarrassing the victim, isolating the victim from friends or family, or controlling money or economic resources are termed *psychological or emotional violence.* The working group for this report decided that emotional abuse occurs if there has been prior physical or sexual abuse or the threat of this abuse.

According to the CDC definition, an intimate partner is a current or former spouse, dating partner, boyfriend, or girlfriend.[14] Despite the CDC's attempts to advance consistent measurement, IPV is still understood, defined, and measured in numerous ways, and violence definitions are always evolving. For example, in 2000 a definitions and measurements working group recommended that the term **"violence and abuse against women" (VAAW)** be used because it more clearly includes physical actions and psychological abuse and trauma.[21] They recommended that the term *VAAW* include physical violence, sexual violence, threats of physical or sexual violence, stalking, and psychological abuse, with the first 3 components comprising a narrower category of violence against women, to try to distinguish between more serious forms of violence. When reviewing and comparing violence surveillance statistics, it is critically important to consider *who* defined violence, *how* violence was defined, and for what outcomes and purposes. Definition and measurement controversies are critical to the study of IPV, because definitions set parameters for research and influence the results and conclusions, meaning that by whom and how IPV is defined ultimately determines who will be labeled a victim or a perpetrator of violence and receive corresponding services.[20,22,23,24] Inconsistent surveillance strategies have limited the public health response to IPV by contributing to conflicting conclusions about the incidence and prevalence of violence, limited comparisons of the magnitude of IPV with other public health problems, poor identification of risk groups in need of specific intervention services, and inconclusive descriptions of the changes in IPV over time.[14]

RATES OF INTIMATE PARTNER VIOLENCE AGAINST WOMEN IN THE UNITED STATES

Rates of lifetime experiences of IPV against women in the United States span from 22% to 54%, depending on the way violence is conceptualized, the measures used, and the population sampled.[2,25-31] Annual rates of IPV against women are lower and span from 1.3% to 8%.[2,26,29,31,32] The National Violence Against Women Survey (NVAWS), which includes a probability sample of women and men across the United States, found that women were more likely than men to report being victimized by an intimate partner.[26] Women were 22.5 times more likely to report being raped, 2.9 times more likely to report being physically assaulted, and 8.2 times more likely to report being stalked, when compared with men.[33] Crime studies and national studies that measure emergency department visits and homicides corroborate these findings that women suffer more serious violence and more injuries from violence compared to men.[33-37]

RATES OF INTIMATE PARTNER VIOLENCE AGAINST MEN IN THE UNITED STATES

Several national family violence surveys, including the National Family Violence Survey, the National Survey of Families and Households, and the National Couples Survey, conclude that female violence against men is just as prevalent as male violence against women.[34] These findings have generated controversy by suggesting that men and women are equal victims of IPV. These findings, however, contrast the findings from shelter-based surveys, hospital records, and court records. Some feminist researchers have argued that gender symmetric findings must indicate a measurement error or the use of measures like the Conflict Tactics Scale (CTS), which counts acts of violence but ignores gender inequities; the context of violent acts; sexual assault; violence by former partners; violence initiation, intention, and motivation; the nature of the relationship; retaliation; and the consequences of violence.[38] Johnson, however, has argued that the 2 groups of researchers use different sampling strategies, which assess types of violence differing in respect to their treatment of gender.[3,4,17,18] For example, while shelter studies sample women who have experienced the most severe forms of violence, broad survey studies often do not reach men who are very violent towards their wives because they refuse to participate. Johnson argued that there are qualitatively 2 different forms of IPV: intimate terrorism and common couple violence. If surveys do not distinguish between which type of violence they are studying, the results are meaningless.[3,4,17,18] Men do suffer from intimate terrorism. For example, the NVAWS found that 0.3% of men reported being raped, 7.4% of men reported physical assault, and 0.6% of men reported stalking by former or current intimate partners in their lifetime.[33] But, for the most part, women suffer from intimate terrorism, and it is common couple violence that is gender symmetric.[3,4,17,18] Intimate terrorism is more harmful; its victims suffer more frequent and more injurious violence, and are more likely to experience posttraumatic stress disorder (PTSD), use painkillers, and miss work.[39] This controversy exemplifies the importance of understanding how violence is defined and measured before interpreting research results.

INTIMATE PARTNER VIOLENCE AND SAME-SEX RELATIONSHIPS

It is possible that models developed to understand IPV among heterosexual couples can provide insight into the dynamics of abuse in same-sex couples. The same gender dynamics, however, are obviously not at play. While we recognize that same-sex relationships are different from heterosexual relationships, we want to clarify that violence is not limited to heterosexual couples. Existing research indicates that interpersonal violence between same-sex partners is high.[40-44] In a probability-based sample of 2881 men who have sex with men (MSM),* 34% endured psychological abuse, 22% suffered physical abuse, and 5% were victims of sexual abuse by intimate male partners.[44] Similarly, the NVAWS found that men with male partners experienced more IPV than men with female partners. Almost 15% of men with male partners reported being raped, physically assaulted, or stalked by a male partner, versus 7% of men with female partners. On the other hand, women living with female intimate partners (11%) experienced less IPV than women with male partners (30%).[45] It is hypothesized, however, that violence is even more underreported in same-sex relationships because of homophobia and of prevailing beliefs that men (not women or lesbians) are violent.[40]

CHILDREN AND INTIMATE PARTNER VIOLENCE

Approximately 15.5 million children live in homes where violence occurs.[46] Unfortunately, research suggests that children of abused mothers are 57 times more likely to be harmed by parental IPV, compared with children of nonabused mothers.[47] Children may be harmed by their mother's abuser, and parents who are victims of domestic violence may neglect their children because they cannot give the child attention or because of their own fears.[48] Children in violent homes face the risk of watching traumatic events, being abused themselves, and being neglected.

EXTENT AND IMPACT OF INTIMATE PARTNER VIOLENCE

The financial impact of IPV against women exceeds $5.5 billion, which includes direct costs of physical and mental health care and indirect costs of lost productivity and work time.[49] There are numerous important medical consequences of IPV. They include bruises, knife wounds, pelvic pain, headaches, back pain, broken bones, gynecological disorders, pregnancy difficulties, sexually transmitted infections including human immunodeficiency virus/acquired immunodeficiency syndrome, gastrointestinal disorders, symptoms of PTSD, heart problems, depression, suicidal behavior, anxiety, low self-esteem, inability to trust, and fear of intimacy.[2,25,26,30,50-53] Intimate partner violence is associated with negative health behaviors that present additional health risks, including high risk sexual behavior, substance abuse, and unhealthy diet-related behaviors.[25,54-57]

Children are especially vulnerable. Children who are exposed to adverse experiences, including witnessing or experiencing violence, suffer a range of health problems and unhealthy behaviors in adult life. These include depression, suicide attempts, multiple sexual partners, sexually transmitted infections, smoking, alcohol use,[58] illicit drug use,[59] sexual risk behaviors among women,[60] poor self-rated health, physical inactivity, obesity, heart disease, cancer, lung disease, fractures, and liver disease.[61]

SUMMARY

Intimate partner violence harms individuals and families in numerous ways. Available surveillance data reveal that prevention activities should prioritize violence perpetrated by *men*. Women are more likely to experience severe IPV and suffer related injuries,

---

* The term MSM is inappropriate because it defines a group of people by their sexual behavior only.[43] However, this term is being used because it is used by the research reports that are summarized.

though IPV researchers need to know more about same-sex partner violence. Everyone who is hurt by violence is more likely to suffer a range of negative health outcomes. While the outcomes of violence are clear, surveillance mechanisms are still hindered by a lack of consensus regarding how to define and measure violence and distinguish between different types of violence.[3,4,17,18] Improving the consistency of IPV measurement strategies is critical to advancing the public health approach to IPV prevention; surveillance informs all of the steps in the approach.

Step Two: Identify Risk and Protective Factors

In step 2 of the public health approach to IPV prevention, researchers identify the causes of IPV by analyzing the risk and protective factors for perpetration and victimization. While the first step determines who, when, where, and how, this step investigates *why* violence occurs. This is important because it identifies modifiable factors that can be addressed in prevention interventions.[10,12]

Not surprisingly, no single factor explains violence. Feminist researchers have historically supported explanations for violence that are based on the ways that male privilege perpetuates gender-based abuse; however, male privilege alone fails to explain the occurrence of IPV against women.[62] Ecological models explain that violence is caused by the relationship between multiple factors. Ecosocial applications to violence vary, but they all share the concept that there are multiple and embedded levels of

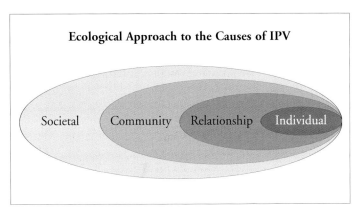

Ecological Approach to the Causes of IPV

Societal   Community   Relationship   Individual

causality.[62] The ecosocial model complements the public health approach, which also acknowledges that social, behavioral, and environmental factors lead to IPV. The model generally examines the risk of being a perpetrator or victim of violence by dividing risk factors into 4 levels: individual, relationship, community, and societal. These are demonstrated graphically in **Figure 15-1**.[62]

Figure 15-1. The ecological approach to understanding the causes of IPV.

The individual level of risk identifies personal history factors such as age, race, gender, income, education, substance abuse, and aggression history. The relationship level describes the ways that risk is connected to close relationships, such as relationships with family members or the influence of friends. The third level explains how community contexts in which relationships occur, such as schools, homes, or workplaces, influence behavior. The fourth level considers how broad societal factors create a climate that encourages or inhibits IPV, including social or cultural norms or social policies. The levels overlap because the factors at each level are strengthened by factors at another.[2]

The World Health Organization's (WHO) *World Report on Violence and Health* summarized the risk factors for violence victimization and perpetration at all 4 levels, which are described in **Table 15-3**.[63,64] The WHO report described the magnitude and impact of violence throughout the world.[63,64] The findings of the world report are supported by a large body of research and numerous reviews and summaries of risk and protective factors.[2,50,62,65,66] As **Table 15-3** indicates, numerous risk factors are associated with perpetrating violence and, of the individual-level factors, only experiencing or witnessing child abuse consistently explains being a victim of violence. Community and

Table 15-3. The Risk Factors for Intimate Violence Perpetration and Victimization

RISK FACTOR	RISK OF BECOMING A...
Individual Level	
Male	Perpetrator
Low intelligence quotient/poor school performance	Perpetrator
Young age	Perpetrator
Victim/witness of child abuse and neglect	Perpetrator/Victim
Problem-drinking/substance abuse	Perpetrator
Psychological/personality disorder	Perpetrator
Relationship Level	
Male-dominated household	Perpetrator
Poor parental monitoring	Perpetrator
Marital discord	Perpetrator
Parental conflict involving violence	Perpetrator
Sexually/physically violent peers	Perpetrator
Community Level	
Poverty	Perpetrator/Victim
Low social capital	Perpetrator/Victim
Weak community response to IPV	Perpetrator/Victim
Inadequate victim care	Perpetrator/Victim
Societal Level	
Economic inequality	Perpetrator/Victim
Gender inequality	Perpetrator/Victim
Culture supporting violence	Perpetrator/Victim
Policies that increase inequity	Perpetrator/Victim

societal influencing factors create an environment in which violence is more likely to occur. Inconsistent measurement confuses the identification of risk and protective factors in the same way that it hinders surveillance. Research studies do not consistently define violence in similar ways or analyze risk and protective factors in the same groups of individuals, leading to different results. For example, Vezina and Herbert[66] reviewed 61 empirical studies published between 1986 and 2006 that investigated the risk factors for psychological, sexual, and physical violence in intimate relationships of girls and adult women aged 12 to 24. While researchers do not consistently measure first-time or repeated victimization, the following factors, in addition to prior victimization, were associated with being a victim: coming from a broken family; living in a rural area; having a depressive disorder; believing that violence is justified and acceptable; having a conduct disorder, participating in risky sexual practices; reporting an adolescent pregnancy; dropping out of school; reporting inadequate parenting; and having an older partner.[66]

The risk factors identified in the table also begin to demonstrate the relationship between all types of oppression. Intimate partner violence occurs more often in families facing distress and even more often when those families are in disadvantaged neighborhoods.[67] Because more African Americans face economic distress, they are more likely to experience IPV than whites, but these differences disappear when controlling for income variables.[67] Intimate partner violence is more common among low income women, low income couples, women whose male partners are unemployed, and couples who report financial strain.[27,28,31,50,67] Poor women are also more likely to experience severe violence.[67] It is not exactly clear how income relates to violence, but it is likely that poverty causes stress, crowding, and hopelessness that exacerbate violence.[62]

These factors are associated with perpetration or victimization but will not always lead to violence. For example, not all abused children are perpetrators and/or victims.[68] It is important to note, however, that the strong link between witnessing or being hurt by violence as a child and becoming a perpetrator and/or victim of violence as an adult creates a cycle of violence that is difficult to escape.[2,26,50,62,65,69] The mechanisms that link witnessing violence to abusive behavior in adulthood are unclear, but social learning theory suggests that children learn to use violence to get their way and that abusive homes can lead to psychological disturbances that combine with other factors to lead to violence.[70]

IPV is caused by the complex interplay between individual, relationship, community, and societal factors. This step of the public health approach is essential because it identifies risk and protective factors for intervention. Some risk and protective factors, such as depression, are more easily modifiable than others, and these may be prioritized in interventions. It is important to recognize, however, that, at its root, violence is driven by more difficult-to-change societal-level forces, including gender inequity, widespread poverty, and policies that overtly or covertly support these inequities. These constraints rob individuals of their opportunities, make them more vulnerable to experiencing violence, and create greater challenges to escaping violence. Below, the concrete ways that social forces lead to violence are explored so that professionals will be able to better integrate these complex determinants into IPV prevention.

STEP THREE: DEVELOP AND EVALUATE PREVENTION STRATEGIES

In the third step of the public health approach to IPV prevention, researchers and service providers work together to develop, implement, and evaluate the effectiveness of interventions to prevent IPV. Interventions must be evaluated so that communities can devote resources toward those that are scientifically proven to work. Interventions can be evaluated by randomized controlled trials, comparisons of different populations for the occurrence of IPV, and observational studies.[10,12]

Public health prevention initiatives for victims and perpetrators are described by the phase of the problem and the level of response. Primary, secondary, and tertiary prevention describe prevention according to the phase of the problem.† Primary prevention approaches aim to prevent IPV before it occurs, through education and policies that introduce new values, information, and skills. Secondary prevention approaches focus on services for groups who possess specific risk factors for IPV victimization or perpetration, to reduce risk factors or increase protective factors. Tertiary approaches aim to minimize

---

† Alternate definitions for primary, secondary, and tertiary prevention exist, though they do not differ greatly from the way they are defined in this document. For example, the CDC (2004) defines primary prevention as approaches that take place before violence has occurred to prevent initial perpetration or victimization, secondary prevention as immediate responses after violence has occurred to manage the short-term consequences of violence, and tertiary prevention as long-term responses after violence has occurred to manage the long-term consequences of violence.[71]

the harm caused by IPV after it has occurred and usually focus on long-term responses, including rehabilitation and therapy.[2,70] While primary prevention programs can be delivered universally to entire populations, such as all schools in a particular district, secondary and tertiary prevention services are *usually* delivered to selected groups of people at risk for violence perpetration and victimization.[2]

Step 3, developing and evaluating prevention programs, directly follows the principles of the public health approach to IPV prevention, surveillance data (step 1) and information about risk and protective factors (step 2). Therefore, IPV prevention strategies do the following:

— Address all 4 levels of ecological risk: individual, relationship, community, and societal risk factors

— Focus on preventing violence perpetration by holding the perpetrator accountable

— Prioritize strategies to prevent male perpetrated violence

— Represent a range of strategies tailored to all stages of human development

Table 15-4 identifies a variety of key IPV prevention strategies. There are numerous kinds of IPV interventions. While explaining each of these strategies in detail is beyond the scope of this chapter, an example of one strategy that responds to each risk level of the ecological model is explained in further detail below.[63]

INDIVIDUAL-LEVEL APPROACHES TO PREVENTION: BATTERER COUNSELING PROGRAMS

Individual-level prevention strategies generally encourage and promote nonviolent behaviors and attitudes in children and young adults or individuals who have already displayed violent behavior and need information and skills to change their actions. These strategies focus on changing individuals' behavior. For example, individual approaches include antiviolence education programs for school students, social development or antibullying programs, batters or victim's counseling or treatment programs.[2,12,62,63,65]

Batterer interventions are an example of an individual-level, tertiary prevention strategy that aims to prevent IPV by stopping men who have been arrested for IPV from acting violently again. The majority of program participants are referred to batterers' programs as a condition of their prosecution or probation. Batterer programs generally use education, counseling, and case management to help men stop their violent behaviors. Many programs use a group format to assist batterers to help each other learn to be nonviolent, decrease batterers' sense of isolation, and improve their communication and interpersonal skills.[72,73]

Batterer programs differ based on the way they define the nature of domestic violence. For example, 3 theoretical approaches direct batterer intervention programs. Social and cultural theories understand violence to be a result of cultural values that legitimize male control over their partners, family-based theories understand violence as a result of family interactions, and individual-based theories explain that violence results from psychological problems, such as personality disorders.[74] Batterer programs generally aim to promote safety, justice and rehabilitation, depending on their understanding of violence. Safety-oriented programs work closely with battered women's shelters and focus on helping batterers to understand their patterns of control and abuse; justice-oriented programs view their services as an extension of actions taken by the criminal justice system; and rehabilitation programs focus on treating individual

Table 15-4. Key IPV Prevention Strategies

Ecological Context	Prevention Strategy	Response Phase
Individual	— School education programs	Primary, secondary
	— Peace education programs	Primary
	— Efforts to reduce unintended pregnancies and provide prenatal/postnatal care	Primary
	— Counseling for victims	Tertiary
	— Medical care for victims	Tertiary
	— Batterer counseling programs*	Tertiary
	— Antidrug and anti-alcohol education programs	Primary
	— Drug and alcohol treatment	Secondary, tertiary
Relationship	— Mentoring programs*	Secondary
	— Home visiting	Secondary, tertiary
	— Parenting training	Secondary, tertiary
Community	— Coordinated community interventions*	Tertiary
	— Community shelters	Tertiary
	— After-school programs	Secondary, tertiary
	— Community policing	Secondary, tertiary
	— Training for medical providers, police, and criminal justice staff	Secondary, tertiary
Societal	— Public education campaigns to change social and cultural norms*	Primary
	— Laws to punish IPV perpetrators	Primary, secondary
	— Laws to promote gender equity	Primary, secondary
	— Antipoverty, work promotion laws	Primary, secondary

* Explained in further detail in the text.

psychopathology, with substance abuse treatment, and counseling. One approach does not work for every batterer or violent situation, and many programs focus on multiple goals.[72-74] While they are common to certain batterer programs, certain approaches, including anger management and couples counseling, are controversial components of batterer programs, because they rely on a single focus or aspect of the violence versus the underlying causes, misattribute violence as anger, and may be dangerous for the abused partner.[74]

The effectiveness of batterer programs is undetermined. Several reviews[75,76] and metaanalyses[77] suggest that these programs have a minimal effect on IPV recidivism. It is difficult to measure program success, because it is often difficult to collect accurate information about whether or not the batterer has continued to harm his partner. Complications such as different standards and goals for programs, varied measures of success, biased analyses that do not account for the participants that drop out of counseling, and different measurement time frames hinder program evaluation.[72,77,78] In addition to mixed results regarding their success, batterer programs are controversial because many victim advocates believe it is unfair to use public funds for batterers while public financial support is declining for women's social services and shelters.[72]

Example Program: Abusive Men Exploring New Direction

Abusive Men Exploring New Direction (AMEND) is a counseling program for abusive men in Denver, Colorado.[79] The program's mission is to help men break the cycle of violence. The program began as a way to provide needed intervention services to men whose partners sought shelter. The 3 main components of the program include counseling services, advocacy services, and community education. Counseling aims to help batterers stop hurting their partners with physical, verbal, and emotional abuse by helping men to identify and take responsibility for their actions as well as to build their self-esteem, anger management, and communication skills. Individual and group counseling sessions focus on addiction, beliefs, gender stereotypes, and family of origin discussions. Advocacy services coordinate with victim advocates to ensure that the batterer does not continue to harm his partner or children. Community education activities aim to give the community information about the root causes of violence.

RELATIONSHIP-LEVEL APPROACHES TO PREVENTION: PEER PROGRAMS

Relationship approaches focus mainly on influencing victims' and perpetrators' relationships, addressing problems within families (eg, marital conflict) or among peers (eg, negative peer influences). These programs include mentoring programs, family and couple therapy programs, home visiting programs, or relationship skills training.[2,12,62,63,65]

Intimate partner violence prevention strategies based on peer influence aim predominantly to modify the behaviors of men at risk for perpetrating violence, and, therefore, exemplify a secondary IPV prevention strategy. These programs, however, can also be used to prevent violence from occurring in the first place and can be primary prevention strategies. Peer-based strategies are common among youth and as a part of school education and skill-building programs.[80,81] Peer programs are based on the philosophy that suggestions from peers may be more acceptable than those of adults.[82] Peer-based programs focus on the protective factors of positive peer relationships[83-85] and the power of the influence of peers to help prevent, intervene, or stop violent behavior.[83-85] More peer programs need to be evaluated, but existing data indicate that these programs may reduce fighting at school and modify students' attitudes about conflict.[82]

Example Program: Mentors in Violence Prevention

Mentors in Violence Prevention (MVP) is a school violence prevention approach that encourages young men and women to assume leadership roles in their communities.[84] Various school systems in different states use the program, which utilizes a bystander approach to prevent violence, focusing on empowering male bystanders to confront their abusive peers and support their abused peers. Classes and workshops use real-life scenarios to give bystanders ideas about how to confront their peers about abusive behaviors.

The sessions explore and challenge cultural norms that violence against women is acceptable, and the mixed gender courses discuss why some men physically and sexually assault their girlfriends, and how cultural definitions of manhood contribute to sexual and domestic violence. The focus of the program is on the nonacceptance of peers' violent behavior and the challenges of standing up to violent peers. The program is delivered by students who receive specific training. The curriculum has been evaluated and has demonstrated an increase in peer ability to discourage violent behavior.

COMMUNITY-LEVEL APPROACHES TO PREVENTION: COORDINATED COMMUNITY RESPONSES

Community approaches raise public awareness about IPV. For example, community-level approaches include public education campaigns or environmental changes, such as improved lighting; extracurricular activities for young people; training for police, health, and medical professionals; efforts to coordinate community level services for victims and perpetrators; and community policing.[2,12,62,63,65]

Coordinated community responses (CCRs) are formal and informal efforts to engage the community to prevent and respond to IPV. These examples are often secondary or tertiary prevention strategies because they focus on coordinating efforts once violence has already occurred, though CCRs can also prevent violence before it occurs.[86] Coordinated community responses usually include *coordinated* efforts between diverse stakeholders such as public health practitioners, law enforcement agents, judges, probation officers, counselors, nurses and doctors, child protection agencies, battered women's advocates. Coordinated community responses generally focus on assisting victims and holding batterers accountable once violence has occurred.[86-88] Some of the common components of CCRs include pro-arrest policies; shelter, advocacy, and treatment for victims; aggressive and prompt persecution; batterer programs; and monitoring of statewide response to domestic violence cases.[87]

Domestic violence shelters are a critical component of any community prevention strategy. Shelters are based on an empowerment philosophy that prioritizes the needs of abused women. Not surprisingly, shelter residents identify shelters as supportive resources.[89] In addition to providing safe housing, research reports that shelters and the advocacy services received there increase women's level of information, decision-making and coping skills, feelings of safety,[90] social support,[90,91] quality of life, and sense of power[92] and alleviate women's psychological distress[90,91] and emotional attachment to their abusive partner.[92] However, when they leave a shelter women have many needs that often include the need for legal assistance, employment, and housing,[93] proving that victims of IPV need numerous and coordinated services to escape violence.

Coordinated community responses are based on the notion that a coordinated and consistent effort is required to stop violence against women and that coordination is necessary to prevent IPV because the effectiveness of one response depends on the effectiveness of another. For example, a protection order is only effective if the police enforce it, and emergency shelter is only helpful if women can find permanent and safe housing. Different actors meet victims at different stages, and diverse members of the community can work together to add different perspectives to the response. For example, a woman may be reluctant to seek shelter and to talk to a victim advocate but willing to talk to a nurse or a doctor. A comprehensive community response can address related problems that challenge battered women such as shelter, food, and medical needs.[88]

Communities have developed different ways to coordinate IPV prevention strategies. The predominant strategies include community intervention projects, criminal justice reforms, and coordinating councils. Community intervention projects are rooted in the domestic violence movement and focus on reforming, improving, and coordinating institutional responses to domestic violence within a community. Criminal justice approaches focus on coordinating services through local prosecutors' offices. Coordinating councils are task forces that provide a forum for collaboration and communication.[88]

The majority of CCR evaluations have focused on individual components of interventions versus the collective community response. Individual evaluations are inconclusive as well as complex because success in one area, such as increased arrests, may not actually be associated with an increase in victim safety. Changing a community's response to domestic violence can take a long time.[94] While a small number of existing studies indicate combined approaches reduce further violence, it remains challenging to evaluate larger system responses because of the different agencies involved, the different goals, different responses, and other methodological problems.[87]

Example Program: Duluth Abuse Intervention Project
The Duluth Abuse Intervention Project (DAIP) is a national and international model of CCR.[95] The Duluth Abuse Intervention Project is a collaboration between the local women's shelter, batterer's program, and the criminal justice and medical systems. For example, police officers communicate with victim advocates so that they can follow up with victims after arrest, explain the legal process, and accompany victims to court. Women are offered support services such as shelter, counseling, and parenting groups. When a defendant pleads guilty, he attends enters a DAIP batterer intervention program, where the counselors interact with victims advocates to ensure that the batterer is not continuing to hurt his partner. In addition, all 911 emergency medical transcripts are given to DAIP staff so that they can contact victims by telephone. The DAIP also tracks 911 calls so that they can discuss them at interagency meetings to update, develop, and revise protocols.

SOCIETAL-LEVEL APPROACHES TO PREVENTION: PUBLIC EDUCATION CAMPAIGNS

Societal-level prevention strategies focus on the cultural, social, and economic factors related to violence and emphasize changes in legislation and the larger social environment. These approaches include legislation and judicial remedies, policy changes to reduce poverty, and efforts to change social and cultural norms.[2,12,62,63,65]

Intimate partner violence has changed from a private household matter to an issue of public concern. As a result, the media now addresses IPV in radio spots, posters, and flyers. Public education campaigns are examples of primary IPV prevention strategies, because they aim to stop IPV before it happens. These approaches, however, can also respond to violence once it has occurred and act as secondary and tertiary responses. These mechanisms are challenged to move their audiences from awareness of IPV to action. They are generally guided by health behavior models that suggest that behavior is influenced by others, that specific behavior factors (like severity of risk) influence risk taking, and that people need confidence to assume skills to change their behaviors.[96]

Example Programs: "There's No Excuse for Domestic Violence"; "Coaching Boys into Men"
"There's No Excuse for Domestic Violence" aimed to alter the environment that permitted abuse to occur in the first place. The campaign specifically encouraged people to act when they heard or saw violence, intervene to ask a friend whether they were okay, and call domestic violence hotlines for further help and support.[97] The campaign generated more than $100 million of donated time and space in 22 000 media outlets. Campaign evaluation indicated that people in media markets with high exposure were more likely to recall the advertisements and report action against domestic violence, call domestic violence an important social issue, and believe that perpetrators should be arrested, when compared with media markets with lower exposure.[96] The Family Violence Prevention Fund (FVPF) recently began another

campaign targeted towards boys called "Coaching Boys into Men." The purpose of this campaign is to encourage men to mentor their sons, grandsons, nephews, and brothers to give them advice about how to behave toward girls. The basis of the campaign is that boys are overwhelmed with negative influences from their friends, neighborhoods, and televisions about being a tough and controlling man and need help learning that there is no place for violence in a relationship **(Figure 15-2)**.[97]

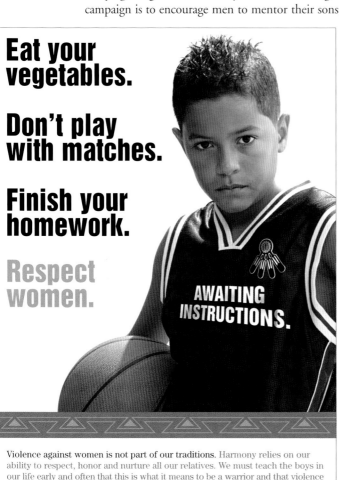

Eat your vegetables.

Don't play with matches.

Finish your homework.

Respect women.

AWAITING INSTRUCTIONS.

Violence against women is not part of our traditions. Harmony relies on our ability to respect, honor and nurture all our relatives. We must teach the boys in our life early and often that this is what it means to be a warrior and that violence never equals strength. A safer world is in their hands, help them grasp it.

www.endabuse.org **Family Violence Prevention Fund**

Funded by the U.S. Department of Health and Human Services, Administration for Children and Families, Administration on Children, Youth and Families. Points of view or opinions in this document do not necessarily represent the official position or policies of the U.S. Department of Health and Human Services.

Figure 15-2

Figure 15-2. The Family Violence Prevention Fund's ad campaign to prevent male violence. Photo credit: Getty Images

SUMMARY

There are multiple approaches to IPV prevention. Because the causes of IPV are complex, intervention is necessary at individual, relationship, community, and societal levels. Likewise, it is important to stop violence before it happens, but also to intervene with those at risk for violence and to help victims. Treatment is also prevention because it helps to stop the cycle of violence. Finally, many current strategies are in need of further evaluation. While it is important to implement prevention programs, it is equally important to evaluate them to understand which programs are effective. Evaluating IPV programs can be challenging because of lack of funds or time to focus on anything but services for victims or perpetrators, but program evaluation will advance the field of IPV prevention by identifying programs that work.[11,98,99]

STEP FOUR: DISSEMINATING EFFECTIVE IPV PREVENTION PROGRAMS

Step 4 includes widespread dissemination of effective projects for community use. This is a critical step in the cycle, because all of the other steps are irrelevant if communities do not actually *implement* effective programs and share in their benefits. Several online and print materials are currently available to help communities implement proven approaches.[11]

— *The Greenbook project* (http://www.thegreenbook.info/). Partnership between the CDC and other federal agencies to fund community projects to implement violence prevention recommendations designed to improve how the court system handles cases of abused women and children, to increase the effectiveness of the child protective system, and to enhance services for victims of domestic violence.

— *The National Online Resource Center on Violence Against Women* (VAWnet) (http://www.vawnet.org). Provides a collection of full-text, searchable resources on IPV, sexual violence, and prevention.

— *Prevention connection* (http://www.calcasa.org). National project that conducts Web trainings and moderates a listserv with information and discussions regarding violence prevention.

— *Blueprints for violence prevention* (http://www.colorado.edu/cspv/blueprints/model/overview.html). National violence prevention initiative to identify effective prevention programs.

— *Substance Abuse and Mental Health Services Administration* (SAMSHA) (http://model programs.samhsa.gov/). Registry of evidence-based effective substance abuse and mental health programs.

USING A HUMAN RIGHTS-BASED APPROACH TO ADVANCE PREVENTION

Existing prevention strategies respond to the immediate causes of violence perpetration, such as anger and stress, and react to victims' and perpetrators' short-term needs, such as housing. To truly prevent IPV, however, it is necessary to uproot the structural factors, such as gender-based inequities and men's unequal access to power, that make someone more vulnerable to becoming a victim and or a perpetrator in the first place. Public health researchers and practitioners who focus on the social and ecological determinants of health often call this type of primary prevention "precursor prevention" and suggest the primary venue through which to implement precursor prevention is the human rights approach.[100] Using a human rights framework to analyze IPV prevention policies and programs can identify the ways in which these initiatives promote or deny social and gender equity and suggest areas for improvement. Addressing the socioeconomic and structural factors that lead to IPV risk expands the public health approach to prevention by focusing on reducing *both IPV risk and vulnerability*.[101] This approach is a form of *precursor* prevention because it goes beyond stopping the violence in the first place (primary prevention) to stopping the factors that *underlie* violence.[102]

VIOLENCE AS A HUMAN RIGHTS PROBLEM

All people are entitled to certain basic human rights. These rights have been enshrined by the international community in the Universal Declaration of Human Rights (UDHR) of 1948,[103] and have been reiterated, clarified, and expanded upon in several more specific international covenants and treaties.[104] Basic rights include the right to an adequate standard of living, health, education, equality, and nondiscrimination.[103] What makes the human rights framework very powerful is that it establishes a consensus understanding that violence is wrong for everyone, no matter what the circumstance, no matter who they are. Human rights hold governments and all people accountable for upholding such rights. The imperative to do so is not only morally binding, but can also be legally binding. Governments can freely decide to become parties to international human rights treaties, which are binding to governments that sign and ratify them. Governments that hold themselves accountable to such treaties are obliged to protect, respect, and fulfill the human rights of their citizens—especially those specific to the document ratified. There are international covenants that defend civil and political rights, social, economic, and cultural rights, and, more specifically, the rights of women, the rights of the child, and nondiscrimination based on race or ethnicity. The United States has signed and ratified the international covenant of civil and political rights, and on nondiscrimination based on race or ethnicity. While the United States is legally bound to adhere to the treaties that it has ratified, it is also responsible for abiding by the conditions stated in other nonbinding declarations, because these conditions reflect binding standards in customary international law.[104]

Violence is recognized as a human rights violation in several key human rights documents, which state that governments should not commit acts of violence; ensure that victims have access to services and redress; and ensure that all citizens enjoy peace and safety.[2] These are described in **Table 15-5**. Violence is particularly problematic because it is both a violation to human rights and a cause of further rights violations. For example, inequality towards women is a human rights violation that results in violence. In turn, violence violates women's right to safety, adequate health, housing, and many other rights. Another reason to incorporate a human rights framework into the public health approach is to help decisionmakers understand how people are made vulnerable by the experience of rights violations, such as discrimination, violence, or a deprived standard of living in terms of food and housing. Indeed, a woman who is abused becomes more *vulnerable* to poor health, to low self-esteem, to losing her job, to depression, and ultimately to more violence. These vulnerabilities make her more likely to participate in risky behaviors, to be exposed to risky situations, and may lead to even poorer health outcomes that also translate to poor health outcomes for her children.

Table 15-5. Right to Be Free from Violence in Key Human Rights Documents

Document	Text Summary
Universal Declaration of Human Rights (UDHR), 1948; International Covenant on Civil and Political Rights (ICCPR), 1966/1976	Everyone has the right to life, liberty, and security of person. No one should be subjected to cruel treatment.[103,106]
Convention on the Elimination of All Forms of Discrimination Against Women (CEDAW), 1979	States the steps that Parties shall take in all fields, in particular in the political, social, economic and cultural fields, all appropriate measures, including legislation, to ensure the full development and advancement of women.[107]
Beijing Declaration and Platform for Action, 1995	All forms of violence against women and girls should be prevented and eliminated.[108]
Vienna Declaration and Program of Action, 1993	Gender-based violence and all forms of sexual harassment and exploitation, including those resulting from cultural prejudice and international trafficking, are incompatible with the dignity and worth of the human person, and must be eliminated.[109]
Declaration on the Elimination of Violence against Women, 1994	States should condemn violence against women and should not invoke any custom, tradition, or religious consideration to avoid their obligations with respect to its elimination. States should pursue by all appropriate means and without delay a policy of eliminating violence against women.[110]

The human rights framework helps us understand how political and economic systems and relationships make people more vulnerable, as well as how the systems and relationships can also protect, respect and fulfill people's right to a dignified life.

APPLYING A RIGHTS-BASED APPROACH TO THE ANALYSIS OF INTIMATE PARTNER VIOLENCE POLICIES

The rights-based approach to health involves assessing the degree to which violations of human rights have health consequences, the ways that health policies can violate human rights, and how vulnerability to ill health can be reduced by taking steps to protect, respect, and fulfill human rights.[104] Policy development and implementation is a mechanism by which nations can ensure the human rights of their citizens. For example, social policy can improve social equity by increasing access to early childhood care, improving access to education, reducing unemployment, and creating stronger safety net programs. The violation of these basic human rights directly relates to IPV risk factors such as gender inequality, substance abuse, and weak social safety nets.[105] Similarly, gender-oriented policy can help alleviate inequities by securing equal treatment in the law, equal rights, and equal opportunities for men and women.[2]

Documenting how state acts violate rights can translate into improved IPV prevention strategies.[111] For example, sometimes US laws actually perpetuate gender inequity and IPV. For instance, criminal justice reforms such as mandatory arrest and no-drop prosecution laws may put victims in more danger by provoking retaliation.[112] In addition, custody laws may force battered women to participate in unsafe visitation with the man who hurt them and their children.[111,113] On another level, policies unrelated to family violence and child custody can also feed IPV. The work requirements of some welfare laws may lead women's partners to be threatened by their partner's participation in education and training, and inspire them to retaliate with violence.[114] From the human rights perspective on health, the US federal, state, and city government must attend to the impact such policies have on the perpetuation of violence. They also must ensure that they have carried out a full analysis of the violence and human rights impact of the implementation of new policies on health, safety, and well being.[115] If they do not, then the United States could be held accountable for not taking adequate steps to protect and fulfill the right to safety and health, or worse, for not respecting the right to safety by perpetuating violence.

EXAMPLE PROGRAM: THE BATTERED WOMEN'S JUSTICE PROJECT

The Battered Women's Justice Project (BMJP) is an example of a program that applied the human rights framework to analyze custody laws for victims of IPV in Massachusetts to identify weaknesses in the policy and to suggest areas for improvement. Researchers interviewed battered mothers who experienced unfair family court litigation, advocates who worked with battered women in court litigation, and interviews with state actors who worked in the court system.[111,113] They found that 6 intersecting human rights violations resulted from specific action, inaction, and attitudes by state actors and the court system. These included failure to protect battered women and children from abuse, discrimination and bias against battered women, degrading treatment of battered women, denial of due process of battered women, allowing the batterer to continue abuse through family courts, and failure to respect the economic rights of battered women and children.[111,113] As a result of their research and human rights documentation, Massachusetts has taken several steps to improve services for victims. These include mandatory domestic violence training for child custody court personnel, more advocates for battered women who need legal support, new standards to guide child custody investigations, and a process to investigate women's complaints.[113]

Summary

The human rights approach adds to the public health approach to prevent IPV by focusing on policy analysis and government accountability. Human rights documentation powerfully exposes the way the government fails to promote gender equity and protect women from violence. The approach also allows IPV to be described in new and heightened ways, increasing the likelihood of policy reform and legal recourse. It addresses the intersecting injustices and multiple oppressions that battered women face. Most importantly, it reveals new opportunities to create policies and programs that do promote social and gender equality and effectively addresses the structural factors that lead to IPV.[111,113]

Conclusion

The public health approach to prevent IPV consists of surveillance, risk and protective factor identification, and program development, evaluation, and dissemination. This method is critical in the effort to prevent IPV because it focuses our attention and efforts on the ways that we can prevent violence at each level: individual, social relationships, community and society. The public health approach continues to evolve, as is evidenced by the variety of case examples presented above. Improving consistency in measurement and strengthening program evaluation will better our efforts to understand how to prevent violence and provide a blueprint for ways to implement effective prevention strategies. While the public health approach aims to respond to the causes of violence, the human rights framework expands this effort to address IPV risk *and* vulnerability, by providing a lens through which to determine whether IPV policies promote or deny gender inequality and other societal conditions that lead to violence. Broadening our prevention perspectives will have a greater impact on prevention solutions and ultimately on the harms of IPV. We cannot prevent nor stop violence solely through our work as medical and health professionals, but we must also move beyond our own professions and work with coalitions that include unusual partners such as law enforcement and youth groups. We must inform policymakers and legislators about the individual community and societal costs of IPV, and we must engage with young people who are just forming their values and solidifying their negotiation skills in personal relationships. The public health and human rights approaches help us to have a broad structural, political, and social understanding of IPV that was previously considered to be an intimate, household problem. This broad understanding also allows us to develop effective programs and develop cross-cutting strategies to prevent violence and its devastating and unacceptable consequences.

References

1. Centers for Disease Control and Prevention (CDC). *Intimate Partner Violence: Overview*. Available at: http://www.cdc.gov/ncipc/factsheets/ipvoverview.htm. Accessed May 1, 2007.

2. Krug E, Dahlberg L, Mercy J, Zwi A, Lozano R. World report on violence and health. Available at: http://www.who.int/violence_injury_prevention/violence/world_report/en/full_en.pdf. Accessed July 1, 2006.

3. Johnson MP. Patriarchal terrorism and common couple violence: two forms of violence against women. *J Marriage Fam.* 1995;57:283-294.

4. Johnson MP, Ferraro KJ. Research on domestic violence in the 1990s: making distinctions. *J Marriage Fam.* 2000;62:948-963.

5. Graffunder C, Noonan R, Cox P, Wheaton J. Through a public health lens, preventing violence against women: an update from the US Centers for Disease Control and Prevention. *J Womens Health.* 2004;13:5-14.

6. Institute of Medicine (IOM). *The future of the public's health in the 21st century.* Washington, DC: The National Academies Press; 2002:1-536. Available at: http://www.nap.edu/catalog/10548.html. Accessed January 1, 2007.

7. Harrell J, Baker E. The essential services of public health. Available at: http://www.apha.org/ppp/science/10ES.htm. Accessed January 1, 2007.

8. US Department of Health and Human Services (DHHS). *Healthy People 2010: Understanding and Improving Health.* Washington, DC: US Government Printing Office; 2000;017-001-001-00-550-9:1-76. Available at: http://www.healthy people.gov/Document/pdf/uih/2010uih.pdf. Accessed January 1, 2007.

9. Family Violence Prevention Fund. Intimate partner violence and Healthy People 2010 fact sheet. Available at: http://www.endabuse.org/hcadvd/2003/tier4.pdf. Accessed January 5, 2007.

10. Saltzman L, Green Y, Marks J, Thacker S. Violence against women as a public health issue, comments from the CDC. *Am J Prev Med.* 2000;19:325-329.

11. Centers for Disease Control and Prevention (CDC). *Intimate Partner Violence: CDC Activities.* Available at: http://www.cdc.gov/ncipc/factsheets/ipvactivities.htm. Accessed January 1, 2007.

12. Mercy J, Rosenberg M, Powell K, Broome C, Roper W. Public health policy for preventing violence. *Health Affairs.* 1993;Winter:7-29.

13. Centers for Disease Control and Prevention (CDC). *Injury Fact Book 2001-2002.* Available at: www.cdc.gov/ncipc/fact_book/factbook.htm. Accessed January 16, 2006.

14. Saltzman L, Fanslow J, McMahon P, Shelley G. *Intimate Partner Violence Surveillance Uniform Definitions and Recommended Data Elements, Version 1.0.* Available at: http://www.cdc.gov/ncipc/pub-res/ipv_surveillance/Intimate%20Partner%20 Violence.pdf. Accessed January 17, 2006.

15. Gelles R, Strauss M. *Intimate Violence: The Definitive Study of the Causes and Consequences of Abuse in the American Family.* New York: Simon and Schuster; 1988.

16. Minnesota Program Development. Wheel gallery. Available at: http://www.duluth-model.org/. Accessed February 2, 2007.

17. Johnson MP. Conflict and control: gender symmetry and asymmetry in domestic violence. *Violence Against Women.* 2006;12:1003-1018.

18. Johnson MP. Domestic violence: It's not about gender—or is it? *J Marriage Fam.* 2005;67:1126-1130.

19. Kilpatrick DG. What is violence against women? Defining and measuring the problem. *J Interpersonal Violence.* 2004;19:1209-1234.

20. DeKerseredy WS, Schartz MD. Definitional Issues. In: Renzetti CM, Edleson JL, Kennedy Bergen R, eds. *Sourcebook on Violence Against Women.* London: Sage Publications; 2001: 23-34.

21. Centers for Disease Control and Prevention (CDC). Morbidity and mortality weekly report (MMWR) recommendations and reports: building data systems for monitoring and responding to violence against women—recommendations from a workshop. Atlanta, Ga: Centers for Disease Control and Prevention; 2000;RR-11:1-18.

22. Muehlenhard CL, Powch IG, Phelps JL, Giusti LM. Definitions of rape-scientific and political implications. *J Social Issues*. 1992;48:23-44.

23. Muehlenhard CL, Kimes LA. The social construction of violence: the case of sexual and domestic violence. *Pers Soc Psychol Rev*. 1999;3:234-245.

24. Mahoney P, Williams L, and West C. Violence against women by intimate partner relationships. In: Renzetti CM, Edleson JL, Kennedy Bergen R, eds. *Sourcebook on Violence Against Women*. London: Sage Publications; 2001:143-178.

25. Coker AL, Davis KE, Arias I, et al. Physical and mental health effects of intimate partner violence for men and women. *Am J Prev Med*. 2002;23:260-268.

26. Tjaden P, Thoennes N. *Full Report of the Prevalence, Incidence, and Conse-quences of Violence Against Women: Findings from the National Violence against Women Survey*, November 2000. Available at: http://www.ncjrs.gov/pdffiles1/nij/183781.pdf. Accessed January 16, 2007.

27. Collins KS, Schoen C, Joseph S, Duchon L, Simantov E, Yellowitz M. Health concerns across a woman's lifespan: the commonwealth fund 1998 survey of women's health. 1999:1-13. Available at: http://www.cmwf.org/publications/publications_show.htm?doc_id=221554. Accessed January 16, 2007.

28. Buehler J, Toomey K. Lifetime and annual incidence of intimate partner violence and resulting injuries, Georgia, 1995. *MMWR Morb Mortal Wkly Rep*. 1998;47: 849-852.

29. Bensley L, MacDonald S, Van Eenwyk J, Wynkoop Simmons K, Ruggles D. *MMWR Morb Mortal Wkly Rep*. 2000;49:589-592.

30. Coker AL, Smith PH, Bethea L, King MR, Mckeown RE. Physical health conse-quences of physical and psychological intimate partner violence. *Arch Family Med*. 2000;9:451-457.

31. Thompson RS, Bonomi AE, Anderson M, et al. Intimate partner violence: prevalence, types, and chronicity in adult women. *Am J Prev Med*. 2006;30:447-457.

32. McFarlane JM, Groff JY, O'Brian JA, Watson K. Prevalence of partner violence against 7,443 African American, White, and Hispanic women receiving care at urban public primary care clinics. *Public Health Nurs*. 2005;22:98-107.

33. Tjaden P, Thoennes N. Prevalence and consequences of male to female and female to male intimate partner violence measured by the national violence against women survey. *Violence Against Women*. 2000;6:142-161.

34. Field CA, Caetano R. Intimate partner violence in the U.S. general population. *J Interpers Violence*. 2005;20:463-469.

35. Bureau of Justice Statistics (BJS). *Crime Characteristics, Summary Findings, 2005*. Available at: http://www.ojp.usdoj.gov/bjs/evict_c.htm. Accessed January 17, 2006.

36. Davis KE, Coker AL, Sanderson M. Physical and mental health effects of being stalked for men and women. *Violence Vict*. 2002;17:429-443.

37. Hale-Carlson G, Hutton B, Fuhrman J, McNutt L. Physical violence and injuries in intimate relationships—New York behavioral risk factor surveillance system, 1994. *MMWR Morb Mortal Wkly Rep*. 1996;45:765-767.

38. Kimmel MS. "Gender symmetry" in domestic violence. *Violence Against Women*. 2002;8:1332-1363.

39. Johnson MP, Leone JM. The differential effects of intimate terrorism and situational couple violence: findings from the national violence against women survey. *J Family Issues*. 2005;26:322-349.

40. Burke LK, Follingstad DR. Violence in lesbian and gay relationships: theory, prevalence, and correlational factors. *Clin Psychol Rev*. 1999;19:487-512.

41. Cameron P. Domestic violence among homosexual partners. *Psychol Rep*. 2003; 93:410-416.

42. Balsam KF, Rothblum ED, Beauchaine TP. Victimization over the life span: a comparison of lesbian, gay, bisexual, and heterosexual siblings. *J Consult Clin Psychol*. 2005;73:477-487.

43. Young R, Meyer I. The trouble with "MSM" and "WSW": erasure of the sexual minority person in public health discourse. *Am J Public Health*. 2005;95:1144-1149.

44. Greenwood GL, Reif MV, Huang B, Pollack LM, Canchola JA, Catania JA. Battering victimization among a probability-based sample of men who have sex with men. *Am J Public Health*. 2002;92:1964-1969.

45. Tjaden P, Thoennes N. *Extent, Nature, and Consequences of Intimate Partner Violence*. Available at: http://www.ncjrs.gov/pdffiles1/nij/181867.pdf. Accessed January 17, 2006.

46. McDonald R, Jouriles EN, Ramisetty-Mikler S, Caetano R, Green CE. Estimating the number of American children living in partner-violent families. *J Family Psychol*. 2006;20:137-142.

47. Parkinson GW, Adams RC, Emerling FG. Maternal domestic violence screening in an office-based pediatric practice. *Pediatrics*. 2001;108(3):43.

48. National Clearinghouse on Child Abuse and Neglect Information. In harm's way: domestic violence and child maltreatment. Available at: http://www.calib.com/dvcps/facts/harm.htm. Accessed December 18, 2006.

49. Centers for Disease Control and Prevention (CDC). *Costs of Intimate Partner Violence Against Women*. Available at: http://www.cdc.gov/ncipc/pub-res/ipv_cost/IPVBook-Final-Feb18.pdf. Accessed January 17, 2006.

50. Centers for Disease Control and Prevention — National Center for Injury Prevention and Control. *Intimate Partner Violence: Fact Sheet*. Available at: http://www. cdc.gov/ncipc/factsheets/ipvfacts.htm. Accessed March 7, 2005.

51. Campbell JC, Jones AS, Dienemann J, et al. Intimate partner violence and physical health consequences. *Arch Intern Med*. 2002;162:1157-1163.

52. Carbone-Lopez K, Kruttschnitt C, Macmillan R. Patterns of intimate partner violence and their associations with physical health, psychological distress, and substance use. *Public Health Rep*. 2006;121:382-392.

53. Silverman JG, Decker MR, Reed E, Raj A. Intimate partner violence victimization prior to and during pregnancy among women residing in 26 U.S. states: associations with maternal and neonatal health. *Am J Obstet Gynecol*. 2006; 195:140-148.

54. Lemon SC, Verhoek-Oftedahl W, Donnelly EF. Preventive healthcare use, smoking, and alcohol use among Rhode Island women experiencing intimate partner violence. *J Womens Health Gender Based Med*. 2002;11:555-562.

55. Weinsheimer RL, Schermer CR, Malcoe LH, Balduf LM, Bloomfield LA. Severe intimate partner violence and alcohol use among female trauma patients. *J Trauma-Injury Infect Crit Care.* 2005;58:22-29.

56. Silverman JG, Raj A, Clements K. Dating violence and associated sexual risk and pregnancy among adolescent girls in the United States. *Pediatrics.* 2004;114:220-225.

57. Silverman JG, Raj A, Mucci LA, Hathaway JE. Dating violence against adolescent girls and associated substance use, unhealthy weight control, sexual risk behavior, pregnancy, and suicidality. *JAMA.* 2001;286:572-579.

58. Dube SR, Felitti VJ, Dong M, Chapman DP, Giles WH, Anda RF. Childhood abuse, neglect, and household dysfunction and the risk of illicit drug use: the adverse childhood experiences study. *Pediatrics.* 2003;111:564-572.

59. Dube SR, Felitti VJ, Dong M, Giles WH, Anda RF. The impact of adverse childhood experiences on health problems: Evidence from four birth cohorts dating back to the 1900. *Prev Med.* 2003;37:268-277.

60. Hillis SD, Anda RF, Felitti VJ, Marchbanks PA. Adverse childhood experiences and sexual risk behaviors in women: a retrospective cohort study. *Fam Plann Perspect.* 2001;33:206-211.

61. Felitti VJ, Anda RF, Nordenberg D, et al. Relationship of childhood abuse and household dysfunction to many of the leading causes of death in adults. The adverse childhood experiences (ACE) study. *Am J Prev Med.* 1998;14:245-258.

62. Heise L. Violence against women, an integrated ecological framework. *Violence Against Women.* 1998;4:262-290.

63. Butchart A, Cerda M, Villaveces A, Sminkey L. Framework for interpersonal violence prevention, framework development document. 2002:1-28. Available at: http://www.who.int/entity/violence_injury_prevention/media/en/407.pdf. Accessed January 1, 2007.

64. World Health Organization (WHO). Preventing violence: a guide to implementing the recommendations of the World report on violence and health. Available at: http://whqlibdoc.who.int/publications/2004/9241592079.pdf. Accessed February 8, 2007.

65. Heise L, Ellsberg M, Gottemoeler M. Ending violence against women, population reports. 1999;Series L, No. 11:1-44. Available at: http://www.infoforhealth.org/pr/l11edsum.shtml. Accessed January 1, 2007.

66. Vezina J, Herbert M. Risk factors for victimization in romantic relationships of young women, a review of empirical studies and implications for prevention. *Trauma Violence Abuse.* 2007;8:33-66.

67. Benson L, Litton Fox G. When violence hits home: How economics and neighborhoods play a role. 2004;NCJ 205004:1-12.

68. Caesar P. Exposure to violence in the families of origin among wife abusers and maritally violent men. *Violence Vict.* 1988;3:49-63.

69. Ashcroft J, Daniels D, Hart S. Violence against women: Identifying risk factors. 2004;NCJ 197019:1.

70. Wolfe DA, Jaffe PG. Prevention of domestic violence and sexual assault. 2003:1-8. Available at: http://www.vawnet.org/DomesticViolence/Research/VAWnetDocs/AR_Prevention.pdf. Accessed January 1, 2007.

71. Centers for Disease Control and Prevention (CDC). *Sexual Violence Prevention: Beginning the Dialogue*. Atlanta, Ga: Centers for Disease Control and Prevention; 2004:1-13.

72. Bennet LW, Williams OJ. Intervention programs for men who batter. In: Renzetti CM, Edleson JL, Kennedy Bergen R, eds. *Sourcebook on Violence Against Women*. London: Sage Publications; 2001:261-278.

73. Jackson S, Feder L, Forde D, Davis R, Maxwell C, Taylor B. Batterer intervention programs, where do we go from here? 2003;NCJ 195078:1-30. Available at: http://www.ncjrs.gov/pdffiles1/nij/195079.pdf. Accessed January 1, 2007.

74. Healey K, Smith C, O'Sullivan C. *Batterer Intervention: Program Approaches and Criminal Justice Strategies*. US Department of Justice, Office of Justice Programs, National Institute of Justice; 1998:1-30.

75. Rosenfeld BD. Court-ordered treatment of spouse abuse. *Clin Psychol Rev*. 1992;12:205-226.

76. Davis RC, Taylor BG. Does batterer, treatment reduce violence? A synthesis of the literature. *Women Crim Justice*. 1999;10:69-93.

77. Babcock JC, Green CE, Robie C. Does batterers' treatment work? A meta-analytic review of domestic violence treatment. *Clin Psychol Rev*. 2004;23:1023-1053.

78. Eckhardt CI, Black MC, Suhr L. Intervention programs for perpetrators of intimate partner violence conclusions from a clinical research perspective. *Public Health Rep*. 2006;121:369-381.

79. AMEND. AMEND, Breaking the cycle of violence. Available at: http://www.amendinc.org/index.htm. Accessed January 31, 2007.

80. O'Brien M. School-based education and prevention programs. In: Renzetti CM, Edleson JL, Kennedy Bergen R, eds. *Sourcebook on Violence Against Women*. London: Sage Publications; 2001:387-416.

81. Mytton JA, DiGuiseppi C, Gough DA, Taylor RS, Logan S. School-based violence prevention programs: systematic review of secondary prevention trials. *Arch Pediatr Adolesc Med*. 2002;156:752-762.

82. Powell K, Muir-McClain L, Halasyamani K. A review of selected school based conflict resolution and peer mediation projects. *J School Health*. 1995;65:426-534.

83. Griffin JP. The building resiliency and vocational excellence (BRAVE) program: a violence-prevention and role model program for young, African American males. *J Health Care Poor Underserved*. 2005;16:78-88.

84. Katz J. Mentors in Violence Prevention (MVP), gender violence prevention and education. Available at: http://www.jacksonkatz.com/mvp.html. Accessed January 5, 2007.

85. Farrel AD, Meyer AL, White KS. Evaluation of responding in peaceful and positive ways (RIPP): a school-based prevention program for reducing violence among urban adolescents. *J Child Clin Psychol*. 2001;30:451-461.

86. Centers for Disease Control and Prevention (CDC). *Domestic Violence Prevention Enhancement and Leadership through Alliances (DELTA)*. Available at: www.cdc. gov/ncipc/DELTA/default.htm. Accessed January 8, 2007.

87. Shepard M. Evaluating coordinated community responses to domestic violence. 1999:1-8. Available at: http://new.vawnet.org/Assoc_Files_VAWnet/AR_ccr.pdf. Accessed January 1, 2007.

88. Stop Violence Against Women (StopVAW). Coordinated community response. Available at: http://www.stopvaw.org/Coordinated_Community_Response.html. Accessed January 9, 2007.

89. Sullivan CM and Gillum T. Shelters and other community based services for battered women and their children. In: Renzetti CM, Edleson JL, Kennedy Bergen R, eds. *Sourcebook on Violence Against Women*. London: Sage Publications; 2001:387-416.

90. Bennett L, Riger S, Schewe P, Howard A, Wasco S. Effectiveness of hotline, advocacy, counseling, and shelter services for victims of domestic violence: a statewide evaluation. *J Interpers Violence*. 2004;19:815-829.

91. Constantino R, Kim Y, Crane PA. Effects of a social support intervention on health outcomes in residents of a domestic violence shelter: a pilot study. *Issues Ment Health Nurs*. 2005;26:575-590.

92. Sullivan CM, Campbell R, Angelique H, Eby KK, Davidson WS. An advocacy intervention program for women with abusive partners: six-month follow-up. *Am J of Comm Psychol*. 1994;22:101-122.

93. Sullivan CM, Basta J, Tan C, Davidson WS. After the crisis: a needs assessment of women leaving a domestic violence shelter. *Violence Vict*. 1992;7:267-275.

94. Clark S, Burt M, Schulte M, Maguire K. Coordinated community responses to domestic violence in six communities. 1996:1-86. Available at: http://aspe.hhs. gov/hsp/cyp/domvilnz.htm. Accessed January 1, 2007.

95. Pence E, McMahon M. A coordinated community response to domestic violence. 1997:1-20. Available at: http://www.stopvaw.org/Coordinated_Community_ Response.html. Accessed January 1, 2007.

96. Ghez, M. Getting the message out: using media to change social norms on abuse. In: Renzetti CM, Edleson JL, Kennedy Bergen R, eds. *Sourcebook on Violence Against Women*. London: Sage Publications; 2001:417-438.

97. Family Violence Prevention Fund (FVPF). Public education programs. Available at: http://www.endabuse.org/programs/publiceducation/. Accessed January 6, 2007.

98. Carlson B. The most important things learned about violence and trauma in the past 20 years. *J Interpers Violence*. 2005;20:119-126.

99. Rhatigan D, Moore T, Street A. Reflections on partner violence, 20 years of research and beyond. *J Interpers Violence*. 2005;20:82-88.

100. Krieger N, Gruskin S. Frameworks matter: ecosocial and health and human rights perspectives on disparities in women's health: the case of tuberculosis. *J Am Med Womens Assoc*. 2001;56:137-142.

101. UNAIDS. The global strategy framework on HIV/AIDS. Available at: http://data. unaids.org/Publications/IRC-pub02/JC637-GlobalFramew_en.pdf. Accessed February 8, 2007.

102. Mann J. Health and human rights. Philadelphia: 1998; lecture on health and human rights at Drexel University. Personal communication, May 28, 1998.

103. Universal Declaration of Human Rights (UDHR), G.A. Res. 217A (III), UN Doc. A/810 (1948).

104. WHO, 25 *Questions and Answers on Health and Human Rights.* Available at: http://www.who.int/hhr/activities/en/25_questions_hhr.pdf. Accessed January 6, 2007.

105. Teti M, Chilton M, Lloyd L, Rubinstein S. Identifying the links between intimate partner violence and HIV/AIDS: Human Rights and Ecosocial frameworks offer insight in US prevention policy. *Int J Health Human Rights.* 2007;9:40-61.

106. International Covenant on Civil and Political Rights (ICCPR), G.A. Res. 2200 (XXI), UN Doc. A/6316 (1966).

107. Committee on the Elimination of All Forms of Discrimination Against Women (CEDAW), UN Doc. A/45/38 (1990).

108. Platform for Action of the Fourth World Conference on Women, UN Doc. A/CONF.177/20 (1995).

109. Vienna Declaration and Programme of Action, UN Doc. A/CONF.157/23 (1993).

110. Declaration on the Elimination of Violence against Women, UN Doc. A/RES/48/104 (1994).

111. Silverman J, Mesh C, Cuthbert C, Slote K, Bancroft L. Child custody determinations in cases involving intimate partner violence: A human rights analysis. *Am J Public Health.* 2004;94:951-957.

112. Goodman L, Epstein D. Refocusing on women: a new direction for policy and research on intimate partner violence. *J Interpers Violence.* 2005;20:479-487.

113. Slote K, Cuthbert C, Mesh C, Driggeɪs M, Bancroft L, Silverman J. Battered mothers speak out. *Violence Against Women.* 2005;11:1367-1395.

114. Raphael J. Domestic violence as welfare to work barrier: Research and theoretical issues. In: Renzetti CM, Edleson JL, Kennedy Bergen R, eds. *Sourcebook on Violence Against Women.* London: Sage Publications; 2001:443-456.

115. Hunt P, McNaughton G. Impact assessments, poverty and human rights: a case study using the right to the highest attainable standard of health. UNESCO, May 2006. Available at: http://www.humanrightsimpact.org/fileadmin/hria_resources/unesco_hria_paper.pdf. Accessed February 15, 2007.

INDEX

A

G